PCF2

PALLIATIVE CARE FORMULARY

Robert Twycross

Andrew Wilcock

Sarah Charlesworth

Andrew Dickman

Radcliffe Medical Press

Radcliffe Medical Press Ltd
18 Marcham Road
Abingdon
Oxon OX14 1AA
United Kingdom

www.radcliffe-oxford.com
The Radcliffe Medical Press electronic catalogue and online ordering facility.
Direct sales to anywhere in the world.

PCF1 1998

Every effort has been made to ensure the accuracy of this text, and that the best information available has been used. This does not diminish the requirement to exercise clinical judgement, and neither the publishers nor the authors can accept any responsibility for its use in practice.

British Library Cataloguing in Publication Data

A catalogue record for this book is available from the British Library.

ISBN 1 85775 511 1

Typeset by Advance Typesetting Ltd, Oxon.
Printed and bound by TJ International Ltd, Padstow, Cornwall

PALLIATIVE CARE FORMULARY

Robert Twycross DM, FRCP, FRCR
Emeritus Clinical Reader in Palliative Medicine,
Oxford University
Director, WHO Collaborating Centre for Palliative Care, Oxford
Academic Director, Oxford International Centre for Palliative Care
Director, palliativedrugs.com Ltd.

Andrew Wilcock DM, FRCP
Macmillan Clinical Reader in Palliative Medicine and Medical Oncology,
Nottingham University
Consultant Physician, Hayward House Macmillan Specialist Palliative Care Unit,
Nottingham City Hospital NHS Trust,
Director, palliativedrugs.com Ltd.

Sarah Charlesworth BPharm (Hons) MRPharmS
Specialist Senior Pharmacist in Palliative Care, palliativedrugs.com Ltd.
Hayward House Macmillan Specialist Palliative Care Unit,
Nottingham City Hospital NHS Trust

Andrew Dickman BSc (Hons) MSc MRPharmS
Specialist Principal Pharmacist in Palliative Care
Whiston Hospital, Willowbrook Hospice and Marie Curie Centre,
Liverpool

Contents

Preface

The Palliative Care Formulary (*PCF2*) is intended for qualified medical and other health professionals, to be used as an information resource. However, readers should satisfy themselves as to the suitability and appropriateness of any information in *PCF2* before using it. *PCF2* often refers to possible uses of drugs which are outside the scope of their marketing licence. The use of drugs in this way has implications for the prescriber and these are discussed elsewhere (see p.vi).

With over 22 000 copies already sold, the PCF has been used to satisfy the NHS National Cancer Standards requirement for specialist palliative care services within a Cancer Centre and Network to have a core palliative care drug formulary.

The main sections in *PCF2* generally follow the systematic order of the *British National Formulary* (*BNF*). The appendices deal with themes that transcend the drug monographs, e.g. important drug interactions, named patient suppliers, the use of nebulised drugs. Drugs marked with an asterisk (*) should generally be used only by, or after consultation with, a specialist palliative care service. Drug prices are net prices based on those in the *BNF* No. 43 (March 2002). *PCF2* does not replace the *BNF* or books on pain and symptom management; it is for use alongside them. *Symptom Management in Advanced Cancer* (3e) (Twycross and Wilcock 2001, Radcliffe Medical Press, Oxford) should be seen as the companion book to *PCF2*, and www.palliativedrugs.com as providers of the companion CD-ROM and website. The latter provides more than 5000 members with drug information, a bulletin board for questions, debate and sharing of experiences and a regular newsletter which highlights particular areas of interest relating to the use of drugs in palliative care. Inside the back cover of *PCF2*, there is a tear-out **red card** and **green card**. The red card is for reporting syringe driver compatibilities and incompatibilities which are not listed in Appendix II. The green card is for making suggestions for additional drugs to be included in the next edition of *PCF*. We hope that readers of *PCF2* will make appropriate use of these cards.

We are grateful to colleagues at Sir Michael Sobell House and Hayward House, and elsewhere, for their advice and support, particularly Ray Corcoran, Vincent Crosby, Andrew Davies, Mellar Davis, Caroline Hare, Andrew Hughes, Aslög Malmberg, Mary Miller, Michael Minton and John Moyle. We are also grateful to the Pharmacy Department at The Royal Marsden Hospital for permission to publish Box A and to the Association for Palliative Medicine and the Pain Society of Great Britain and Ireland for permission to publish Box B in *Using licensed drugs for unlicensed purposes*, p.ix and p.x respectively. Thanks are also due to Karen Allen (Sobell House) and Karen Isaacs (Hayward House) for their respective parts in preparing the typescript, to Meg Roberts for library assistance, and to Susan Brown for her invaluable contribution as copy editor.

Robert Twycross
Andrew Wilcock
Sarah Charlesworth
Andrew Dickman
July 2002

Using licensed drugs for unlicensed purposes

In palliative care, up to a quarter of all prescriptions are for licensed drugs given for unlicensed indications and/or via an unlicensed route,[1,2] and this is reflected in the recommendations contained in *PCF2*. The symbol † is used to draw attention to such use. However, it is impossible to highlight every example of unlicensed use. Often it is simply a matter of the route or dose being different from the manufacturer's licence (see *Data Sheets* and *Summaries of Product Characteristics*). For example, haloperidol is widely used PO as an anti-emetic, whereas the licence for use as an anti-emetic is restricted to the IM route. It is important therefore to understand that the licensing process for drugs *regulates the activities of pharmaceutical companies and not a doctor's prescribing practice*. The Medicines Act 1968 specifically safeguards a doctor's clinical freedom. Further, drugs prescribed outside the licence can be dispensed by pharmacists[3] and administered by nurses or midwives.[4]

The licensing process

A marketing licence is necessary in the UK for a product for which therapeutic claims are made. After receiving satisfactory evidence of quality, safety and efficacy, the Licensing Authority (working through the Medicines Control Agency) grants a licence, called the Marketing Authorisation. This allows a pharmaceutical company to market and supply a product for the specific indications listed in its *Data Sheet* or *Summary of Product Characteristics*. (Alternatively, since 1995, drugs can be licensed through the European Union). Restrictions are imposed by the Licensing Authority if evidence of safety and efficacy is unavailable in particular patient groups, e.g. children. Once a product is marketed, further clinical trials and experience may reveal other indications. For these to become licensed, additional evidence needs to be submitted. The considerable expense of this, perhaps coupled with a small market for the new indication, often means that a revised application is not made.

Prescribing outside the licence

In the UK, a doctor may legally:

- prescribe unlicensed medicines
- in a named patient, use unlicensed products specially prepared, imported or supplied
- use or advise a licensed medicine for indications or in doses or by routes of administration outside the licensed recommendations
- supply another doctor with an unlicensed medicine
- override the warnings and precautions given in the licence
- use unlicensed drugs in clinical trials.

The responsibility for the consequences of these actions lies with the doctor.[5] In addition to clinical trials such prescriptions may be justified:

- when prescribing generic formulations (for which indications are not described)
- with established drugs for proven but unlicensed indications
- with drugs for conditions for which there are no other treatments (even in the absence of strong evidence)
- when using drugs in individuals not covered by the licence, e.g. children.

Prescription of a drug (whether licensed use/route or not) requires a doctor, in the light of published evidence, to balance both the potential good and the potential harm which might ensue. Doctors have a duty to act with reasonable care and skill in a manner consistent with the practice of professional colleagues of similar standing. Thus, when prescribing outside the terms of a licence, doctors must be fully informed about the actions and uses of the drug, and be assured of the quality of the particular product. It is possible to draw a hierarchy of degrees of reasonableness relating to the use of unlicensed drugs (Figure 1).[6] The more dangerous the medicine and the more flimsy the evidence the more difficult it is to justify its prescription.

It has been recommended that when prescribing a drug outside its licence, a doctor should:[4–7]

- record in the patient's notes the reasons for the decision to prescribe outside the licensed indications
- where possible explain the position to the patient (and family as appropriate) in sufficient detail to allow them to give informed consent; the Patient Information Leaflet obviously does not contain information about unlicensed indications
- inform other professionals, e.g. pharmacist, nurses, general practitioner, involved in the care of the patient to avoid misunderstandings.

However, in palliative care, the use of drugs for unlicensed uses or by unlicensed routes is so widespread that such an approach is impractical. Indeed, in the UK, a survey showed that few (<5%) palliative medicine consultants *always* obtain verbal or written consent, document in the notes or inform other professionals when using licensed drugs for unlicensed purposes/routes.[8] Concern was expressed that not only would it be impractical to do so, but it would be burdensome for the patient, increase anxiety and might result in refusal of beneficial treatment. Some half to two-thirds indicated that they would *sometimes* obtain verbal consent (53%), document in the notes (41%) and inform other professionals (68%), when using treatments which are not widely used within the specialty, e.g. ketamine (see p.289), octreotide (see p.230), ketorolac (see p.154).

This is a grey area and each doctor must decide how explicit to be. Some NHS trusts have policies in place and some centres have produced information cards or leaflets for patients and carers (Box A). A position statement from the Association for Palliative Medicine and the Pain Society has recently been produced (Box B).

---

1 Atkinson C and Kirkham S (1999) Unlicensed uses for medication in a palliative care unit. *Palliative Medicine.* **13**: 145–152.

2 Todd J and Davis A (1999) Use of unlicensed medication in palliative medicine. *Palliative Medicine.* **13**: 466.

3 Royal Pharmaceutical Society of Great Britain (2000) *Professional standards directorate fact sheet: five. The use of unlicensed medicines in pharmacy.*

4 Anonymous (1992) Prescribing unlicensed drugs or using drugs for unlicensed indications. *Drug and Therapeutics Bulletin.* **30**: 97–99.

5 Tomkins C (1988) Drugs without a product licence. *Journal of the Medical Defence Union.* **Spring**: 7.

6 Ferner R (1996) Prescribing licensed medicines for unlicensed indications. *Prescribers' Journal.* **36**: 73–79.

7 Cohen P (1997) Off-label use of prescription drugs: legal, clinical and policy considerations. *European Journal of Anaesthesiology.* **14**: 231–235.

8 Pavis H and Wilcock A (2001) Prescribing of drugs for use outside their licence in palliative care: survey of specialists in the United Kingdom. *British Medical Journal.* **323**: 484–485.

9 Seydel C (2001) Personal communication.

	Status	*The drug*	*Published data*	*The illness*
Most reasonable	Licensed for the intended indication	Well known; generally safe	Recommended in standard textbooks	Life-threatening
↓	Licensed for another indication; other related products licensed for the intended indication	Well known, but some clear undesirable effects	Well-documented studies in peer-reviewed journals	Severe
		Well known; has serious undesirable effects *or* Little studied; no clear undesirable effects	Only poor quality studies reported	Mild
	A licensed product; not licensed for the intended indication, nor are similar medicines	Little studied; has serious undesirable effects	Only anecdotal evidence published	
Least reasonable	Drug/product not licensed at all	Not studied	No published data available	Trivial

Figure 1 Factors influencing the reasonableness of prescribing decisions.[6]

Box A Example of a patient information leaflet relating to the use of medicines outside their licence[9]

USE OF MEDICINES OUTSIDE THEIR LICENCE

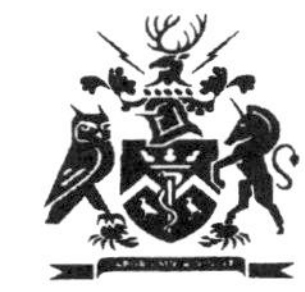

THE ROYAL MARSDEN

This leaflet contains important information about your medicines, please read it carefully.

Medicines prescribed by your doctor or bought over-the-counter from a pharmacist are licensed for use by the Medicines Control Agency.

When a manufacturer markets a new medicine they must obtain a licence from the Medicines Control Agency. The licence restricts the way in which the medicine can be used, the conditions it can be used to treat, the doses to be used and the age of the patient it is given to.

Manufacturers are obliged to include with their medicines a Patient Information Leaflet. The information in it must by law reflect the product licence and must be given to you.

Medicines are often, however, used by hospital doctors in ways, for conditions or ages that are not specified on the product licence. This is true for a lot of medicines used in a cancer hospital or in children.

If you are prescribed a drug treatment at The Royal Marsden your doctor will have carefully thought about the best medicine for you. Medicines are only used outside the product licence when there is research and/or experience to back up such use. Every patient at The Royal Marsden is given this leaflet. This is because pharmacists can not always tell when they dispense a medicine outside the licence, as the reason for prescribing is not stated on the prescriptions.

Your medicines may all be prescribed according to the product licence. You will know if one of your medicines is **not** when you read the Patient Information Leaflet supplied by the manufacturer. You will then notice that the information in it is not relevant to how you are taking the medicine.

Medicines used very commonly outside the product licence include some antidepressants and anti-epileptics (anti-convulsants) which are used to relieve some types of pain. Also, because this is more comfortable and convenient for you, some medicines are often injected subcutaneously (under the skin) instead of being injected into a vein or muscle.

If you have any queries or concerns and would like to discuss this further, your doctor or pharmacist will be happy to help.

You may contact your Doctor or Nurse at:

The Royal Marsden Hospital Chelsea
Fulham Road
London, SW3 6JJ

Tel. 020 7352 8171

or

The Royal Marsden Hospital Sutton
Downs Road, Sutton
Surrey, SM2 5PT

Tel. 020 8642 6011

or

Pharmacy Medicines Information For Patients

Tel. 020 8770 3821

The department is open between 9am and 5pm Monday to Friday.
You can leave a message at any time.

Box B The recommendations of the Association for Palliative Medicine and the Pain Society

The use of drugs beyond licence in palliative care and pain management

1 This statement should be seen as reflecting the views of a responsible body of opinion within the clinical specialties of palliative care and pain management.

2 The use of drugs beyond licence should be seen as a legitimate aspect of clinical practice.

3 The use of drugs beyond licence in palliative care and pain management practice is currently both necessary and common.

4 Choice of treatment requires partnership between patients and healthcare professionals, and informed consent should be obtained, whenever possible, when prescribing any drug. Patients should be informed of any identifiable risks and details of any information given should be recorded. It is often necessary to take additional steps when recommending drugs beyond licence.

5 Patients, carers and healthcare professionals need accurate, clear and specific information that meets their needs. The Association for Palliative Medicine and the Pain Society should work in conjunction with pharmaceutical companies to design accurate information for patients and their carers about the use of drugs beyond licence.

6 Health professionals involved in prescribing, dispensing and administering drugs beyond licence should select those drugs that offer the best balance of benefit against harm for any given patient.

7 Health professionals should inform, change and monitor their practice with regard to drugs used beyond licence in the light of evidence from audit and published research.

8 The Department of Health should work with health professionals and the pharmaceutical industry to enable and encourage the extension of product licences where there is evidence of benefit in circumstances of defined clinical need.

9 Organisations providing palliative care and pain management services should support therapeutic practices that are underpinned by evidence and advocated by a responsible body of professional opinion.

10 There is urgent need for the Department of Health to assist healthcare professionals to formulate national frameworks, guidelines and standards for the use of drugs beyond licence. The Pain Society and the Association for Palliative Medicine should work with the Department of Health, NHS Trusts, voluntary organisations, and the pharmaceutical industry to design accurate information for staff, patients and their carers in clinical areas where drugs are used off label. Practical support is necessary to facilitate and expedite surveillance and audit which are essential to develop this initiative.

Guidance about prescribing in palliative care

Drugs are not the total answer for the relief of pain and other symptoms. For many symptoms, the concurrent use of non-drug measures is equally important, and sometimes more important. Further, drugs must always be used within the context of a systematic approach to symptom management, namely:

- evaluation
- explanation
- management
- monitoring
- attention to detail.

In palliative care, the axiom 'diagnosis before treatment' still holds true. Even when the cancer is responsible, a symptom may be caused in different ways, e.g. in lung cancer vomiting may be caused by hypercalcaemia or by raised intracranial pressure, to name but two possible causes. Treatment often varies according to the cause.

Attention to detail includes *precision in taking a drug history*. Thus, if a patient says, 'I take morphine every 4 hours', the doctor should say, 'Tell me, when do you take your first dose?' 'And your second dose?' etc. When this is done, it often turns out that the patient is taking morphine q.d.s. rather than q4h, and possibly p.r.n. rather than prophylactically. On one occasion, 'every 4 hours' meant 0800, 1200, 1600, 2000h. It was not surprising, therefore, that this patient woke in excruciating pain at about 0300h – so much so that she dreaded going to bed at night.

Attention to detail also means *providing clear instructions for drug regimens*. 'Take as much as you like, as often as you like', is a recipe for anxiety and poor symptom relief. The drug regimen should be written out in full for the patient and his family to work from (Figures 2 and 3). This should be in an ordered and logical way, e.g. analgesics, anti-emetics, laxatives, followed by other drugs. Times to be taken, name of drugs, reason for use ('for pain', 'for bowels', etc.) and dose (x ml, y tablets) should all be stated. The patient should also be advised how to obtain further supplies, e.g. from the general practitioner.

When prescribing an additional drug, it is important to ask:

'What is the treatment goal?'
'How can it be monitored?'
'What is the risk of adverse effects?'
'What is the risk of drug interactions?'
'Is it possible to stop any of the current medications?'

Good prescribing is a skill, and makes the difference between poor and excellent symptom control. It extends to considering size, shape and taste of tablets and solutions; and avoiding 'bastard' doses which force:

- patients to take more tablets than would be the case if doses were 'rounded up' to a more convenient tablet size. For example, it is better to prescribe m/r morphine 60mg (a single tablet) rather than 50mg (3 tablets: 30mg + 10mg + 10mg)
- nurses to spend more time refilling syringes for 24h infusions. For example, in the UK, prescribing diamorphine 100mg (a single ampoule) instead of 90mg (60mg ampoule + 30mg ampoule).

It is necessary to be equally thorough when monitoring treatment. It is often difficult to predict the optimum dose of a symptom relief drug, particularly opioids, laxatives and psychotropic drugs. Further, undesirable effects put drug compliance in jeopardy. Arrangements must be made, therefore, for continuing supervision and adjustment of medication.

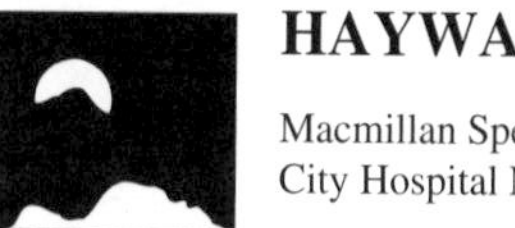

HAYWARD HOUSE

Macmillan Specialist Palliative Care Unit
City Hospital NHS Trust, Nottingham

Medication Information Chart

Patient details/Identification label
Mr Albert Brown
1 Park Road
Anytown AB1 2CD

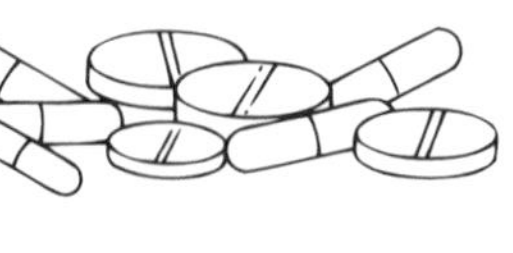

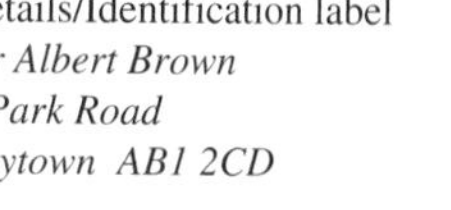

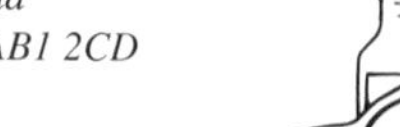

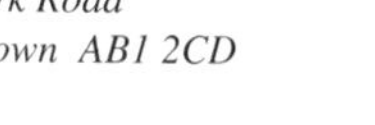

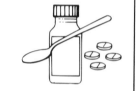

General advice

- Keep this chart with you so you can show your doctor or nurse a list of your medications.
- If you need a further supply, give your GP at least *48 hours* notice.
- If your chemist has difficulty in obtaining your medicines, please ask him to contact the palliative care pharmacist, on (0115) 962 7619 or in the evening/at weekends contact the on-call pharmacist at City Hospital via the switchboard on (0115) 969 1169.
- Occasionally your medication may be supplied in different strengths or presentations. If you have any concerns about this, check with your local pharmacist or district nurse.
- If you need to see a doctor, telephone your GP first unless advised otherwise.
- If you, or your family doctor, need any advice, please ring (0115) 962 7619 and ask to speak to a *red team nurse*.

Figure 2 Side 1 of patient's Medication Information Chart.

Regular medication Description	(Trade name)	Strength	Reason	When to take ON WAKING		LUNCH 2pm	TEA 6pm		BED TIME
MORPHINE SULPHATE MR Purple tablet	(MST)	30mg	PAIN RELIEF *take 12 hours apart*	1					1
DICLOFENAC Round brown tablet		50mg	BONE PAIN	1		1			1
SODIUM VALPROATE Lilac tablet	(Epilim)	200mg	NERVE PAIN						2
CODANTHRAMER Orange liquid		strong	FOR BOWELS				TWO 5ml spoons		
DOMPERIDONE Small white tablet	(Motilium)	10mg	STOP SICKNESS	2		2	2		2
As needed									
MORPHINE SOLUTION Clear liquid	(Oramorph)	10mg in 5ml	Breakthrough pain	Take ONE 5ml spoon every 2–4 hours if needed					
ASILONE Suspension White liquid			Indigestion	Take TWO 5ml spoonfuls FOUR times a day					

Completed by: S THORP Nurse/Pharmacist (Pharmacist circled) Checked by: M SMITH On: 24-2-98

Figure 3 Side 2 of patient's Medication Information Chart.

Finally, it may be necessary to compromise on complete relief in order to avoid unacceptable undesirable effects. For example, antimuscarinic effects such as dry mouth or visual disturbance may limit dose escalation and, with inoperable bowel obstruction, it may be better to aim to reduce the incidence of vomiting to once or twice a day rather than to seek to abolish it altogether.

Drug names

PCF2 uses recommended International Non-proprietary Names (rINNs). For about 150 drugs, the rINN differs from the British Approved Name (BAN). Following a European Union directive, the use of BANs will be phased out and all drugs marketed in the UK will eventually be known by their rINNs. For drugs where there is a high risk of confusion, there will be a transition period during which both the BAN and the rINN must be used (Table 1). In the case of adrenaline (BAN), an exception has been made; in the UK, it will continue to have priority over epinephrine (rINN), i.e. will be prescribed as *adrenaline (epinephrine)*.

Table 1 Drugs relevant to palliative care for which both rINN and BAN must be used in the UK

rINN	*BAN*
Alimemazine	Trimeprazine
Bendroflumethiazide	Bendrofluazide
Calcitonin (salmon)	Salcatonin
Chlorphenamine	Chlorpheniramine
Dicycloverine	Dicyclomine
Dosulepin	Dothiepin
Epinephrine	*Adrenaline*
Furosemide	Frusemide
Levomepromazine	Methotrimeprazine
Lidocaine	Lignocaine
Mitoxantrone	Mitozantrone
Norepinephrine	*Noradrenaline*
Procaine benzylpenicillin	Procaine penicillin
Tetracaine	Amethocaine
Trihexyphenidyl	Benzhexol

For many drugs, the change is slight (e.g. danthron → dantron) but for others the rINN is very different (e.g. methotrimeprazine → levomepromazine). Certain general rules apply:

- 'ph' become 'f' (e.g. cephradine → cefradine)
- 'th' becomes 't' (e.g. indomethacin → indometacin)
- 'y' becomes 'i' (e.g. napsylate → napsilate).

However, there are many exceptions. Other affected drugs relevant to palliative care are listed in Table 2.

Outside Europe it is important to note several differences between rINNs and USANs, i.e. names used in the USA (Table 3). Note also that:

- diamorphine (available only in the UK) = di-acetylmorphine = heroin
- hyoscine = scopolamine
- liquid paraffin = mineral oil.

Table 2 Other drugs relevant to palliative care affected by European Union Directive

rINN	*BAN*
Amobarbital	Amylobarbitone
Amoxicillin	Amoxycillin
Beclometasone	Beclomethasone
Benorilate	Benorylate
Benzathine benzylpenicillin	Benzathine penicillin
Benzatropine	Benztropine
Cefalexin (etc.)	Cephalexin (etc.)
Ciclosporin	Cyclosporin
Clomethiazole	Chlormethiazole
Dantron	Danthron
Dexamfetamine	Dexamphetamine
Dienestrol	Dienoestrol
Diethylstilbestrol	Stilboestrol
Dimeticone	Dimethicone
Estradiol	Oestradiol
Guaifenesin	Guaiphenesin
Indometacin	Indomethacin
Levothyroxine	Thyroxine
Methenamine hippurate	Hexamine hippurate
Oxetacaine	Oxethazine
Phenobarbital	Phenobarbitone
Retinol	Vitamin A
Sodium cromoglicate	Sodium cromoglycate
Sulfasalazine	Sulphasalazine
Sulfathiazole	Sulphathiazole

Table 3 Important differences between rINNs and USANs

rINN	*USAN*
Dextropropoxyphene	Propoxyphene
Dimeticone[a]	Simethicone
Paracetamol	Acetaminophen
Pethidine	Meperidine

a. in some countries, dimeticone is called (di)methylpolysiloxane.

List of abbreviations

General	
*	specialist use only
†	unlicensed use
BNF	British National Formulary
BP	British Pharmacopoeia
CSM	Committee on Safety of Medicines (UK)
IASP	International Association for the Study of Pain
IDIS	International Drug Information Service
MCA	Medicines Control Agency (UK)
rINN	recommended International Non-proprietary Name
SPC	Summary of Product Characteristics
UK	United Kingdom
USA	United States of America
USP	United States Pharmacopoeia
WHO	World Health Organization
Medical	
ADH	antidiuretic hormone (vasopressin)
β_2	beta 2 adrenergic (receptors)
CNS	central nervous system
COX	cyclo-oxygenase; alternative, prostaglandin synthase
COPD	chronic obstructive pulmonary disease
CSF	cerebrospinal fluid
CT	computed tomography
δ	delta-opioid (receptors)
D_2	dopamine type 2 (receptors)
DIC	disseminated intravascular coagulation
ECG	electrocardiogram
FEV_1	forced expiratory volume in 1 second
FRC	functional residual capacity
FVC	forced vital capacity of lungs
H_1, H_2	histamine type 1, type 2 (receptors)
Ig	immunoglobulin
INR	International normalised ratio
κ	kappa-opioid (receptors)
MAOI(s)	mono-amine oxidase inhibitor(s)
MRI	magnetic resonance imaging
MSU	mid-stream specimen of urine
μ	mu-opioid (receptors)
NMDA	N-methyl D-aspartate
NSAID(s)	non-steroidal anti-inflammatory drug(s)
$PaCO_2$	arterial partial pressure of carbon dioxide
PaO_2	arterial partial pressure of oxygen
PCA	patient-controlled analgesia
PG(s)	prostaglandin(s)
PPI(s)	proton pump inhibitor(s)
RIMA(s)	reversible inhibitor(s) of mono-amine oxidase type A
SSRI(s)	selective serotonin re-uptake inhibitor(s)
Tlco	transfer factor of the lung for carbon monoxide

UTI	urinary tract infection
VIP	vaso-active intestinal polypeptide

Drug administration

a.c.	ante cibum (before food)
amp	ampoule containing a single dose (cp. vial)
b.d.	bis die (twice daily); alternative, b.i.d.
CD	preparation subject to prescription requirements under The Misuse of Drugs Act (UK); for regulations see BNF
CIVI	continuous intravenous infusion
CSCI	continuous subcutaneous infusion
e/c	enteric-coated
ED	epidural
IM	intramuscular
IT	intrathecal
IV	intravenous
IVI	intravenous infusion
m/r	modified release; alternative, slow release, controlled release
~~NH~~S	not prescribable on NHS prescriptions
o.d.	omni die (daily, once a day)
o.m.	omni mane (in the morning)
o.n.	omni nocte (at bedtime)
OTC	over-the-counter (can be obtained without a prescription)
p.c.	post cibum (after food)
PO	per os, by mouth
POM	prescription only medicine
PR	per rectum
p.r.n.	pro re nata (as needed, when required)
PV	per vaginum
q.d.s.	quater die sumendus (four times a day); alternative, q.i.d.
q4h	quarta quaque hora (every 4 hours)
SC	subcutaneous
SL	sublingual
stat	immediately
t.d.s.	ter die sumendus (three times a day); alternative, t.i.d.
vial	sterile container with a rubber bung containing either a single or multiple doses (cp. amp)
WFI	water for injections

Units

cm	centimetre(s)
cps	cycles per sec
dl	decilitre(s)
g	gram(s)
Gy	Gray(s), a measure of radiation
h	hour(s)
Hg	mercury
kg	kilogram(s)
L	litre(s)
mg	milligram(s)
ml	millilitre(s)
mm	millimetre(s)
mmol	millimole(s)
min	minute(s)
mosmol	milli-osmole(s)
nm	nanometre(s)
nmol	nanomole(s); alternative, nM
sec	second(s)

1: GASTRO-INTESTINAL SYSTEM

Antacids
Alginic acid
Dimeticone
Oxetacaine

Antimuscarinics
Hyoscine butylbromide
Propantheline

Prokinetics
Cisapride

H_2-receptor antagonists

Misoprostol

Proton pump inhibitors

Loperamide

Laxatives
Ispaghula husk
Contact (stimulant) laxatives
Docusate
Lactulose
Macrogol (polyethylene glycol)
Magnesium salts
Rectal preparations (enemas)

Preparations for haemorrhoids

Pancreatin

ANTACIDS — BNF 1.1

Antacids taken by mouth to neutralise gastric acid include:

- sodium bicarbonate
- magnesium salts
- aluminium hydroxide
- hydrotalcite/aluminium magnesium carbonate
- calcium carbonate.

Magnesium salts *are laxative and can cause diarrhoea;* ***aluminium salts*** *constipate.* Most proprietary antacids contain a mixture of **magnesium salts** and **aluminium salts** so as to have a neutral impact on intestinal transit. With doses of 100–200ml/24h or more, the effect of **magnesium salts** increasingly overrides the constipating effect of **aluminium**.

The sodium content of some antacids may be detrimental in patients with hypertension or cardiac failure; Gaviscon® liquid and **magnesium trisilicate mixture** both contain >6mmol/10ml compared with 0.1mmol/10ml in Asilone®. Regular use of **sodium bicarbonate** may cause sodium loading and metabolic alkalosis. Regular use of **calcium carbonate** may cause hypercalcaemia, particularly if taken with **sodium bicarbonate**.

Aluminium hydroxide binds dietary phosphate. It is of benefit in patients with hyperphosphataemia in renal failure. Long-term complications of phosphate depletion and osteomalacia are not an issue in advanced cancer. **Hydrotalcite** binds bile salts and is of specific benefit in patients with bile salt reflux, e.g. after certain forms of gastroduodenal surgery.

Note:

- *the administration of antacids should be separated from the administration of e/c tablets*; direct contact between e/c tablets and antacids may result in damage to the enteric coating with consequential exposure of the drug to gastric acid, and of the stomach mucosa to the drug

- apart from **sodium bicarbonate**, antacids delay gastric emptying and may thereby modify drug absorption
- some proprietary preparations contain peppermint oil which masks the chalky taste of the antacid and helps belching by decreasing the tone of the lower oesophageal sphincter
- most antacid tablets feel gritty when sucked; some patients dislike this
- some proprietary preparations are fruit-flavoured, e.g. Tums® (chewable tablet) and Remegel® (chewing gum)
- the cheapest preparations are **Magnesium Trisilicate** BP and **Aluminium Hydroxide Gel** BP given alone or as a mixture
- some antacids contain additional substances for use in specific situations, e.g. **alginic acid** (see below), **dimeticone** (see p.3), **oxetacaine** (see p.3).

Nowadays, antacids are generally taken p.r.n.; H_2-receptor antagonists (see p.10) and PPIs (see p.13) are used instead when gastric acid reduction is indicated.

ALGINIC ACID — BNF 1.1.3

Class: Alginate.

Indications: Acid reflux ('heartburn').

Pharmacology

Alginic acid prevents oesophageal reflux pain by forming an inert low-density raft on the top of the acidic stomach contents. Both acid and air bubbles are necessary to produce the raft. Alginic acid preparations may therefore be less effective if used with an H_2-receptor antagonist or a proton pump inhibitor (reduces acid) and/or an antiflatulent (reduces air bubbles). Gaviscon®, a proprietary alginic acid preparation, is a weak antacid; most of the antacid content adheres to the alginate raft. This neutralises acid which seeps into the oesophagus around the raft but does nothing to correct the underlying causes, e.g. lax lower oesophageal sphincter, hyperacidity, delayed gastric emptying, obesity. Indeed, alginic acid preparations are no better than dimeticone-containing antacids in the treatment of acid reflux.[1] Alginic acid preparations have been largely superseded by acid suppression with H_2-receptor antagonists and PPIs.
Onset of action <5min.
Duration of action 1–2h.

Cautions

Gaviscon® liquid contains Na^+ 6mmol/10ml and it should not be used in patients with fluid retention or heart failure.

Dose and use

Several preparations are available but none is recommended. For patients already taking Gaviscon® and who are reluctant to change to Asilone® (or other option), prescribe Gaviscon® 1–2 tablets or Gaviscon® liquid 10–20ml p.c. & o.n., and p.r.n.

Supply

Compound alginic acid preparations
Gaviscon® (Reckitt Benckiser 01482 326151)
Tablets (alginic acid 500mg, dried **aluminium hydroxide** 100mg, **magnesium trisilicate** 25mg, **sodium bicarbonate** 170mg) peppermint or lemon flavour, contain 2mmol Na^+/tab, 28 days @ 1 q.d.s. = £4.20.
Oral suspension sugar-free (sodium alginate 250mg, **sodium bicarbonate** 133.5mg, **calcium carbonate** 80mg/5ml) peppermint or aniseed flavour, contains 3mmol Na^+/5ml, 28 days @ 10ml q.d.s. = £6.05.

Oral suspension (sugar-free) sodium alginate 500mg, **potassium bicarbonate** 100mg/5ml, contains 2.3mmol Na^+/5ml, 28 days @ 5ml q.d.s. = £7.21.

1 Pokorny C *et al.* (1985) Comparison of an antacid/dimethicone mixture and an alginate/antacid mixture in the treatment of oesophagitis. *Gut.* **26**: A574.

DIMETICONE — BNF 1.1.1 & 1.1.3

Class: Antifoaming agent.

Indications: Acid dyspepsia (including acid reflux), gassy dyspepsia, †hiccup (if associated with gastric distension).

Pharmacology

Dimeticone (dimethylpolysiloxane) is an antifoaming agent present in several proprietary antacids, e.g. Asilone®. By facilitating belching, dimeticone eases flatulence, distension and postprandial gastric discomfort. Dimeticone-containing antacids are as effective as Gaviscon® in the treatment of acid reflux.[1] Asilone® should be used in preference to Gaviscon® because it is cheaper and contains almost no sodium.
Onset of action <5min.
Duration of action 1–2h.

Cautions

Although Asilone® contains both **aluminium** and **magnesium**, if large amounts are used, e.g. 30–60ml q.d.s., the laxative effect of **magnesium** will override the constipating effect of **aluminium**.[2]

Dose and use

- starting dose Asilone® suspension 5ml p.r.n., or 5ml q.d.s. & p.r.n.
- if necessary, double dose to 10ml.

Supply

Asilone® (Thornton & Ross 01484 842217)
Oral suspension (sugar-free) activated dimeticone 135mg, dried **aluminium hydroxide** 420mg, light **magnesium oxide** 70mg/5ml (low Na^+), 28 days @ 5ml q.d.s. = £2.18; use within 28 days of opening.

1 Pokorny C *et al.* (1985) Comparison of an antacid/dimethicone mixture and an alginate/antacid mixture in the treatment of oesophagitis. *Gut.* **26**: A574.
2 Morrissey J and Barreras R (1974) Antacid therapy. *New England Journal of Medicine.* **290**: 550–554.

OXETACAINE

Class: Local anaesthetic.

Indications: Odynophagia (painful swallowing) caused by oesophagitis, including postradiation.

Pharmacology

Like **lidocaine** (lignocaine) and **bupivacaine**, oxetacaine is a local anaesthetic of the amide type. It produces a reversible loss of sensation by preventing or diminishing the conduction of sensory nerve impulses near the site of its application. Because the mode of action decreases the

permeability of the nerve cell membrane to sodium ions, local anaesthetics are said to have a membrane stabilising effect. Oxetacaine is effective when applied topically, and is a constituent in some ointments and suppositories for the relief of pain from haemorrhoids.
Onset of action 5min.
Duration of action 2–3h.

Dose and use

For short-term symptomatic treatment while specific treatment of the underlying condition (hyperacidity, candidiasis) permits healing of the damaged mucosa:

- Mucaine® suspension 5–10ml (without fluid) 15min a.c. & o.n., and p.r.n. before drinks.

The production of Mucaine® was discontinued in the UK in May 2002. There is no comparable proprietary alternative. Consider extemporaneous preparation comprising lidocaine viscous 2% mixed in equal parts with an aluminium-magnesium antacid (co-magaldrox, e.g. Maalox®).

Supply

Mucaine® (Wyeth Australia and Canada; not UK)

ANTIMUSCARINICS — BNF 1.2

Antimuscarinics (anticholinergics) are used principally as smooth muscle antispasmodics and antisecretory drugs. They comprise the natural belladonna alkaloids (**atropine** and **hyoscine**) and synthetic and semisynthetic derivatives. The derivatives are divided into tertiary amines, e.g. **dicycloverine** (dicyclomine), and quaternary ammonium compounds, e.g. **hyoscine *butylbromide***, **glycopyrronium** and **propantheline**. The quaternary ammonium compounds are less lipid-soluble than the natural alkaloids, are less likely to cross the blood-brain barrier but are also less well absorbed from the gut. Central antimuscarinic-like effects (e.g. delirium) are therefore not a problem but peripheral antimuscarinic effects are characteristic (Box 1.A).

Box 1.A Peripheral antimuscarinic effects

Visual Mydriasis Loss of accommodation	} blurred vision	**Gastro-intestinal** Dry mouth Heartburn Constipation
Cardiovascular Palpitations Extrasystoles Arrhythmias	} also related to noradrenaline (norepinephrine) potentiation and a quinidine-like action	**Urinary tract** Hesitancy of micturition Retention of urine

Some other drugs used in palliative care also have antimuscarinic properties (Box 1.B). Antimuscarinic effects may be a limiting factor in their use. The concurrent use of two antimuscarinics should generally be avoided.

Cautions

Antimuscarinics block the final common (cholinergic) pathway through which prokinetics act: *the two types of drugs should not be prescribed concurrently.*[1] Antimuscarinics relax the lower oesophageal sphincter and, if possible, should be avoided in patients with symptomatic acid reflux. Antimuscarinics should be avoided in paralytic ileus. Glaucoma may be precipitated in those at risk, particularly the elderly.

Box 1.B Antimuscarinic drugs used in palliative care

Antihistamines
- chlorphenamine (chlorpheniramine)
- cyclizine
- dimenhydrinate
- promethazine

Antiparkinsonians
- orphenadrine
- procyclidine

Antispasmodics
- mebeverine
- oxybutynin
- propantheline

Belladonna alkaloids
- atropine
- hyoscine

Glycopyrronium

Phenothiazines
- chlorpromazine
- levomepromazine (methotrimeprazine)
- prochlorperazine
- thioridazine

Tricyclic antidepressants

1 Schuurkes JAJ *et al.* (1986) Stimulation of gastroduodenal motor activity: dopaminergic and cholinergic modulation. *Drug Development Research.* **8**: 233–241.

HYOSCINE BUTYLBROMIDE — BNF 1.2

Class: Antimuscarinic.

Indications: Intestinal colic, genito-urinary colic, dysmenorrhoea, †inoperable bowel obstruction, †drying secretions (e.g. sialorrhoea, drooling, death rattle).

Contra-indications: Narrow-angle glaucoma (unless moribund).

Pharmacology

Hyoscine *butylbromide* is an antimuscarinic (see p.4) and has both smooth muscle relaxant (antispasmodic) and antisecretory properties. Unlike **hyoscine *hydrobromide***, hyoscine *butylbromide* does not cross the blood-brain barrier and therefore does not have a central anti-emetic action or cause drowsiness. Because they are poorly absorbed, tablets of hyoscine *butylbromide* are of limited use, except perhaps for mild-to-moderate bowel colic. In healthy volunteers a bolus injection of 20mg has a maximum antisecretory duration of action of 2h;[1] however, the same dose by CSCI is often effective for 24h in 'death rattle'. Hyoscine *butylbromide* and **hyoscine *hydrobromide*** act faster than **glycopyrronium** in death rattle,[2] but the overall efficacy is generally the same[3] with death rattle reduced in 1/2–2/3 of patients.
Bio-availability 8–10% PO.
Onset of action <10min SC/IM/IV; 1–2h PO.
Time to peak plasma concentration 1–2h PO.
Plasma halflife 5–6h.
Duration of action <2h in volunteers; probably longer in moribund patients.

Cautions

As for all antimuscarinics (see p.4). Blocks the final common (cholinergic) pathway through which prokinetics act;[4] avoid concurrent use.

Dose and use

Inoperable bowel obstruction with colic[5,6]

- 20mg SC stat
- 60mg/24h CSCI
- increase to 120mg/24h if response inadequate
- maximum dose 300mg/24h.

For patients with obstructive symptoms without colic, **metoclopramide** (see p.113) should be tried before hyoscine butylbromide because the obstruction may well be functional rather than organic.

Death rattle

- 20mg SC stat
- 20–40mg/24h CSCI; some suggest 60–120mg/24h CSCI[7]
- repeat 20mg SC p.r.n.

Some centres use **hyoscine *hydrobromide*** (see p.118) or **glycopyrronium** (see p.287) instead.[7]

Supply

Buscopan® (Boehringer Ingelheim 01344 424600)
Tablets 10mg, 28 days @ 20mg q.d.s. = £10.36.
Injection 20mg/ml, 1ml amp = £0.20.

1 Herxheimer A and Haefeli L (1966) Human pharmacology of hyoscine butylbromide. *Lancet.* **ii**: 418–421.
2 Back I *et al.* (2001) A study comparing hyoscine hydrobromide and glycopyrrolate in the treatment of death rattle. *Palliative Medicine.* **15**: 329–336.
3 Hughes A *et al.* (2000) Audit of three antimuscarinic drugs for managing retained secretions. *Palliative Medicine.* **14**: 221–222.
4 Schuurkes JAJ *et al.* (1986) Stimulation of gastroduodenal motor activity: dopaminergic and cholinergic modulation. *Drug Development Research.* **8**: 233–241.
5 De-Conno F *et al.* (1991) Continuous subcutaneous infusion of hyoscine butylbromide reduces secretion in patients with gastrointestinal obstruction. *Journal of Pain and Symptom Management.* **6**: 484–486.
6 Baines M (1997) ABC of palliative care: nausea, vomiting and intestinal obstruction. *British Medical Journal.* **315**: 1148–1150.
7 Bennett M *et al.* Using anti-muscarinic drugs in the management of death rattle: evidence based guidelines for palliative care. *Palliative Medicine.* **16**: In press.

PROPANTHELINE — BNF 1.2

Class: Antimuscarinic.

Indications: Intestinal smooth muscle spasm, urinary frequency, †paraneoplastic sweating.

Pharmacology

Propantheline is a typical antimuscarinic (see p.4). It doubles gastric emptying half-time[1] and slows gastro-intestinal transit generally, with variable effects on drug absorption (e.g. the *rate* of absorption of **paracetamol** is reduced). Propantheline is extensively metabolised in the small bowel before absorption. *If taken with food, the effect of propantheline by mouth is almost abolished.*[2]

Bio-availability <50% PO.
Onset of action 30–60min.
Time to peak plasma concentration no data.
Plasma halflife 3–4h.
Duration of action 4–6h.

Cautions and undesirable effects

For full list, see manufacturer's SPC.
As for all antimuscarinics (see p.4).

Dose and use

Intestinal colic

- usual dose 15mg t.d.s. *1h a.c.* & 30mg o.n.
- maximum dose 30mg q.d.s.

Urinary frequency: same as for colic; largely superseded by **oxybutynin** (see p.242) and **amitriptyline** (see p.94).

Sweating: 15–30mg b.d.–t.d.s.; largely superseded by **thioridazine** (see p.79), **propranolol** (see BNF 2.4) and **thalidomide** (see p.237).

Supply

Pro-Banthine® (Hansam 0870 241 3019)

Tablets 15mg, 28 days @ 15mg t.d.s. & 30mg o.n. = £19.15.

1 Hurwitz A *et al.* (1977) Prolongation of gastric emptying by oral propantheline. *Clinical Pharmacology and Therapeutics.* **22**: 206–210.

2 Ekenved G *et al.* (1977) Influence of food on the effect of propantheline and L-hyoscyamine on salivation. *Scandinavian Journal of Gastroenterology.* **12**: 963–966.

PROKINETICS — BNF 1.2

Prokinetics accelerate gastro-intestinal transit by a neurohumoral mechanism. The term is restricted to drugs which co-ordinate antroduodenal contractions and accelerate gastroduodenal transit (Table 1.1). This excludes other drugs which enhance intestinal transit such as bulk-forming agents and other laxatives, and drugs which cause diarrhoea by increasing gut secretions, e.g. **misoprostol**. Some drugs increase contractile motor activity but not in a co-ordinated fashion, and so do not reduce transit time, e.g. **bethanechol**. Such drugs are promotility but not prokinetic. **Erythromycin** is the only readily available motilin agonist. Its action is mainly limited to the stomach; tolerance often develops after a few days.

Apart from **erythromycin**, prokinetics act by triggering a cholinergic system in the gut wall. This action is impeded by opioids (Figure 1.1). On the other hand, antimuscarinics block the cholinergic receptors on the intestinal muscle fibres.[2] Thus, drugs with antimuscarinic properties will block the action of prokinetic drugs to a greater or lesser extent. *Prokinetics and antimuscarinics should not be prescribed concurrently.* However, **domperidone** and **metoclopramide** will still exert an antagonistic effect at the dopamine receptors in the area postrema (see p.108).

Prokinetics are used in various conditions in palliative care (Table 1.2). D_2-receptor antagonists block the dopaminergic 'brake' on gastric emptying induced by stress, anxiety and nausea from any cause. In contrast, $5HT_4$-receptor agonists have a direct excitatory effect which in theory gives them an advantage over the D_2-receptor antagonists particularly for patients with gastric stasis or functional bowel obstruction. However, when used for dysmotility dyspepsia, **metoclopramide** is no more potent than **domperidone** in standard doses.[3,4] **Cisapride** is several times more potent; unlike **metoclopramide** and **domperidone**, it has no central effect.[5,6]

Table 1.1 Gastro-intestinal prokinetics[1]

Class	*Examples*	*Site of action*
D_2-receptor antagonist	Domperidone Metoclopramide	Stomach Stomach
$5HT_4$-receptor agonist	Metoclopramide Cisapride	Stomach → jejunum Stomach → colon
Motilin agonist	Erythromycin	Stomach

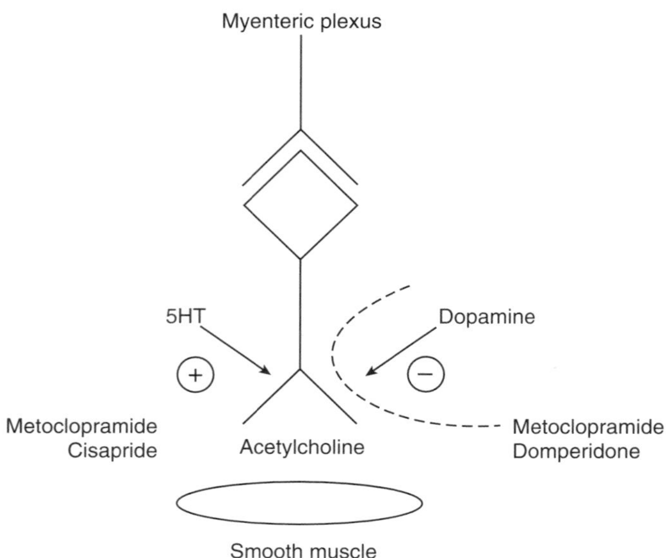

Figure 1.1 Schematic representation of drug effects on antroduodenal co-ordination via a postganglionic effect on the cholinergic nerves from the myenteric plexus.

⊕ stimulatory effect of 5HT triggered by metoclopramide and cisapride; ⊖ inhibitory effect of dopamine; – – – blockade of dopamine inhibition by metoclopramide and domperidone. (The licence for cisapride has been suspended.)

Table 1.2 Indications for prokinetics in palliative care

Gastro-oesophageal reflux	Functional bowel obstruction
Gastroparesis	cancer of head of pancreas
dysmotility dyspepsia	drug-induced
drug-induced	neoplastic
paraneoplastic autonomic neuropathy	Constipation (cisapride only)
spinal cord compression	Irritable bowel syndrome (cisapride only)
diabetic autonomic neuropathy	

1 Debinski H and Kamm M (1994) New treatments for neuromuscular disorders of the gastrointestinal tract. *Gastrointestinal Journal Club.* **2**: 2–11.
2 Schuurkes JAJ *et al.* (1986) Stimulation of gastroduodenal motor activity: dopaminergic and cholinergic modulation. *Drug Development Research.* **8**: 233–241.
3 Loose FD (1979) Domperidone in chronic dyspepsia: a pilot open study and a multicentre general practice crossover comparison with metoclopramide and placebo. *Pharmatheripeutica.* **2**: 140–146.
4 Moriga M (1981) A multicentre double blind study of domperidone and metoclopramide in the symptomatic control of dyspepsia. In: G Touse (ed) *Progress with Domperidone. A gastrokinetic and anti-emetic agent.* Royal Society of Medicine, London, pp.77–79.
5 McHugh S *et al.* (1992) Cisapride vs metoclopramide: an acute study in diabetic gastroparesis. *Digestive Diseases and Science.* **37**: 997–1001.
6 Fumagalli I and Hammer B (1994) Cisapride versus metoclopramide in the treatment of functional dyspepsia: a double-blind comparative trial. *Scandinavian Journal of Gastroenterology.* **29**: 33–37.

CISAPRIDE

Class: Prokinetic, $5HT_4$-receptor agonist.

Indications: †Dyspepsia or nausea associated with delayed gastric emptying unresponsive to **metoclopramide** (e.g. paraneoplastic autonomic neuropathy), †nausea caused by SSRIs and **venlafaxine**,[1,2] †functional bowel obstruction, †constipation (as a 'co-laxative').

Contra-indications: Concurrent administration with oral or parenteral (but not topical) forms of imidazole antifungals (**fluconazole**, **ketoconazole**, **itraconazole**, **miconazole**), **erythromycin** and **clarithromycin**.

Pharmacology

Cisapride is a $5HT_4$-receptor agonist with a strong prokinetic action. It is 2–4 times more potent than **metoclopramide**.[3,4] It has a diffuse prokinetic effect ('panprokinetic' compared with 'gastrokinetic') and reverses opioid-induced delayed gastric emptying more completely. To explain the beneficial effect of cisapride in nausea caused by SSRIs and **venlafaxine**, it has been postulated that $5HT_4$-receptor activation reduces the release of 5HT from enterochromaffin cells.[5] At high plasma concentrations cisapride causes prolongation of the QT interval which predisposes to ventricular arrhythmias (see Prolongation of the QT interval in palliative care, p.327). Because of this, the licence for cisapride in the UK has been suspended.
Bio-availability <50% (fasting), 65% (with food) PO; PR <50% of PO.
Onset of action 0.5–1h.
Time to peak plasma concentration 1–2.5h PO.
Plasma halflife 10h.
Duration of action 12–16h.

Cautions

Serious drug interactions: rare cases of serious (occasionally fatal) cardiac arrhythmias, including ventricular arrhythmias and *torsade de pointes* associated with QT prolongation have been reported in patients taking cisapride in combination with imidazole antifungals (**fluconazole**, **ketoconazole**, **itraconazole**, **miconazole**), **erythromycin** or **clarithromycin**. The interaction relates to inhibition of one of the liver cytochrome P450 enzymes which results in an increase in plasma concentrations of cisapride (see Cytochrome P450, p.331). Most of those affected were receiving several other medications and had pre-existing cardiac disease or risk factors for arrhythmias. The original reports were of **ketoconazole** given in daily doses of *600–1200mg* in patients with prostate cancer. Partly because it is given in smaller doses, **fluconazole** has less effect on the enzyme than **ketoconazole**. The likelihood of this interaction occurring with **fluconazole** 50–100mg o.d. is infinitesimal.[6]

The elderly, hepatic and renal impairment, cardiac disorders.

Undesirable effects

For full list, see manufacturer's SPC.
Colic and diarrhoea, occasional headaches and lightheadedness. Liver function abnormalities (and possibly cholestasis) also reported.

Dose and use

Even though often given q.d.s. (e.g. 15–30min a.c. t.d.s. & o.n.), administration b.d. is generally satisfactory:

- starting dose 10mg b.d.
- maximum dose 20mg b.d.

If causes colic or diarrhoea, halve the dose or give half the dose more frequently.

Supply

Licence suspended by the UK Medicines Control Agency as a result of increasing concerns relating to rare but life-threatening ventricular arrhythmias. (Available from Janssen-Cilag as a named patient supply only; see Special orders and named patient supplies, p.349.)

Prepulsid® (Janssen-Cilag 01494 567567)
Tablets 10mg, 28 days @ 10mg b.d. = £13.16.
Oral suspension 1mg/ml, 28 days @ 10mg b.d. = £17.47.

1 Bergeron R and Blier P (1994) Cisapride for the treatment of nausea produced by selective serotonin reuptake inhibitors. *American Journal of Psychiatry.* **151**: 1084–1086.
2 Russel J (1996) Relatively low doses of cisapride in the treatment of nausea in patients treated with venlafaxine for treatment of refractory depression. *Journal of Clinical Psychopharmacology.* **16**: 357.
3 McHugh S *et al.* (1992) Cisapride vs metoclopramide: an acute study in diabetic gastroparesis. *Digestive Diseases and Science.* **37**: 997–1001.
4 Fumagalli I and Hammer B (1994) Cisapride versus metoclopramide in the treatment of functional dyspepsia: a double-blind comparative trial. *Scandinavian Journal of Gastroenterology.* **29**: 33–37.
5 Gebauer A *et al.* (1993) Modulation by 5HT3 and 5HT4 receptors of the release of 5-hydroxytryptamine from the guinea-pig small intestine. *Naunyn Schmiedebergs Archives of Pharmacology.* **347**: 137–140.
6 Twycross R and Wilcock A (2001) *Symptom Management in Advanced Cancer* (3e). Radcliffe Medical Press, Oxford.

H2-RECEPTOR ANTAGONISTS — BNF 1.3.1

Class: Ulcer-healing drugs.

Indications: Acid dyspepsia (including acid reflux) and peptic ulceration.

Pharmacology

H_2-receptor antagonists reduce both gastric acid output and the volume of gastric secretions. **Ranitidine** is more effective if taken o.n. rather than with the evening meal.[1] In patients taking NSAIDs, **ranitidine** is less effective than PPIs in healing gastroduodenal ulcers (63% vs 80% at 8 weeks) and in preventing relapse (59% vs 72% over 6 months).[2] **Cimetidine** does not alter the metabolism of **morphine** in humans.[3] **Famotidine, nizatidine** and **ranitidine** do not share the drug metabolism inhibitory properties of **cimetidine**; **ranitidine** is recommended for use instead, even though more expensive (see Cytochrome P450, p.331).
Bio-availability **cimetidine** 75% PO; **ranitidine** 50% PO.
Onset of action <1h.
Time to peak plasma concentration **cimetidine** 45–90min PO, 15min IM; **ranitidine** 2–3h PO.
Plasma halflife **cimetidine** 2h; **ranitidine** 2–3h.
Duration of action **cimetidine** 7h; **ranitidine** 8–12h.

Cautions

Serious drug interactions: **cimetidine** binds to microsomal cytochrome P450 and inhibits the metabolism of **diazepam, methadone, phenytoin, theophylline** and **warfarin.**

Hepatic impairment, renal impairment. **Cimetidine** causes a transient rise in the plasma concentrations of **carbamazepine**. Cumulation of **diazepam** and **methadone** can cause drowsiness and delirium.[4]

Undesirable effects

For full list, see manufacturer's SPC.

Dizziness, drowsiness or fatigue and rash occur occasionally; rare reports of headache, liver dysfunction and blood disorders. **Cimetidine** occasionally also causes gynaecomastia; rare reports of impotence and myalgia.

Dose and use

H_2-receptor antagonists have been largely superseded by PPIs (see p.13). The dose and duration of treatment is least with duodenal ulceration and most with reflux oesophagitis (Table 1.3). For any indication, the dose should be doubled if the initial response is poor. Parenteral formulations are available for IM and for IV use if treatment is considered necessary in a patient with severe nausea and vomiting (see BNF section 1.3.1).

Table 1.3 Recommended dose regimens for H_2-receptor antagonists

Indication	*Cimetidine*	*Ranitidine*
Duodenal ulcer	400mg b.d. *or* 800mg o.n. for 4+ weeks	150mg b.d. *or* 300mg o.n. for 4–8 weeks
Gastric ulcer	400mg b.d. *or* 800mg o.n. for 6+ weeks	150mg b.d. *or* 300mg o.n. for 4–8 weeks
NSAID-associated ulcer	400mg b.d. *or* 800mg o.n. for 8+ weeks	150mg b.d. *or* 300mg o.n. for 8 weeks
Reflux oesophagitis	400mg q.d.s. *or* 800mg b.d. for 8+ weeks	150mg b.d. *or* 300mg o.n. for 8–12 weeks
Reduction of degradation of pancreatin supplements	400mg *1h a.c.*	150mg *1h a.c.*

Supply

Cimetidine (non-proprietary)
Tablets 400mg, 800mg, 28 days @ 400mg b.d. or 800mg o.n. = £5.21 and £5.33 respectively.

Tagamet® (GSK 0800 221441)
Tablets 400mg, 800mg, 28 days @ 400mg b.d. or 800mg o.n. = £21.11.
Tablets effervescent 400mg, 28 days @ 400mg b.d. = £19.19.
Oral syrup 200mg/5ml, 28 days @ 400mg b.d. = £26.59.
Injection 100mg/ml, 2ml amp = £0.36.

Dyspamet® (Goldshield 020 8649 8500)
Oral suspension sugar-free 200mg/5ml, 28 days @ 400mg b.d. = £22.47.

Ranitidine (non-proprietary)
Tablets 150mg, 300mg, 28 days @ 150mg b.d. or 300mg o.n. = £7.60.

Zantac® (GSK 0800 221441)
Tablets 150mg, 300mg, 28 days @ 150mg b.d. or 300mg o.n. = £18.22 and £17.92 respectively.
Tablets effervescent 150mg, 300mg, 28 days @ 150mg b.d. or 300mg o.n. = £26.02 and £25.59 respectively.
Oral syrup 75mg/5ml, 28 days @ 150mg b.d. = £41.66.
Injection 25mg/ml, 2ml amp = £0.64.

1 Johnston DA and Wormsley KG (1988) The effect of food on ranitidine-induced inhibition of nocturnal gastric secretion. *Alimentary Pharmacology and Therapeutics*. **2**: 507–511.
2 Yeomans N *et al.* (1998) A comparison of omeprazole with ranitidine for ulcers associated with nonsteroidal anti-inflammatory drugs. Acid suppression trial. *New England Journal of Medicine*. **338**: 719–726.

3 Mojaverian P *et al.* (1982) Cimetidine does not alter morphine disposition in man. *British Journal of Clinical Pharmacology.* **14**: 809–813.
4 Sorkin E and Ogawa C (1983) Cimetidine potentiation of narcotic action. *Drug Intelligence and Clinical Pharmacy.* **17**: 60–61.

MISOPROSTOL **BNF 1.3.4**

Class: Prostaglandin analogue.

Indications: Prevention or healing of NSAID-induced gastroduodenopathy.

Contra-indications: Pregnancy (misoprostol increases uterine tone).

Pharmacology

Misoprostol is a synthetic PG analogue with gastric antisecretory and protective properties which, after oral administration, is rapidly de-esterified to its free acid. It helps prevent NSAID-related gastroduodenal erosions and ulcers.[1,2] However, misoprostol is no more effective than a PPI in the treatment of NSAID-related gastroduodenal injury, and maintenance therapy with a PPI is associated with a lower relapse rate (PPI 61%; misoprostol 48%; placebo 27%).[3] Colic and diarrhoea may limit the use of misoprostol. NSAID-associated ulcers may be treated with an H_2-receptor antagonist, a PPI or misoprostol; the causal NSAID need not be discontinued during treatment.[3,4]
Bio-availability 90% PO.
Onset of action <30min.
Time to peak plasma concentration 30min.
Plasma halflife 1–2h for free acid.
Duration of action 2–4h.

Cautions

Conditions where hypotension might precipitate severe complications, e.g. cerebrovascular disease, cardiovascular disease.

Undesirable effects

For full list, see manufacturer's SPC.
Diarrhoea (may necessitate stopping treatment), colic, dyspepsia, flatulence, nausea and vomiting, abnormal vaginal bleeding (intermenstrual bleeding, menorrhagia, postmenopausal bleeding), rashes, dizziness.

Dose and use

Prophylaxis against NSAID-induced ulcers
- 200microgram b.d.–q.d.s. taken with the NSAID.

NSAID-associated ulceration
- 200microgram t.d.s. with meals & o.n. *or*
- 400microgram b.d. (breakfast and bedtime) for 4–8 weeks.[1]

If causes diarrhoea, give 200microgram t.d.s. & o.n. and avoid **magnesium salts**.

Supply

Cytotec® (Pharmacia 01908 661101)
Tablets 200microgram 28 days @ 200microgram b.d. = £10.40.

1 Bardhan KD *et al.* (1993) The prevention and healing of acute NSAID-associated gastroduodenal mucosal damage by misoprostol. *British Journal of Rheumatology.* **32**: 990–995.
2 Silverstein FE *et al.* (1995) Misoprostol reduces serious gastrointestinal complications in patients with rheumatoid arthritis receiving nonsteroidal anti-inflammatory drugs. *Annals of Internal Medicine.* **123**: 241–249.

3 Hawkey C *et al.* (1998) Omeprazole compared with misoprostol for ulcers associated with nonsteroidal anti-inflammatory drugs. *New England Journal of Medicine.* **338**: 727–734.
4 Hawkins C and Hanks G (2000) The gastroduodenal toxicity of nonsteroidal anti-inflammatory drugs. A review of the literature. *Journal of Pain and Symptom Management.* **20**: 140–151.

PROTON PUMP INHIBITORS BNF 1.3.5

Class: Ulcer-healing drug.

Indications: Acid dyspepsia (including acid reflux), peptic ulceration.

Pharmacology

Proton pump inhibitors (PPIs) reduce gastric acid output but, in contrast to H_2-receptor antagonists, do not reduce the volume of gastric secretions. Because **lansoprazole, omeprazole** and **pantoprazole** are all rapidly degraded by acid, they are formulated as e/c granules or tablets. These dissolve in the duodenum where the drug is rapidly absorbed to be selectively taken up by gastric parietal cells and converted into active metabolites. These irreversibly inhibit the proton pump (H^+/K^+-ATPase) and thereby block gastric acid secretion. Elimination is predominantly by metabolism in the liver to inactive derivatives excreted mainly in the urine. The plasma halflives of PPIs are all <2h but, because they irreversibly inhibit the proton pump, the antisecretory activity continues for several days until new proton pumps are synthesised.

When treating peptic ulceration **lansoprazole** 30mg o.d. is as effective as **omeprazole** 40mg o.d., and **pantoprazole** 40mg o.d. is as effective as **omeprazole** 20mg o.d.[1] However, **omeprazole** shows a dose-response curve above the standard dose of 20mg o.d., whereas no further benefit is seen by increasing the dose of **lansoprazole** and **pantoprazole** above 30mg and 40mg o.d. respectively.[2,3] Thus, **omeprazole** 40mg o.d. is superior to **lansoprazole** 60mg o.d. and **pantoprazole** 80mg o.d. in the management of severe gastro-oesophageal reflux disease (oesophagitis and stricture).[4] The bio-availability of **lansoprazole** is reduced by food and the manufacturer recommends that it should be given o.m. *1h before breakfast* (see SPC). However, the reduced bio-availability appears not to reduce efficacy.[5–7] In one study of **lansoprazole** given after food, acid suppression was comparable after 7 days even though there was a significant difference on day 1.[8] For administration by nasogastric tube, the e/c granules of **lansoprazole** or **omeprazole** can be removed from the capsule and dissolved in sodium bicarbonate (see Administering drugs via feeding tubes, p.355).

Bio-availability **lansoprazole** 80–90% PO; **omeprazole** 65% PO; **pantoprazole** 77% PO.
Onset of action <2h.
Time to peak plasma concentration **lansoprazole** 1.5–2h PO; **omeprazole** 3–6h PO; **pantoprazole** 2.5h PO.
Plasma halflife **lansoprazole** 1–2h; **omeprazole** 0.5–1h; **pantoprazole** 1–2h (increases to 7–9h in hepatic cirrhosis).
Duration of action >24h.

Cautions

Serious undesirable drug reactions: ocular damage,[9] impaired hearing, angina, hypertension. Most cases of ocular damage have been reported with IV **omeprazole.**[10] PPIs possibly cause vasoconstriction by blocking potassium-hydrogen ATPase. Because the retinal artery is an end-artery, anterior ischaemic optic neuropathy may result. If the PPI is stopped, visual acuity may improve. Some patients have become permanently blind, *in some instances after 3 days*. Impaired hearing and deafness have also been reported, again mostly with IV **omeprazol**e. A similar mechanism may be responsible for the angina and hypertension included as undesirable effects in the USA Data Sheet on **omeprazole.** (IV **omeprazole** is available only on a named patient basis.)

PPIs are metabolised by the cytochrome P450 family of liver enzymes (see Cytochrome P450, p.331). However, clinically important interactions are rare with all three drugs.[11,12] **Omeprazole** increases the bio-availability of digoxin by 10%. The SPC for **omeprazole** advises caution when using the drug in patients taking **warfarin**, **phenytoin** or **diazepam**, and the

SPC for **lansoprazole** advises caution with **oral contraceptives**, **warfarin**, **phenytoin**, **carbamazepine** and **theophylline**. No significant interactions between **pantoprazole** and other drugs have been identified.[13]

Undesirable effects

For full list, see manufacturer's SPC.
Headache and diarrhoea occur in about 3% of patients; more so with **lansoprazole** than **omeprazole**. Dizziness, nausea, constipation, abdominal pain, pruritus and rashes. Occasional cases of acute interstitial nephritis have been reported, sometimes with eosinophilia ± a rash.[14]

Dose and use

PPIs are increasingly used in preference to H_2-receptor antagonists to treat hyperacidity. PPIs are used in combination with antibiotics for the eradication of *Helicobacter pylori* (see BNF 1.3), and for the treatment of NSAID-induced uclers.
Lansoprazole
- 30mg o.m. for 4 weeks, followed by 15mg o.m. indefinitely
- some patients may need 30mg o.m. for 8 weeks.

A higher dose, i.e. 30mg b.d., is recommended only when **lansoprazole** is being used with antibiotics to eradicate *Helicobacter pylori*. The Data Sheet for **lansoprazole** states that administration should be o.m., a.c. in order to achieve 'optimal acid inhibition'. However, published data show that this precaution is unnecessary.[7,8] For patients with obstructive dysphagia and acid dyspepsia or with severe gastritis and vomiting, the rectal route can be used.[15]
Omeprazole
- 20mg o.m.
- 40mg o.m. in reflux oesophagitis if poor response to standard dose.

Supply

Omeprazole (non-proprietary)
Capsules (enclosing e/c granules) 10mg, 20mg, 40mg, 28 days @ 20mg o.d. = £28.55.
Tablets e/c 10mg, 20mg, 40mg, 28 days @ 20mg o.d. = £28.56.

Losec® (AstraZeneca 0800 783 0033)
Tablets dispersible (MUPS®) 10mg, 20mg, 40mg, 28 days @ 20mg o.d. = £28.56.
Capsules (enclosing e/c granules) 10mg, 20mg, 40mg, 28 days @ 20mg o.d. = £28.56.

Lansoprazole
Zoton® (Wyeth 01628 604377)
Capsules (enclosing e/c granules) 15mg, 30mg, 28 days @ 30mg o.d. = £23.75.
Oral suspension 30mg/sachet, 28 days @ 30mg o.d. = £34.14.

Pantoprazole
Protium® (Abbott 01628 773355)
Tablets e/c 20mg, 40mg, 28 days @ 40mg o.d. = £23.65.

---

1 Anonymous (1997) Pantoprazole – a third proton pump inhibitor. *Drug and Therapeutics Bulletin*. **35**: 93–94.
2 Dammann H *et al.* (1993) The effects of lansoprazole, 30 or 60mg daily, on intragastric pH and on endocrine function in healthy volunteers. *Alimentary Pharmacology and Therapeutics*. **7**: 191–196.
3 Koop H *et al.* (1996) Intragastric pH and serum gastrin during administration of different doses of pantoprazole in healthy subjects. *European Journal of Gastroenterology and Hepatology*. **8**: 915–918.
4 Jaspersen D *et al.* (1998) A comparison of omeprazole, lansoprazole and pantoprazole in the maintenance treatment of severe reflux oesophagitis. *Alimentary Pharmacology and Therapeutics*. **12**: 49–52.
5 Delhotal-Landes B *et al.* (1991) The effect of food and antacids on lansoprazole absorption and disposition. *European Journal of Drug Metabolism and Pharmacokinetics*. **3**: 315–320.
6 Andersson T (1990) Bioavailability of omeprazole as enteric coated (EC) granules in conjunction with food on the first and seventh days of treatment. *Drug Investigations*. **2**: 184–188.

7 Moules I *et al.* (1993) Gastric acid inhibition by the proton pump inhibitor lansoprazole is unaffected by food. *British Journal of Clinical Research.* **4**: 153–161.
8 Brummer RJM and Geerling BJ (1995) Acute and chronic effect of lansoprazole and omeprazole in relation to food intake. *Gut.* **37**: 127.
9 Schonhofer P *et al.* (1997) Ocular damage associated with proton pump inhibitors. *British Medical Journal.* **314**: 1805.
10 Schonhofer P (1994) Intravenous omeprazole and blindness. *Lancet.* **343**: 665.
11 Andersson T (1996) Pharmacokinetics, metabolism and interactions of acid pump inhibitors. Focus on omeprazole, lansoprazole and pantoprazole. *Clinical Pharmacokinetics.* **31**: 9–28.
12 Tucker G (1994) The interaction of proton pump inhibitors with cytochrome P450. *Alimentary Pharmacology and Therapeutics.* **8**: 33–38.
13 Steinijans W (1996) Lack of pantoprazole drug interactions in man: an updated review. *International Journal of Clinical Pharmacology and Therapeutics.* **34**: S31–S50.
14 Assouad M *et al.* (1994) Recurrent acute interstitial nephritis on rechallenge with omeprazole. *Lancet.* **344**: 549.
15 Zylicz Z and Sorge Av (1998) Rectal omeprazole in the treatment of reflux pain in esophageal cancer. *Journal of Pain and Symptom Management.* **15**: 144–145.

LOPERAMIDE — BNF 1.4.2

Class: Antimotility, antidiarrhoeal.

Indications: Acute and chronic diarrhoea,† ileostomy (to improve faecal consistency).

Pharmacology

Loperamide is a highly potent μ-opioid receptor agonist.[1] Although well absorbed from the gut, it is almost completely metabolised by the liver where it is conjugated and excreted via the bile. Further, although highly lipophilic,[2] loperamide is a substrate for the efflux membrane transporter, P-glycoprotein, in the blood-brain barrier and it is actively excluded from the CNS.[3,4] Consequently, loperamide acts almost exclusively via a local effect in the gastro-intestinal tract[1] and the maximum therapeutic impact may not manifest for 16–24h, which has implications for dosing.[4] Like **morphine** and other μ-receptor agonists, loperamide decreases propulsive intestinal activity and increases non-propulsive activity.[2,6] It also has an intestinal antisecretory effect mediated by calmodulin antagonism, which is a property not shared by other opioids.[7–9] Paradoxically, loperamide also reduces sodium-dependent uptake of glucose and other nutrients from the small bowel.[10] Tolerance does not occur. Unlike **diphenoxylate**, loperamide has no analgesic effect in therapeutic and supratherapeutic doses. CNS effects have been observed rarely in children under 2 years of age who received excessive doses.[11,12] Loperamide is about 3 times more potent than **diphenoxylate** and 50 times more potent than **codeine**.[13] It is longer acting and, if used regularly, generally needs to be given only b.d. The following regimens are approximately equivalent:

loperamide 2mg b.d.
diphenoxylate 2.5mg q.d.s. (in **co-phenotrope**)
codeine phosphate 60mg q.d.s.

In very severe diarrhoea, e.g. AIDS-related, loperamide may need to be supplemented by **morphine** PO or **diamorphine/morphine** by CSCI to achieve control; **morphine** and **diamorphine** have both peripheral and central constipating effects.
Bio-availability 10% PO.
Onset of action about 1h; maximum effect 16–24h.[5]
Time to peak plasma concentration 2.5h (syrup); 5h (capsules).[14]
Plasma halflife 11h.[14]
Duration of action up to 3 days.[15]

Cautions

Ensure that the diarrhoea is not secondary to faecal impaction.
Inhibitors of P-glycoprotein will result in increased movement across the blood-brain barrier.[3] Thus, CNS effects are potentially possible if loperamide is taken regularly in association with **ketoconazole**, **quinidine** or **verapamil**.

Undesirable effects

For full list, see manufacturer's SPC.

Abdominal bloating, paralytic ileus, faecal impaction, overflow diarrhoea.

Dose and use

For acute diarrhoea:

- starting dose 4mg PO stat
- followed by 2mg after each loose bowel action for up to 5 days
- maximum dose 16mg/24h.

For chronic diarrhoea for which symptomatic treatment is appropriate, the same initial approach is used for 2–3 days, after which a prophylactic b.d. regimen is instituted based on the needs of the patient during the previous 24h, plus 2mg after each loose bowel action. The effective dose varies widely. In palliative care, it is occasionally necessary to increase the dose to as much as 32mg/24h; *this is twice the recommended maximum daily dose.*

Supply

Loperamide (non-proprietary)
Capsules 2mg, 28 days @ 2mg q.d.s. = £7.24.

Imodium® (Janssen-Cilag 01494 567567)
Capsules 2mg, 28 days @ 2mg q.d.s. = £4.55.
Oral syrup 1mg/5ml, 28 days @ 2mg q.d.s. = £11.76.

1 Shannon HE and Lutz EA (2002) Comparison of the peripheral and central effects of the opioid agonists loperamide and morphine in the formalin test in rats. *Neuropharmacology.* **42**: 253–261.

2 Ooms L *et al.* (1984) Mechanisms of action of loperamide. *Scandinavian Journal of Gastroenterology.* **19 (suppl 96)**: 145–155.

3 Heykants J *et al.* (1974) Loperamide (R 18553), a novel type of antidiarrheal agent. Part 5: The pharmacokinetics of loperamide in rats and man. *Arzneimittel-Forschung.* **24**: 1649–1653.

4 Sadeque A *et al.* (2000) Increased drug delivery to the brain by P-glycoprotein inhibition. *Clinical Pharmacology and Therapeutics.* **68**: 231–237.

5 Dreverman J and van-der-Poel A (1995) Loperamide oxide in acute diarrhoea: a double-blind placebo-controlled trial. *Alimentary Pharmacology and Therapeutics.* **9**: 441–446.

6 Van-Nueten J *et al.* (1974) Loperamide (R 18553), a novel type of antidiarrheal agent. Part 3: In vitro studies on the peristaltic reflex and other experiments on isolated tissues. *Arzneimittel-Forschung.* **24**: 1641–1645.

7 Daly J and Harper J (2000) Loperamide: novel effects on capacitative calcium influx. *Cellular and Molecular Life Sciences.* **57**: 149–157.

8 Merritt J *et al.* (1982) Loperamide and calmodulin. *Lancet.* **1**: 283.

9 Zavecz J *et al.* (1982) Relationship between anti-diarrheal activity and binding to calmodulin. *European Journal of Pharmacology.* **78**: 375–377.

10 Klaren P *et al.* (2000) Effect of loperamide on Na+/D-glucose cotransporter activity in mouse small intestine. *Journal of Pharmacy and Pharmacology.* **52**: 679–686.

11 Friedli G and Haenggeli C-A (1980) Loperamide overdose managed by naloxone. *Lancet.* **ii**: 1413.

12 Minton N and Smith P (1987) Loperamide toxicity in a child after a single dose. *British Medical Journal.* **294**: 1383.

13 Schuermans V *et al.* (1974) Loperamide (R18553), a novel type of antidiarrhoeal agent. Part 6: clinical pharmacology. Placebo-controlled comparison of the constipating activity and safety of loperamide, diphenoxylate and codeine in normal volunteers. *Arzneimittel-Forschung Drug Research.* **24**: 1653–1657.

14 Killinger J *et al.* (1979) Human pharmacokinetics and comparative bioavailability of loperamide hydrochloride. *Journal of Clinical Pharmacology.* **19**: 211–218.

15 Heel R *et al.* (1978) Loperamide: A review of its pharmacological properties and therapeutic efficacy in diarrhoea. *Drugs.* **15**: 33–52.

LAXATIVES BNF 1.6

Constipation is common in advanced cancer, particularly in immobile patients with small appetites and those receiving constipating drugs such as opioids. Exercise and increased dietary fibre are rarely appropriate options. As a general rule, all patients prescribed **morphine** should also be prescribed a laxative. About 1/3 of patients also need rectal measures, either because of failed oral treatment or electively, e.g. in patients with paraplegia or bedbound debilitated elderly patients. There are several classes of laxatives (Box 1.C).

In contrast to the BNF, **docusate sodium** is classed as a surface-wetting agent, i.e. a faecal softener and not a contact (stimulant) laxative. At doses commonly used, it acts mainly by lowering surface tension, thereby enabling water to percolate into the substance of the faeces.

Opioids cause constipation by decreasing propulsive intestinal activity and increasing non-propulsive activity, and also by enhancing the absorption of fluid and electrolytes.[1] Colonic contact laxatives reduce intestinal ring contractions and thereby facilitate propulsive activity; they provide a logical approach to the correction of opioid-induced constipation. In the UK, a combination of a peristaltic stimulant and a faecal softener is generally prescribed.

Box 1.C Classification of commonly used laxatives

Bulk-forming drugs (fibre)
Ispaghula husk (e.g. Fybogel®, Regulan®)
Methylcellulose
Sterculia (e.g. Normacol®)

Lubricants
Liquid paraffin/mineral oil

Surface-wetting agents
Docusate sodium
Poloxamer 188

Osmotic laxatives
Lactulose syrup
Macrogol (polyethylene glycol) 3350
Liquid paraffin and magnesium hydroxide emulsion BP
Magnesium hydroxide suspension (Milk of Magnesia®)
Magnesium sulphate (Epsom Salts)

Contact (stimulant) laxatives
Bisacodyl
Dantron
Senna
Sodium picosulphate

1 Beubler E (1983) Opiates and intestinal transport: in vivo studies. In: LA Turnberg (ed) *Intestinal Secretion.* Smith Kline & French, Herefordshire, pp.53–55.

ISPAGHULA HUSK BNF 1.6.1

Class: Bulk-forming laxative.

Indications: Colostomy regulation, haemorrhoids, anal fissure, diverticular disease, irritable bowel syndrome (if unprocessed wheat bran unpalatable).

Contra-indications: Dysphagia, intestinal obstruction, colonic atony, faecal impaction.

Pharmacology

Ispaghula is derived from the husks of an Asian plant, *Plantago ovata*. It has very high water-binding capacity, is partly fermented in the colon, and increases bacterial cell mass. Like other bulk-forming laxatives, isphagula stimulates peristalsis by increasing faecal mass. Its water-binding capacity also helps to make loose faeces more formed in some patients with a colostomy.
Onset of action full effect obtained only after several days.
Duration of action best taken regularly to obtain a consistent ongoing effect; may continue to act for 2–3 days after the last dose.

Cautions
Adequate fluid intake should be maintained to avoid intestinal obstruction.

Undesirable effects
For full list, see manufacturer's SPC.
Flatulence, abdominal distension, faecal impaction, intestinal obstruction.

Dose and use
Ispaghula swells in contact with fluid and needs to be drunk quickly before it absorbs water. Stir the granules or powder briskly in 150ml of water and swallow immediately; carbonated water can be used if preferred. Alternatively, the granules can be swallowed dry, or mixed with a vehicle such as jam, and followed by 100–200ml of water. Give 1 sachet o.m.–t.d.s., preferably after meals; not immediately before going to bed.

Supply
Fybogel® (Reckitt Benckiser 01482 326151)
Oral granules plain, orange or lemon flavour 3.5g/sachet (low Na^+, sugar- and gluten-free), 28 days @ 1 sachet b.d. = £3.96.

Regulan® (Procter & Gamble 01932 896000)
Oral powder orange or lemon-lime flavour 3.4g/sachet (sugar- and gluten-free), 28 days @ 1 sachet b.d. = £1.96.

CONTACT (STIMULANT) LAXATIVES — BNF 1.6.2

Indications: The prevention and treatment of constipation.

Contra-indications: Large bowel obstruction.

Pharmacology
Anthranoid laxatives such as **senna** are derived from plants. They are inactive glycosides which pass unabsorbed and unchanged through the small bowel and are hydrolysed by bacterial glycosidases in the large bowel to yield active compounds. Thus, glycosides have no effect on the small bowel but become active in the large bowel. **Dantron**, a synthetic anthranoid, is not a glycoside and has a direct action on the small bowel as well as the large bowel.[1] Absorption of sennosides or any of their metabolites is small; whereas **dantron** is absorbed to some extent from the small bowel with subsequent significant urinary excretion. Active anthranoid compounds have both motor and secretory effects on the bowel. They act by stimulating first the submucosal (Meissner's) plexus and then the myenteric (Auerbach's) plexus. The motor effect precedes the secretory effect, and is the more important laxative action. There is a decrease in segmenting muscular activity and an increase in propulsive waves. Differences in bacterial flora may explain individual differences in responses to anthranoid laxatives.

Polyphenolics such as **bisacodyl** and **sodium picosulphate** have a similar laxative effect to the anthranoids. **Bisacodyl** and **sodium picosulphate** are hydrolysed to the same active metabolite but the mode of hydrolysis differs.[2] **Bisacodyl** is hydrolysed by intestinal enzymes and acts on both the small and large bowels. When applied to the bowel mucosa, **bisacodyl** induces almost immediate powerful propulsive motor activity. In contrast, **sodium picosulphate** is hydrolysed by colonic bacteria and its action is therefore confined to the large bowel. Its activity is more uncertain because it depends on bacterial flora. **Phenolphthalein** is another polyphenolic laxative, present in some proprietary laxatives. It undergoes enterohepatic circulation and can cause a drug rash; it is generally best avoided.

Onset of action
Bisacodyl tablets 10–12h; suppositories 20–60min.
Danthron 6–12h.
Senna 8–12h.
Sodium picosulphate 10–14h.

Cautions

Because very high doses in rodents revealed a carcinogenic risk,[3,4] UK licences for laxatives containing **dantron** are limited to constipation in terminally ill patients.

Undesirable effects

For full list, see manufacturer's SPC.
Intestinal colic, diarrhoea. **Bisacodyl** suppositories may cause local rectal inflammation. **Dantron** discolours urine, typically red but sometimes green or bluish. Prolonged contact with skin (e.g. in urinary or faecally incontinent patients) may cause a dantron burn – a red erythematous rash with a sharply demarcated border which, if ignored, may become excoriated.

Dose and use

The doses recommended here for opioid-induced constipation are higher (often much higher) than those featured in the BNF and the SPC. Because round-the-clock opioids constipate, round-the-clock, b.d. or t.d.s. laxatives may well be necessary, rather than the traditional o.n. (or o.m.) dose.

Bisacodyl

- by mouth 5–20mg o.n.–b.d.
- by suppository 10–20mg o.d.

Dantron

Variable, according to preparation, individual need and patient acceptance (Box 1.D).

Box 1.D Management of opioid-induced constipation

All opioids constipate, although to a varying extent. Morphine is more constipating than methadone and fentanyl.

1 Ask about the patient's past (premorbid) and present bowel habit and use of laxatives; record the date of last bowel action.

2 Palpate for faecal masses in the line of the colon; do a rectal examination if the bowels have not been open for >3 days or if the patient reports rectal discomfort.

3 For inpatients, keep a daily record of bowel actions.

4 Encourage fluids generally, and fruit juice and fruit specifically.

5 When an opioid is prescribed, prescribe co-danthrusate 1 capsule o.n. prophylactically; although occasionally it is appropriate to optimise a patient's existing bowel regimen, rather than change automatically to co-danthrusate.

6 If already constipated, prescribe co-danthrusate 2 capsules o.n.

7 Adjust the dose every few days according to results, up to 3 capsules t.d.s.

8 If the patient prefers a liquid preparation, use co-danthrusate suspension (5ml = 1 capsule).

9 If >3 days since last bowel action, 'uncork' with suppositories, e.g. bisacodyl 10mg and glycerine 4g or a micro-enema. If these are ineffective, administer a phosphate enema and possibly repeat the next day.

10 If co-danthrusate causes intestinal colic, divide the total daily dose into smaller more frequent doses, e.g. change from co-danthrusate 2 capsules b.d. to 1 capsule q.d.s. Alternatively, change to an osmotic laxative, e.g. lactulose 20–40ml o.d.–t.d.s. or magnesium hydroxide + liquid paraffin 25–50ml o.m.–b.d.

11 If the maximum dose of co-danthrusate is ineffective, halve dose and add an osmotic laxative, e.g. lactulose 20ml b.d. or magnesium hydroxide + liquid paraffin 25ml o.m.–b.d.

12 Lactulose may be preferable to co-danthrusate in patients with a history of colic with other colonic stimulants, e.g. senna.

Senna
- starting dose 15mg o.n. or, if taking opioids, 15mg b.d.
- increase if necessary to 15–22.5mg t.d.s.

Sodium picosulphate
- 5–20ml o.n.–b.d.

Supply

Bisacodyl (non-proprietary)
Tablets e/c 5mg, 28 days @ 10mg o.n. = £1.65.
Suppositories 10mg, 28 days @ 10mg o.d. = £1.75.

Dulco-lax® (Boehringer Ingelheim 01344 424600)
Tablets e/c 5mg, 28 days @ 10mg o.n. = £3.30.
Suppositories 10mg, 28 days @ 10mg o.d. = £1.77.

Dantron
(a) **Co-danthramer** (**dantron** and **poloxamer 188**) (non-proprietary)

Co-danthramer suspension 5ml = 1 co-danthramer capsule.

Co-danthramer suspension 15ml = 5ml **strong** co-danthramer suspension.

Strong co-danthramer suspension 5ml = 2 **strong** co-danthramer capsules.

Capsules co-danthramer 25/200 (dantron 25mg, poloxamer 188 200mg), 28 days @ 2 o.n. = £12.00.
Oral suspension co-danthramer 25/200 in 5ml (dantron 25mg, poloxamer 188 200mg/5ml), 28 days @ 10ml o.n. = £10.52.
Strong capsules co-danthramer 37.5/500 (dantron 37.5mg, poloxamer 188 500mg), 28 days @ 2 o.n. = £14.51.
Strong oral suspension co-danthramer 75/1000 in 5ml (dantron 75mg, poloxamer 188 1g/5ml), 28 days @ 5ml o.n. = £14.06.

(b) **Co-danthrusate** (**dantron** and **docusate sodium**) (non-proprietary)
Capsules co-danthrusate 50/60 (dantron 50mg, docusate sodium 60mg), 28 days @ 2 o.n. = £11.96.
Oral suspension co-danthrusate 50/60 (dantron 50mg, docusate sodium 60mg/5ml), 28 days @ 10ml o.n. = £12.25.

Senna (non-proprietary)
Tablets total sennosides 7.5mg, 28 days @ 15mg o.n. = £0.84.

Senokot® (Reckitt Benckiser 01482 326151)
Tablets total sennosides 7.5mg (~~NHS~~), available OTC.
Oral granules total sennosides 15mg/5ml spoonful, 28 days @ 5ml o.n. = £4.09.
Oral syrup total sennosides 7.5mg/5ml, 28 days @ 10ml o.n. = £6.19.

Sodium picosulfate (non-proprietary)
Oral syrup 5mg/5ml, 28 days @ 10ml o.n. = £5.18.

Laxoberal® (~~NHS~~) and Dulco-lax Liquid® (Boehringer Ingelheim 01344 424600)
Oral syrup 5mg/5ml, 28 days @ 10ml o.n. = £5.18.

The proprietary name Laxoberal® (~~NHS~~) and Dulco-lax Liquid® are used for **sodium picosulfate** oral syrup 5mg/5ml, the proprietary name Dulco-lax® is used for **bisacodyl** tablets and suppositories.

1 Lennard-Jones J (1994) Clinical aspects of laxatives, enemas and suppositories. In: M Kamm and J Lennard-Jones (eds) *Constipation.* Wrightson Biomedical Publishing, Petersfield, pp.327–341.

2 Jauch R *et al.* (1975) Bis-(p-hydroxyphenyl)-pyridyl-2-methane: the common laxative principle of bisacodyl and sodium picosulfate. *Arzneimittel-Forschung Drug Research.* **25**: 1796–1800.

3 Mori H *et al.* (1985) Induction of intestinal tumours in rats by chrysazin. *British Journal of Cancer.* **52**: 781–783.

4 Mori H *et al.* (1986) Carcinogenicity of chrysazin in large intestine and liver of mice. *Japanese Journal of Cancer Research (Gann).* **77**: 871–876.

DOCUSATE BNF 1.6.3

Class: Surface-wetting agent (faecal softener).

Indications: Constipation, †partial bowel obstruction.

Pharmacology

Although classified as a stimulant laxative in the BNF, docusate is principally an emulsifying and wetting agent and has a relatively weak effect on bowel transit. Other wetting agents include **poloxamer 188** (in **co-danthramer**). Docusate lowers surface tension, thereby allowing water and fats to penetrate hard, dry faeces. It also stimulates fluid secretion by the small and large bowel.[1,2] Docusate does not interfere with protein or fat absorption.[3] Docusate has been evaluated in several groups of elderly patients; frequency of defaecation increased and the need for enemas decreased almost to zero.[4–6] Given these clinical results, it is surprising that, in a study in normal subjects, docusate did not increase faecal weight.[7] In palliative care, docusate is not recommended as the sole laxative except in patients with partial bowel obstruction.[8] The routine combination of docusate (or alternative surface-wetting agent) and a contact (stimulant) laxative has been criticised because of a lack of published data supporting such a regimen.[9] However, in the UK such a combination is widely used in patients with opioid-induced constipation (see Box 1.D, p.19).

Onset of action 12–72h.

Cautions

Docusate enhances the absorption of **liquid paraffin**;[10] combined preparations of these substances are prohibited in some countries.

Undesirable effects

For full list, see manufacturer's SPC.

Docusate solution may cause an unpleasant aftertaste or burning sensation, minimised by drinking plenty of water after taking the solution.

Dose and use

Docusate is used in combination with **dantron** in **co-danthrusate** as the laxative of choice for opioid-induced constipation (see Box 1.D, p.19). Docusate is used alone for patients with persistent partial bowel obstruction. Dose varies according to individual need:

- usual starting dose 100mg b.d.
- usual maximum dose 200mg b.d.–t.d.s.; *the latter is higher than the BNF maximum dose of 500mg/day.*

Supply

Dioctyl® (Schwarz 01494 797500)
Capsules 100mg, 28 days @ 100mg b.d. = £2.80.

Docusol® (Typharm 01603 735200)
Oral solution 50mg/5ml, 28 days @ 10ml b.d. = £4.63.

1 Donowitz M and Binder H (1975) Effect of dioctyl sodium sulfosuccinate on colonic fluid and electrolyte movement. *Gastroenterology.* **69**: 941–950.

2 Moriarty K *et al.* (1985) Studies on the mechanism of action of dioctyl sodium sulphosuccinate in the human jejunum. *Gut.* **26**: 1008–1013.

3 Wilson J and Dickinson D (1955) Use of dioctyl sodium sulfosuccinate (aerosol O.T.) for severe constipation. *Journal of the American Medical Association.* **158**: 261–263.

4 Cass L and Frederik W (1955) Doxinate in the treatment of constipation. *American Journal of Gastroenterology.* **49**: 691–698.

5 Harris R (1957) Constipation in geriatrics. *American Journal of Digestive Diseases.* **2**: 487–492.

6 Hyland C and Foran J (1968) Dicotyl sodium sulphosuccinate as a laxative in the elderly. *Practitioner.* **200**: 698–699.

7 Chapman R *et al.* (1985) Effect of oral dioctyl sodium sulfosuccinate on intake-output studies of human small and large intestine. *Gastroenterology.* **89**: 489–493.

8 Twycross R and Wilcock A (2001) *Symptom Management in Advanced Cancer* (3e). Radcliffe Medical Press, Oxford.
9 Hurdon V *et al.* (2000) How useful is docusate in patients at risk for constipation? A systematic review of the evidence in the chronically ill. *Journal of Pain and Symptom Management.* **19**: 130–136.
10 Godfrey H (1971) Dangers of dioctyl sodium sulfosuccinate in mixtures. *Journal of the American Medical Association.* **215**: 643.

LACTULOSE BNF 1.6.4

Class: Osmotic laxative.

Indications: Constipation, particularly in patients who experience bowel colic with contact (stimulant) laxatives, or who fail to respond to contact (stimulant) laxatives alone; hepatic encephalopathy.

Contra-indications: Intestinal obstruction, galactosaemia.

Pharmacology

Lactulose is a synthetic disaccharide, a combination of galactose and fructose, which is not absorbed by the small bowel. It is a 'small bowel flusher', i.e. through an osmotic effect, lactulose deposits a large volume of fluid into the large bowel. Lactulose is fermented in the large bowel to acetic and lactic acids, hydrogen and carbon dioxide with an increase in faecal acidity, which also stimulates peristalsis. The low pH discourages the proliferation of ammonia-producing organisms, hence its use in hepatic encephalopathy. Lactulose does not affect the management of diabetes mellitus; 15ml contains 14 calories.
Onset of action up to 48h.

Undesirable effects

For full list, see manufacturer's SPC.
Abdominal bloating, discomfort and flatulence, diarrhoea, intestinal colic.

Dose and use

Solution

- starting dose 15ml b.d. and adjust according to need
- in hepatic encephalopathy, 30–50ml t.d.s.; adjust dose to produce 2–3 soft faecal evacuations per day.

Powder

- starting dose 10g b.d. and adjust according to need
- in hepatic encephalopathy, 20–30g t.d.s.; adjust dose to produce 2–3 soft faecal evacuations per day.

The powder can be placed on the tongue and washed down with water or other liquid, or sprinkled on food, or mixed with water or other liquid before swallowing.

Supply

Lactulose (non-proprietary)
Oral solution 3.1–3.7g/5ml with other ketoses, 28 days @ 15ml b.d. = £4.08.
Oral powder 10g/sachet with other ketoses, 28 days @ 1 sachet b.d. = £5.60.

MACROGOL (POLYETHYLENE GLYCOL) BNF 1.6.4

Class: Osmotic laxative.

Indications: Constipation, faecal impaction.

Contra-indications: Severe inflammatory conditions of the intestines, intestinal obstruction.

Pharmacology

Macrogol 3350 (polyethylene glycol 3350) acts by virtue of an osmotic action in the intestines, thereby producing an increase in faecal volume which induces a laxative effect. Electrolytes present in the formulation ensure that there is virtually no net gain or loss of sodium and potassium In faecal impaction; controlled studies with enemas have not been performed. In a non-comparative study in 27 adult patients, macrogol 3350 had cleared the faecal impaction in 12/27 (44%) after 1 day of treatment; 23/27 (85%) after treatment for 2 days, and 24/27 (89%) by the end of 3 days.[1,2] Macrogol 3350 is unchanged in the gastro-intestinal tract, virtually unabsorbed and has no known pharmacological activity. Any macrogol 3350 that is absorbed is excreted via the urine.
Onset of action 1–2 days for constipation; 1–3 days for faecal impaction.

Undesirable effects

For full list, see manufacturer's SPC.
Uncommon: Abdominal bloating, discomfort, borborygmi, nausea.
Very rare: electrolyte shift (oedema, shortness of breath, dehydration and cardiac failure).

Dose and use

Each sachet is taken in 125ml of water.
Faecal impaction

- 8 sachets on day 1, *to be taken in* $<$*6h*
- patients with cardiovascular impairment should restrict intake to not more than 2 sachets/h
- repeat on days 2 and 3 p.r.n.

Most patients do not need a full second day's dose.
Constipation

- starting dose 1 sachet o.d.
- increase to 1 sachet t.d.s. if necessary.

Although it is more expensive than **lactulose** (another osmotic laxative), it is more effective and better tolerated.[3]

Supply

Movicol® (Norgine 01895 826600)
Oral powder macrogol 3350 (polyethylene glycol 3350 13.125g, **sodium bicarbonate** 178.5mg, **sodium chloride** 350.7mg, **potassium chloride** 46.6mg/sachet, 28 days @ 1 sachet b.d. = £13.94.

1 Culbert P *et al.* (1998) Highly effective oral therapy (polyethylene glycol/electrolyte solution) for faecal impaction and severe constipation. *Clinical Drug Investigation.* **16**: 355–360.
2 Culbert P *et al.* (1998) Highly effective new oral therapy for faecal impaction. *British Journal of General Practice.* **48**: 1599–1600.
3 Attar A *et al.* (1999) Comparison of a low dose polyethylene glycol electrolyte solution with lactulose for treatment of chronic constipation. *Gut.* **44**: 226–230.

MAGNESIUM SALTS BNF 1.6.4

Class: Osmotic laxative.

Indications: Constipation, particularly in patients who experience bowel colic with contact (stimulant) laxatives, or who fail to respond to the latter.

Pharmacology

Magnesium and sulphate ions are poorly absorbed from the gut. Their action is mainly osmotic but other factors may be important, e.g. the release of cholecystokinin.[1,2] Magnesium ions also decrease absorption or increase secretion in the small bowel. Total faecal PGE_2 increases progressively as the dose of magnesium hydroxide is raised from 1.2 to 3.2g daily.[3] Increased PG in the gut lumen has been found with anthranoid laxatives and may have a role in their action. Also see **Magnesium**, p.256.

Dose and use

Magnesium hydroxide mixture contains about 8% of hydrated magnesium oxide and the usual dose is 25–50ml. **Magnesium sulphate** is a more potent laxative which tends to produce a large volume of liquid stool. The compound is not popular with patients because it often leads to a sense of distension and the sudden passage of offensive liquid faeces which is socially inconvenient; it is very difficult to adjust the dose to produce a normal soft stool. The usual dose is 4–10g of crystals dissolved in warm water and taken with extra fluid.

Supply

All the preparations below are available OTC.

Magnesium Hydroxide Mixture BP

Oral suspension (Cream of Magnesia) contains about 8% hydrated magnesium oxide 415mg (7.1mmol elemental magnesium)/5ml, *do not store in a cold place*; available OTC as Milk of Magnesia®.

Magnesium sulphate

Oral powder (Epsom Salts) also Andrews Liver Salts® (magnesium sulphate, **citric acid, sodium bicarbonate**) (NHS).

Oral solution magnesium sulphate (Epsom Salts) 4–5g/10ml prepared extemporaneously.

1 Donowitz M (1991) Magnesium-induced diarrhea and new insights into the pathobiology of diarrhea. *New England Journal of Medicine*. **324**: 1059–1060.

2 Harvey R and Read A (1975) Mode of action of the saline purgatives. *American Heart Journal*. **89**: 810–813.

3 Donowitz M and Rood R (1992) Magnesium hydroxide: new insights into the mechanism of its laxative effect and the potential involvement of prostaglandin E2. *Journal of Clinical Gastroenterology*. **14**: 20–26.

RECTAL PREPARATIONS (ENEMAS) BNF 1.6.2 & 1.6.4

Indications: Constipation if oral laxatives and suppositories are ineffective.

Treatment strategy

One third of patients receiving **morphine** continue to need rectal measures either regularly or intermittently despite oral laxatives.[1,2] These comprise laxative suppositories, enemas and digital evacuation. Sometimes these measures are elective, e.g. in paraplegics and in the very old and debilitated (Box 1.E). Suppositories take about 30min to dissolve after insertion. In patients who defaecate within 5min of the insertion of a **bisacodyl** suppository, the mechanism of action is ano-rectal stimulation and not pharmacological. A response after 20–30min reflects systemic absorption and subsequent hydrolysis to the active metabolite. In the UK, most patients needing laxative suppositories receive both **glycerol** and **bisacodyl**. **Bisacodyl** may result in some delayed rectal discharge or faecal incontinence. Carbalax® is often used by patients with chronic neurological dysfunction, e.g. paraplegia. It is in effect a gas enema and is safer than a large-volume **phosphate** enema.[3]

Osmotic micro-enemas contain mainly sodium lauryl sulpho-acetate and sodium citrate with several excipients, including glycerol and sorbitol. Sodium lauryl sulpho-acetate is a wetting agent (similar to **docusate**) whereas sodium citrate draws fluid into the bowel by osmosis, an action enhanced by sorbitol, and displaces bound water from the faeces. Digital evacuation is the ultimate approach to faecal impaction, but the need for this can be reduced by using **macrogol** (**polyethylene glycol**; see p.23).[4,5]

Box 1.E Rectal measures for the relief of constipation or faecal impaction

Suppositories

Glycerol 4g, has a hygroscopic and lubricant action. Also claimed to be a rectal stimulant but this is unsubstantiated.

Bisacodyl 10mg, after hydrolysis by enteric enzymes, stimulates propulsive activity.[6]

Carbalax, a mixture of sodium bicarbonate and sodium phosphate which reacts in the rectum, releasing 200ml of carbon dioxide and stimulating evacuation by rectal distension.

Enemas

Faecal softener micro-enema containing 90–120mg of docusate sodium/5ml.

Lubricant enema, arachis/peanut oil (130ml), generally instilled and left overnight before giving stimulant laxative suppository or enema.

Osmotic micro-enemas, small volume (5ml) containing sodium citrate, glycerol and sorbitol.

Osmotic standard enemas, large volume (120–130ml) phosphate enemas.

Supply

Suppositories

Glycerol Suppositories BP (glycerin suppositories)
Suppositories gelatin 140mg, glycerol 700mg/1g, 28 days @ 4g o.d. = £1.66.

Bisacodyl (non-proprietary)
Suppositories 10mg, 28 days @ 10mg o.d. = £1.75.

Dulco-lax® (Boehringer Ingelheim 01344 424600)
Suppositories 10mg, 28 days @ 10mg o.d. = £4.14.

Sodium acid phosphate
Carbalax® (Forest 01322 550550)
Suppositories sodium acid phosphate 1.3g, sodium bicarbonate 1.08g, 28 days @ 1 o.d. = £4.99.

Faecal softener enemas
Fletcher's Enemette® (Pharmax 01322 550550), docusate sodium 90mg and glycerol 3.78g, 5ml unit = £0.31.
Norgalax Micro-enema® (Norgine 01895 826600), docusate sodium 120mg in 10g, 10g unit = £0.64.

Lubricant enema
Fletcher's Arachis (peanut) Oil Retention Enema® (Pharmax 01322 550550), in 130ml single-dose disposable pack = £1.02. *Do not use in patients with peanut allergy.*

Osmotic micro-enemas
These all contain sodium citrate, glycerol and sorbitol and are supplied in 5ml single-dose disposable packs with nozzle:
Micolette® (Dexcel-Pharma 01327 312266), 5ml = £0.32.

Micralax® (Celltech 01753 534655), 5ml = £0.33.
Relaxit® (Crawford 01908 262346), 5ml = £0.31.

Osmotic standard enemas
Fleet® Ready-to-use Enema (De Witt 01928 579029), sodium acid phosphate 21.4g and sodium phosphate 9.4g/118ml, single-dose with standard tube = £0.46.
Fletcher's Phosphate Enema® (Forest 01322 550550), sodium acid phosphate 12.8g and sodium phosphate 10.24g/128ml (corresponds to Phosphates Enema Formula B), 128ml with standard tube = £0.44; with long rectal tube = £0.61.

1 Twycross RG and Lack SA (1986) *Control of Alimentary Symptoms in Far Advanced Cancer.* Churchill Livingstone, Edinburgh.
2 Twycross RG and Harcourt JMV (1991) The use of laxatives at a palliative care centre. *Palliative Medicine.* **5**: 27–33.
3 Goldman M (1993) Hazards of phosphate enemas. *Gastroenterology Today.* **3**: 16–17.
4 Culbert P *et al.* (1998) Highly effective oral therapy (polyethylene glycol/electrolyte solution) for faecal impaction and severe constipation. *Clinical Drug Investigation.* **16**: 355–360.
5 Culbert P *et al.* (1998) Highly effective new oral therapy for faecal impaction. *British Journal of General Practice.* **48**: 1599–1600.
6 Roth vW and Beschke vK (1988) Pharmakokinetik und laxierende wirkung von bisacodyl nach gabe verschiedener zubereitungsformen. *Arzneimittel-Forschung Drug Research.* **38**: 570–574.

PREPARATIONS FOR HAEMORROIDS — BNF 1.7

Peri-anal pruritus (often associated with haemorrhoids), soreness and excoriation are best treated by the application of a bland ointment or cream. If associated with the evacuation of hard faeces, the constipation should be corrected (see Laxatives, p.17). Soothing preparations containing mild astringents such as bismuth subgallate, zinc oxide and hamamelis all give symptomatic relief in haemorrhoids. Many proprietary preparations also contain lubricants, vasoconstrictors and antiseptics.

Local anaesthetics relieve pruritus ani as well as pain associated with haemorrhoids. **Lidocaine** (lignocaine) ointment can be used before defaecation to relieve pain associated with an anal fissure. Local anaesthetic ointments are absorbed through the rectal mucosa and could produce a systemic effect if applied excessively. They should be used for only a few days because, apart from **lidocaine**, they can cause contact dermatitis. Corticosteroids can be combined with local anaesthetics and astringents; suitable for short-term use after exclusion of infection, such as *Herpes simplex*. Pain associated with spasm of the internal anal sphincter may be helped by topical **glyceryl trinitrate** ointment (see p.39).

Dose and use

Anusol®
For pruritus ani, haemorrhoids, peri-anal excoriation:
- apply ointment topically b.d. and after defaecation
- insert suppository after defaecation and o.n.

Scheriproct®
For anal pain:
- apply ointment b.d. for 5–7 days (t.d.s.–q.d.s. on first day if necessary), then o.d. for a few days after symptoms have cleared
- insert suppository after defaecation for 5–7 days (in severe cases initially b.d.–t.d.s.).

Supply

Anusol® (Parke Davis 023 8062 0500)
Cream, ointment and ***suppositories*** bismuth oxide, Peru balsam, zinc oxide, all available OTC.

Scheriproct® (Schering Health 01444 232323)
Ointment cinchocaine hydrochloride 0.5%, prednisolone hexanoate 0.19%, 30g = £3.53.
Suppositories cinchocaine hydrochloride 1mg, prednisolone hexanoate 1.3mg, 12 = £1.66.

PANCREATIN BNF 1.9.4

Class: Enzyme supplement.

Indications: *Symptomatic* steatorrhoea caused by biliary and/or pancreatic obstruction, e.g. cancer of the pancreas.

Pharmacology

Steatorrhoea (the presence of undigested faecal fat) often results in increased bowel frequency, typically with pale, bulky, offensive, frothy and greasy faeces which flush away only with difficulty; associated with abdominal distension, increased flatus, loss of weight, and mineral and vitamin deficiency (A, D, E and K).

Pancreatin is a standardised preparation of porcine lipase, protease and amylase. Pancreatin hydrolyses fats to glycerol and fatty acids, degrades protein into amino acids, and converts starch into dextrin and sugars. Because they are inactivated by gastric acid, pancreatin preparations are best taken with food (or immediately before or after food). Gastric acid secretion may be reduced by giving **cimetidine** or **ranitidine** an hour before meals or a PPI o.d. Concurrent use of antacids further reduces gastric acidity. E/c preparations, such as Creon®, Nutrizym GR®, Pancrease®, deliver a higher enzyme concentration in the duodenum provided the granules are swallowed whole without chewing.

Cautions

Fibrotic strictures of the colon have developed in children aged 2–13 years with cystic fibrosis who have used certain high-strength preparations of pancreatin, e.g. Nutrizym 22® and Pancrease HL®. Fibrosing colonopathy has not been reported in adults or in patients without cystic fibrosis. Creon® 25 000 has not been implicated.

Undesirable effects

For full list, see manufacturer's SPC.

Nausea, vomiting and abdominal discomfort. Peri-anal irritation with larger doses.

Dose and use

There are several different proprietary preparations of pancreatin; Creon® capsules are the preparations of first choice. Capsules are taken whole or their contents added to fluid or soft food and swallowed without chewing:

- Creon® 10 000, initially give 1–2 capsules with each meal
- Creon® 25 000, initially give 1 capsule with each meal.

Capsule strength denotes lipase unit content. The dose is adjusted upwards according to size, number, and consistency of stools, so that the patient thrives; extra allowance may be needed if snacks are taken between meals. If a pancreatin preparation continues to seem ineffective, prescribe a PPI or H_2-receptor antagonist.

Supply

Creon® (Solvay 023 8046 7000)

Capsules (enclosing e/c granules) Creon 10 000, 28 days @ 2 t.d.s. = £27.99.

Capsules (enclosing e/c pellets) Creon 25 000, 28 days @ 1 t.d.s. = £32.76.

2: CARDIOVASCULAR SYSTEM

FUROSEMIDE (FRUSEMIDE) BNF 2.2.2

Class: Loop diuretic.

Indications: Oedema, †malignant ascites (with **spironolactone**), †bronchorrhoea.

Contra-indications: Hepatic encephalopathy, anuric renal failure.

Pharmacology

Furosemide inhibits sodium (and hence water) resorption from the ascending limb of the loop of Henle in the renal tubule. It also increases urinary excretion of K^+, H^+, Cl^- and Mg^{2+}. Diuretics such as furosemide are the standard first-line therapy for the treatment of congestive cardiac failure (Figure 2.1).

Furosemide alone has little effect on malignant ascites, even when used in daily doses of 100–200mg PO.[1,2] However, furosemide 100mg CIVI over 24h can have a marked short-term effect with a decrease in girth of up to 10cm and only a modest diuresis (<3L in 24h), suggesting part of the impact is fluid redistribution within the body.[2] Even so, its use in malignant ascites is best limited to when treatment alone with **spironolactone**, an aldosterone antagonist, is insufficient.

Nebulised furosemide attenuates experimentally-induced cough and breathlessness,[3,4] and also allergen-induced asthma,[5] possibly via an effect on vagal sensory nerve endings. Anecdotally, it is of benefit in bronchorrhoea[6] and severe breathlessness.[7] However, unpublished data suggest that, in severe breathlessness, such use could be deleterious (Stone P, personal communication). Use of nebulised furosemide should therefore be restricted to randomised controlled trials.

Bio-availability 60–70%.
Onset of action <1h PO; 2–5min IV.
Time to peak plasma concentration no data.
Plasma halflife 30–120min.
Duration of action 6–8h PO; 2h IV.

Cautions

Increased risk of hypokalaemia with corticosteroids, β_2-adrenoceptor agonists, **theophylline**, **amphotericin** and **carbenoxolone**; increased risk of hyponatreamia with **carbamazepine**, **aminoglutethimide**; increased risk of hypotension with ACE inhibitors and tricyclic antidepressants.
Withdrawal: The elderly frequently receive long-term diuretic therapy for hypertension, congestive cardiac failure and non-cardiac ankle oedema. The withdrawal of diuretics even in normotensive patients with no signs of congestive cardiac failure requires careful monitoring as about half will develop cardiac failure, generally within 4 weeks.[8]

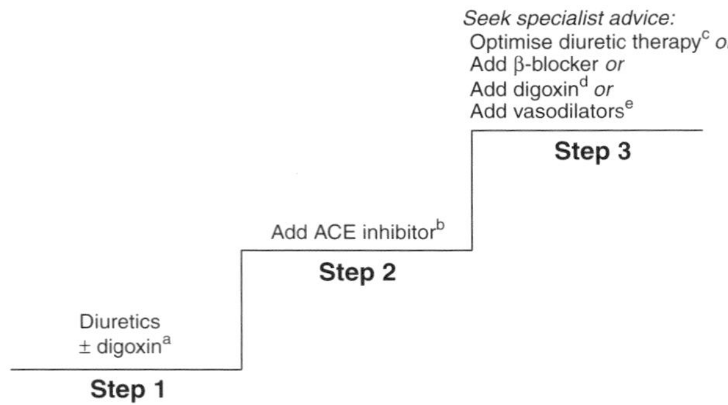

Figure 2.1 Drug treatment for congestive cardiac failure.

a. patients in atrial fibrillation
b. if an ACE inhibitor is not tolerated, substitute an angiotensin-II receptor antagonist, e.g. losartan *or* hydralazine + a nitrate
c. e.g. combine a loop with a thiazide diuretic *or* add spironolactone 25–50mg o.d. *or* add metolazone 2.5–10mg once or twice per week *or* give loop diuretic IV
d. patients in sinus rhythm
e. e.g. hydralazine + a nitrate.

Undesirable effects

For full list, see manufacturer's SPC.

Nausea and gastrointestinal disturbances, hypokalaemia (may precipitate encephalopathy in hepatic failure), hyponatraemia, hyperglycaemia (worsening diabetic control), hyperuricaemia (precipitating gout), urinary retention (in prostatic hypertrophy), hypotension, rashes, photosensitivity, bone marrow depression, tinnitus and deafness, hypocalcaemia, acute pancreatitis.

Dose and use

Congestive cardiac failure

- starting dose 40mg o.m.
- usual maintenance dose 40–80mg o.m.
- usual maximum dose 160mg o.m.

Ascites

Generally used only as a supplement to **spironolactone**.

- starting dose 40mg o.m.
- usual maintenance dose 20–40mg o.m.
- usual maximum dose 80mg o.m.

Bronchorrhoea

- 20mg nebulised q.d.s.

Supply

Furosemide (frusemide) (non-proprietary)

Tablets 20mg, 40mg, 500mg, 28 days @ 20mg, 40mg o.m. = £0.49 and £0.78 respectively.

Oral solution 20mg/5ml, 40mg/5ml, 50mg/5ml, 28 days @ 20mg, 40mg o.m. = £11.98 and £15.47 respectively.

Lasix® (Borg 01462 442993)

Tablets 20mg, 40mg, 500mg, 28 days @ 20mg, 40mg o.m. = £1.57 and £2.27 respectively.

Oral solution Paediatric 5mg/5ml, 28 days @ 20mg o.m. = £13.74.

1 Fogel M *et al.* (1981) Diuresis in the ascitic patient: a randomised controlled trial of three regimens. *Journal of Clinical Gastroenterology.* **3**: 73–80.

2 Amiel S *et al.* (1984) Intravenous infusion of frusemide as treatment for ascites in malignant disease. *British Medical Journal.* **288**: 1041.
3 Bianco S *et al.* (1989) Protective effect of inhaled furosemide on allergen-induced early and late asthmatic reactions. *New England Journal of Medicine.* **321**: 1069–1073.
4 Ventresca P *et al.* (1990) Inhaled furosemide inhibits cough induced by low-chloride solutions but not by capsaicin. *American Review of Respiratory Disease.* **142**: 143–146.
5 Nishino T *et al.* (2000) Inhaled furosemide greatly alleviates the sensation of experimentally induced dyspnea. *American Journal of Respiratory and Critical Care Medicine.* **161**: 1963–1967.
6 Twycross R and Wilcock A (2001) *Symptom Management in Advanced Cancer* (3e). Radcliffe Medical Press, Oxford, pp.162–163.
7 Shimoyama N and Shimoyama M (2002) Nebulized furosemide as a novel treatment for dyspnea in terminal cancer patients. *Journal of Pain and Symptom Management.* **23**: 73–76.
8 Walma E *et al.* (1997) Withdrawal of long term diuretic medication in elderly patients: a double blind randomised trial. *British Medical Journal.* **315**: 464–468.

SPIRONOLACTONE — BNF 2.2.3

Class: Potassium-sparing diuretic; aldosterone antagonist.

Indications: Oedema, malignant ascites.

Contra-indications: Hyperkalaemia, hyponatraemia.

Pharmacology

Spironolactone is a potassium-sparing diuretic which inhibits the action of aldosterone on distal tubules. Hyperaldosteronism is a common concomitant of malignant ascites.[1] Treatment with even very large PO doses of a loop diuretic (e.g. **furosemide** (frusemide) 200mg) generally fails to relieve ascites.[2] On the other hand, spironolactone in a median daily dose of 300mg is successful in about 2/3 of patients.[1,2] Benefit is most likely when ascites is caused by extensive liver metastases rather than peritoneal carcinomatosis or is chylous.[3] Paracentesis is preferable for patients with the last two causes of ascites, for those with a tense distended abdomen, and those unable to tolerate spironolactone. Spironolactone is also used in low dose (25–50mg) in patients with moderate-to-severe congestive cardiac failure (see Figure 2.1, p.30).

Bio-availability 73–90%.
Onset of action 2–4h; maximum diuresis up to 2 weeks.
Time to peak plasma concentration 1–3h PO.
Plasma halflife 80min; active metabolites 12–24h.
Duration of action 16–24h; possibly longer.

Cautions

Serious drug interactions: risk of hyperkalaemia with potassium-sparing diuretics and ACE inhibitors.

Elderly; hepatic impairment, renal impairment. Risk of hyperkalaemia, particularly if prescribed concurrently with an NSAID. Effect reduced by **aspirin** and possibly other NSAIDs. Spironolactone increases the plasma concentration of **digoxin** by up to 25%.

Undesirable effects

For full list, see manufacturer's SPC.
Nausea and vomiting, impotence, gynaecomastia, menstrual irregularities, lethargy, headache, delirium, rashes, hyperkalaemia, hyponatraemia, hepatotoxicity, osteomalacia and blood disorders. Ataxia, impotence and androgenic effects.

Dose and use
- monitor body weight and renal function
- starting dose 100–200mg o.m.; but give in divided dosage if it causes nausea and vomiting
- increase dose by 100mg every 3–7 days to achieve a weight loss of 0.5–1kg/24h
- usual maintenance dose 300mg daily
- usual maximum dose 400–600mg o.d.[1,2]

Elimination of ascites may take 10–28 days. If not achieving the desired weight loss with spironolactone 300–400mg daily, consider adding **furosemide** (frusemide) 40mg o.m.

Supply
Spironolactone (non-proprietary)
Tablets 25mg, 50mg, 100mg, 28 days @ 200mg o.m. = £9.27.
Oral suspension 5mg/5ml, 10mg/5ml, 25mg/5ml, 50mg/5ml and 100mg/5ml. (Unlicensed, available as a special order from Rosemont 0113 244 1999; see Special orders and named patient supplies, p.349.)
Aldactone® (Pharmacia 01908 661101)
Tablets 25mg, 50mg, 100mg, 28 days @ 200mg o.m. = £22.14.

1 Greenway B *et al.* (1982) Control of malignant ascites with spironolactone. *British Journal of Surgery.* **69**: 441–442.
2 Fogel M *et al.* (1981) Diuresis in the ascitic patient: a randomized controlled trial of three regimens. *Journal of Clinical Gastroenterology.* **3**: 73–80.
3 Pockros P *et al.* (1992) Mobilization of malignant ascites with diuretics is dependent on ascitic fluid characteristics. *Gastroenterology.* **103**: 1302–1306.

*FLECAINIDE — BNF 2.3

Class: 1C anti-arrhythmic.

Indications: Cardiac arrhythmias, †neuropathic pain.

Contra-indications: Recent myocardial infarction, heart disease requiring medication, abnormal ECG.

Pharmacology
Flecainide is a chemical congener of **lidocaine** (lignocaine). It is a membrane stabiliser, i.e. it inhibits sodium ion channels in nerve membranes, thereby decreasing excitability and slowing conduction velocity. Flecainide is licensed for use primarily in the treatment of ventricular arrhythmias but is sometimes used as an adjuvant analgesic for nerve injury pain instead of **mexiletine** (see p.33), either as the drug of choice or after treatment failure with a combination of an antidepressant and anti-epileptic. Benefit is reported in about 2/3 of patients with cancer, but there have been no controlled trials.[1–4] Other options include **ketamine** (see p.289), **methadone** (see p.194) and spinal analgesia.

When used as prophylaxis against arrhythmias after myocardial infarction, flecainide was associated with an increased incidence of sudden death.[5] In consequence, when used as an anti-arrhythmic, the manufacturer recommends that treatment is started in hospital. However, at some centres, flecainide for neuropathic pain is started on an outpatient basis without an ECG provided the patient is in normal rhythm, is not in cardiac failure and has no history of myocardial infarction.
Bio-availability 70–95% PO.
Onset of action 0.5–2h as an anti-arrhythmic.
Time to peak plasma concentration 1.5–6h PO.
Plasma halflife 12–27h.
Duration of action 15–23h as an anti-arrhythmic.

Cautions

Hepatic and renal impairment. Risk of myocardial depression increased by β-blockers, calcium-channel blockers and hypokalaemia; risk of arrhythmia if used with a pro-arrhythmic drug, e.g. triyclic antidepressants. Plasma concentration increased by **amiodarone**, **cimetidine**, **fluoxetine**, **propranolol**, **quinine**, decreased by **carbamazepine**, **phenytoin** and **phenobarbital**.

Undesirable effects

For full list, see manufacturer's SPC.
Common: dizziness, double/blurred vision, cardiac arrhythmias or block, nausea, vomiting, abnormal liver function tests.
Rare: dyskinesia, ataxia, peripheral neuropathy, psychosis, delirium.[3,4,6]

Dose and use

Generally, tricyclic antidepressants should be stopped at least 48h before starting flecainide. Initial doses are comparable to those used in cardiology:

- starting dose 50mg b.d.
- usual dose 100mg b.d.
- maximum 200mg b.d.

Some suggest the use of a test dose of **lidocaine** (lignocaine) 2–5mg/kg IVI in order to predict if flecainide or **mexiletine** will be of benefit.[7] However, in patients with cancer, **lidocaine** (lignocaine) 5mg/kg IVI over 30min is no more effective than placebo.[8]

Supply

Flecainide (non-proprietary)
Tablets 50mg, 100mg, 28 days @ 100mg b.d. = £20.73.

Tambocor® (3M 01509 611611)
Tablets 50mg, 100mg, 28 days @ 100mg b.d. = £20.73.

1 Dunlop R *et al.* (1988) Analgesic effects of oral flecainide. *Lancet.* **1**: 420–421.
2 Sinnott C *et al.* (1991) Flecainide in cancer nerve pain. *Lancet.* **337**: 1347.
3 Chong S *et al.* (1997) Pilot study evaluating local anesthetics administered systemically for treatment of pain in patients with advanced cancer. *Journal of Pain and Symptom Management.* **13**: 112–117.
4 Broadley K (1998) Personal communication.
5 Cardiac arrhythmia suppression trial (CAST) (1989) Investigators' preliminary report: effect of encainide and flecainide on mortality in a randomized trial of arrhythmia suppression after myocardial infarction. *New England Journal of Medicine.* **321**: 406–412.
6 Bennett M (1997) Paranoid psychosis due to flecainide toxicity in malignant neuropathic pain. *Pain.* **70**: 93–94.
7 Galer B *et al.* (1996) Response to intravenous lidocaine infusion predicts subsequent response to oral mexiletine: a prospective study. *Journal of Pain and Symptom Management.* **12**: 161–167.
8 Ellemann K *et al.* (1989) Trial of intravenous lidocaine on painful neuropathy in cancer patients. *Clinical Journal of Pain.* **5**: 291–294.

*MEXILETINE — BNF 2.3

Class: 1B anti-arrhythmic.

Indications: Cardiac arrhythmias, †neuropathic pain.

Contra-indications: Heart disease requiring medication; abnormal ECG.

Pharmacology

Mexiletine is a chemical congener of **lidocaine** (lignocaine). It is a membrane stabiliser, i.e. it inhibits sodium ion channels in nerve membranes, thereby decreasing excitability and slowing conduction velocity. Mexiletine is used primarily in the treatment of ventricular arrhythmias. Mexiletine is sometimes used as an adjuvant analgesic for nerve injury pain, either as the drug of choice or after treatment failure with a combination of an antidepressant and an anti-epileptic. Mexiletine is of proven value in pain caused by peripheral nerve injury caused by several conditions but not HIV.[1–4] Benefit is reported in 2/3 of patients with cancer, but there have been no controlled trials.[5,6] Although sometimes used in central poststroke or spinal cord injury pain, it is not of proven benefit.[3,7] Other options include **ketamine** (see p.289), **methadone** (see p.194) and spinal analgesia.

Bio-availability 80–88% PO.

Onset of action 1–3h.

Time to peak plasma concentration 1.5–4h; 7–11h m/r preparation.

Plasma halflife 6–17h.

Duration of action 6–8h.

Cautions

Hepatic impairment. Opioids and antimuscarinics delay absorption. Risk of myocardial depression with other anti-arrhythmics (→ hypotension); risk of arrhythmia if used with a pro-arrhythmic drug, e.g. a tricyclic antidepressant. Effect reduced by drugs causing hypokalaemia (e.g. loop and thiazide diuretics). Plasma concentration of mexiletine increased by **amitriptyline** but decreased by **phenytoin** and **rifampicin**. Mexiletine increases the plasma concentration of **theophylline** (see Cytochrome P450, p.331).

Undesirable effects

For full list, see manufacturer's SPC.

Nausea, vomiting, constipation, bradycardia, hypotension, cardiac arrhythmias, pulmonary infiltrates, intestinal lung disease and pulmonary fibrosis, drowsiness, tremor, delirium, convulsions, altered mood, psychosis, dysarthria, ataxia, paraesthesia, nystagmus, jaundice, hepatitis and blood disorders.

Dose and use

Generally, tricyclic antidepressants should be stopped at least 48h before starting mexiletine. Compared with use in cardiology, the initial dose of mexiletine is low:

- starting dose 50mg t.d.s.
- increase dose by 50mg t.d.s. every 3–7 days to a maximum of 10mg/kg/day.

In the event of undesirable effects, give a smaller dose more frequently p.c. to delay absorption, thereby reducing the maximum plasma concentration.

At one centre, mexiletine is given in high doses (400mg PO stat & 200mg q6h) *with* ***amitriptyline*** to patients with *poststroke central pain* which has failed to respond to antidepressant monotherapy.[8] This is done on an inpatient basis following cardiological review; combined treatment definitely *not* recommended in debilitated cancer patients.

Some suggest the use of a test dose of **lidocaine** (lignocaine) 2–5mg/kg IVI in order to predict if mexiletine or **flecainide** will be of benefit.[9] However, in patients with cancer, **lidocaine** (lignocaine) 5mg/kg IVI over 30min is no more effective than placebo.[10]

Supply

Mexitil® (Boehringer Ingelheim 01344 424600)

Capsules 50mg, 200mg, 28 days @ 200mg t.d.s. = £9.97.

Mexitil PL® (Boehringer Ingelheim 01344 424600)

Perlongets® (= capsules m/r, each enclosing 5 miniature tablets) 360mg, 28 days @ 1 b.d. = £11.97.

1 Dejgard A *et al.* (1988) Mexiletine for treatment of chronic painful diabetic neuropathy. *Lancet.* **1**: 9–11.

2 Chabal C *et al.* (1992) The use of oral mexiletine for the treatment of pain after peripheral nerve injury. *Anaesthesiology.* **76**: 513–517.

3 Kalso E *et al.* (1998) Systemic local-anaesthetic-type drugs in chronic pain: a systematic review. *European Journal of Pain.* **2**: 3–14.
4 Kemper C *et al.* (1998) Mexiletine for HIV-infected patients with painful peripheral neuropathy: a double-blind, placebo-controlled, crossover treatment trial. *Journal of Acquired Immuno-Deficiency Syndromes.* **19**: 367–372.
5 Chong S *et al.* (1997) Pilot study evaluating local anesthetics administered systemically for treatment of pain in patients with advanced cancer. *Journal of Pain and Symptom Management.* **13**: 112–117.
6 Sloan P *et al.* (1999) Mexiletine as an adjuvant analgesic for the management of neuropathic cancer pain. *Anesthesia and Analgesia.* **89**: 760–761.
7 Chiou-Tan F *et al.* (1996) Effect of mexiletine on spinal cord injury dysaesthetic pain. *American Journal of Physical Medicine and Rehabilitation.* **75**: 84–87.
8 Bowsher D (1995) The management of central post-stroke pain. *Postgraduate Medical Journal.* **71**: 598–604.
9 Galer B *et al.* (1996) Response to intravenous lidocaine infusion predicts subsequent response to oral mexiletine: a prospective study. *Journal of Pain and Symptom Management.* **12**: 161–167.
10 Ellemann K *et al.* (1989) Trial of intravenous lidocaine on painful neuropathy in cancer patients. *Clinical Journal of Pain.* **5**: 291–294.

*CLONIDINE — BNF 2.5.2

Class: α-adrenergic agonist.

Indications: Migraine prophylaxis, hypertension, †pain poorly responsive to epidural or intrathecal **diamorphine/morphine** and **bupivacaine**, †spasticity, †diarrhoea or †gastroparesis related to autonomic dysfunction in diabetes mellitus, †sweating.

Pharmacology

Clonidine is a mixed α_1- and α_2-adrenergic agonist (mainly α_2). It reduces the responsiveness of peripheral blood vessels to vasoconstrictor and vasodilator substances, and to sympathetic nerve stimulation.[1] Clonidine can cause a reduction in venous return and mild bradycardia, resulting in a reduced cardiac output. Clonidine attenuates the opioid withdrawal syndrome, indicating an interaction with the opioid system. Reproducible pain relief in some patients with neuropathic pain has been observed, particularly when given via the epidural (ED) or intrathecal (IT) routes.[2–5] ED doses above 300microgram/24h are reported not to yield additional benefit,[6] although high-dose ED clonidine, 10mg/kg bolus, followed by 6mg/kg/h, given alone provides effective postoperative analgesia.[7] ED clonidine is absorbed into the systemic circulation producing significant plasma concentrations (reflected clinically by drowsiness and cardiovascular effects), reaching a peak after 20min. It is debatable whether clonidine has a 'selective' spinal effect.[8] The analgesic effect of clonidine can be reversed by α-adrenergic antagonists but not by **naloxone**.[5] It is probable that clonidine analgesia is mediated by an agonist effect at α_2-adrenergic receptors or imidazoline receptors resulting in:

- peripheral and/or central suppression of sympathetic transmitter release[5,9]
- presynaptic inhibition of nociceptive afferents[10]
- postsynaptic inhibition of spinal cord neurones[11,12]
- facilitation of brain stem pain modulating systems.[13]

The addition of clonidine helps relieve muscle hypertonia and spasms which have failed to respond to maximal doses of **baclofen** in patients with spinal cord injury.[14,15] Clonidine improves chronic diarrhoea in patients with diabetes mellitus, usually with autonomic neuropathy, that may result from loss of adrenergic innervation to the intestinal mucosa. Clonidine, by stimulating α_2-adrenergic receptors on enterocytes, promotes intestinal fluid and electrolyte absorption, inhibits anion secretion and may also modify intestinal motility.[16,17] Clonidine also improves symptoms of diabetic gastroparesis.[18]

Clonidine appears to relieve sweating, with or without 'hot flushes', that occurs with the menopause, or in both men and women as a result of hormonal manipulation by drugs, e.g. tamoxifen, or surgery, e.g. castration.[19,20] However, some trials have found no difference from placebo.[21,22]

About half of a dose of clonidine is excreted unchanged by the kidneys, and most of the remainder is metabolised by the liver to inactive metabolites. Cumulation will occur in renal impairment, extending its halflife up to 40h.

Clonidine can also be given by mouth, as a transdermal patch,[4,23] and by CSCI. Exceptionally, patients have received up to 1.5mg CSCI (10 × 150microgram amp) with increasing effect.[6]

Bio-availability 75–100% PO; 60% TD.[24]
Onset of action 30–60min IV, PO; 2–3 days transdermal.
Time to peak plasma concentration 1.5–5h PO; 20min ED; 2 days TD.
Plasma halflife 12–16h.
Duration of action 8–24h PO; 24h TD.

Cautions

After stopping long-term treatment: agitation, rebound hypertension.

Undesirable effects

For full list, see manufacturer's SPC.
Hypotension (after bolus injection), sedation and dry mouth (initially), dry eyes, dizziness, headache, euphoria, nocturnal restlessness, paraesthesia of extremities, peripheral vasoconstriction, nausea, constipation, rash, depression (long-term use). TD is better tolerated than PO.

Dose and use

Analgesia
ED clonidine is generally given with **diamorphine/morphine** and **bupivacaine**. A typical ED regimen would be:
- a test bolus dose of 50–150microgram in 5ml saline injection over 5min
- if relief obtained, 150–300microgram/24h by infusion.

Clonidine is also used IT. A typical IT regimen would be:
- a test bolus dose of 50microgram in 5ml saline injection over 5min
- if relief obtained, 50–150microgram/24h by infusion.

Spasticity
Generally used as an adjunct to a maximal dose of **baclofen**:
- starting dose, 50microgram b.d.
- increase by 50microgram every 3–7 days
- usual maximum dose 200microgram b.d.

Gastroparesis or diarrhoea related to autonomic dysfunction in diabetes mellitus
- starting dose 50microgram b.d.
- increase by 50microgram every 24h
- usual maintenance dose 150microgram b.d.
- usual maximum dose for diabetic gastroparesis 300microgram b.d.
- usual maximum dose for diabetic diarrhoea 600microgram b.d.

Sweating
- starting dose 50microgram b.d.
- increase by 50microgram every 3–7 days
- usual maintenance dose 50–100microgram b.d.

Supply

Catapres® (Boehringer Ingelheim 01344 424600)
Tablets 100microgram, 300microgram, 28 days @ 100microgram b.d. = £3.14.
Injection 150microgram/ml, 1 amp = £0.29.

Catapres® TTS
Transdermal patch 2.5mg, 5mg, 7.5mg, 1 patch (7 days treatment) = £10.85, £20.11 and £31.50 respectively. (Unlicensed, available as a named patient supply from IDIS 020 8410 0700; see Special orders and named patient supplies, p.349.)

1 Hieble JP and Ruffolo RR (1991) Therapeutic applications of agents interacting with alpha-adrenoceptors. In: RR Ruffolo (ed) *Alpha-adrenoceptors: molecular biology, biochemistry and pharmacology.* Karger, Basel, pp.180–220.

2 Glynn C *et al.* (1988) A double-blind comparison between epidural morphine and epidural clonidine in patients with chronic noncancer pain. *Pain.* **34**: 123–128.
3 Max MB *et al.* (1988) Association of pain relief with drug side effects in postherpetic neuralgia: a single-dose study of clonidine, codeine, ibuprofen and placebo. *Clinical Pharmacology and Therapeutics.* **43**: 363–371.
4 Zeigler D *et al.* (1992) Transdermal clonidine versus placebo in painful diabetic neuropathy. *Pain.* **48**: 403–408.
5 Quan D *et al.* (1993) Clonidine in pain management. *Annals of Pharmacotherapy.* **27**: 313–315.
6 Glynn C (1997) Personal communication.
7 deKock M *et al.* (1999) Epidural clonidine or bupivacaine as the sole analgesic agent during and after abdominal surgery. *Anesthesiology.* **90**: 1354–1362.
8 Wells J and Hardy P (1987) Epidural clonidine. *Lancet.* **i**: 108.
9 Langer SZ *et al.* (1980) Recent developments in noradrenergic neurotransmission and its relevance to the mechanism of action of certain antihypertensive agents. *Hypertension.* **2**: 372–382.
10 Calvillo O and Ghignone M (1986) Presynaptic effect of clonidine on unmyelinated afferent fibers in the spinal cord of the cat. *Neuroscience Letters.* **64**: 335–339.
11 Yaksh T (1985) Pharmacology of spinal adrenergic systems which modulate spinal nociceptive processing. *Pharmacology, Biochemistry and Behaviour.* **22**: 845–858.
12 Michel MC and Insel PA (1989) Are there multiple imidazoline binding sites? *TIPS.* **10**: 342–344.
13 Sagen J and Proudfit H (1985) Evidence for pain modulation by pre- and postsynaptic noradrenergic receptors in the medulla oblongata. *Brain Research.* **331**: 285–293.
14 Weingarden S and Belen J (1992) Clonidine transdermal system for treatment of spasticity in spinal cord injury. *Archives of Physical Medicine and Rehabilitation.* **73**: 876–877.
15 Yablon S and Sipski M (1993) Effect of transdermal clonidine on spinal spasticity: a case series. *American Journal of Physical Medicine and Rehabilitation.* **72**: 154–156.
16 Fedorak R *et al.* (1985) Treatment of diabetic diarrhea with clonidine. *Annals of Internal Medicine.* **102**: 197–199.
17 Fedorak R and Field M (1987) Antidiarrheal therapy prospects for new agents. *Digestive Diseases and Science.* **32**: 195–205.
18 Rosa-Silva L *et al.* (1995) Treatment of diabetic gastroparesis with oral clonidine. *Alimentary Pharmacology and Therapeutics.* **9**: 179–183.
19 Goldberg R *et al.* (1994) Transdermal clonidine for ameliorating tamoxifen-induced hot flashes. *Journal of Clinical Oncology.* **12**: 155–158.
20 Pandya K *et al.* (2000) Oral clonidine in postmenopausal patients with breast cancer experiencing tamoxifen-induced hot flashes: a university of Rochester Cancer Centre community clinical oncology program study. *Annals of Internal Medicine.* **132**: 788–793.
21 Salmi T and Punnonen R (1979) Clonidine in the treatment of menopausal symptoms. *International Journal of Gynaecology and Obstetrics.* **16**: 422–461.
22 Loprinzi C *et al.* (1994) Transdermal clonidine for ameliorating post-orchidectomy hot flashes. *Journal of Urology.* **151**: 634–636.
23 Davis K *et al.* (1991) Topical application of clonidine relieves hyperalgesia in patients with sympathetically maintained pain. *Pain.* **47**: 309–317.
24 Toon S *et al.* (1989) Rate and extent of absorption of clonidine from a transdermal therapeutic system. *Journal of Pharmacy and Pharmacology.* **41**: 17–21.

GLYCERYL TRINITRATE — BNF 2.6

Class: Nitrate.

Indications: Angina, left ventricular failure, †severe smooth muscle spasm pain (particularly of the oesophagus, rectum and anus), †biliary and †renal colic.

Contra-indications: Hypotension, aortic or mitral stenosis, cardiac tamponade, constrictive pericarditis; marked anaemia, cerebral haemorrhage, narrow-angle glaucoma

Pharmacology

Glyceryl trinitrate promotes smooth muscle relaxation in blood vessels and the gastro-intestinal tract and can improve dysphagia and odynophagia caused by oesophagitis and oesophageal spasm.[1] It relieves pain associated with anal fissure and aids healing.[2] It may also relieve rectal tenesmoid pain. If ineffective or poorly tolerated, consider the use of other smooth muscle relaxants, e.g. **nifedipine**, **hyoscine *butylbromide***.

Glyceryl trinitrate produces its smooth muscle relaxant effects via its metabolism to nitric oxide (NO), which stimulates guanylate cyclase. This results in an increase in cyclic guanosine monophosphate which reduces the amount of intracellular calcium available for muscle contraction. NO appears to have an important role in the regulation of distal oesophageal peristalsis and relaxation of the lower oesophageal sphincter. A wider role of NO in pain is evident but is yet to be clarified. NO is produced when the NMDA-receptor is stimulated by excitatory amino acids (see **ketamine**, p.289) and may be important in the development of opioid tolerance as NO synthase inhibitors attenuate the development of analgesic tolerance.[3] Glyceryl trinitrate applied systemically (transdermally) can improve pain in patients with cancer and, as a topical gel, reduces local pain and inflammation.[4–6]

It is rapidly absorbed through the buccal mucosa but orally is inactivated by the gastro-intestinal mucosa and the extensive first-pass metabolism in the liver. Many patients on long-acting or transdermal nitrates develop tolerance; i.e. experience a reduced therapeutic effect. Tolerance is generally prevented if nitrate levels are allowed to fall for 4–8h in every 24h (a 'nitrate holiday'). This may not be possible for patients with persistent pain. If tolerance develops, it will be necessary to increase the dose to restore efficacy.

Bio-availability 40% SL; 60–75% m/r buccal; 75% TD.
Onset of action 1–3min SL; 30–60min ointment or TD patch.
Time to peak plasma concentration 2–5min SL; 3–4h TD.
Plasma halflife 2–30min.
Duration of action 30–60min SL; 8h ointment; 24h TD patch.

Cautions

Severe hepatic or renal impairment, hypothyroidism, malnutrition or hypothermia, recent diagnosis of myocardial infarction. Exacerbates the hypotensive effect of other drugs. Drugs causing a dry mouth may reduce the effect of sublingual nitrates.

Undesirable effects

For full list, see manufacturer's SPC.

Headache, flushing, dizziness, postural hypotension, tachycardia; these generally settle with repeated use.

Dose and use

For dysphagia/odynophagia administer dose 5–15min a.c.

- starting dose 500microgram SL
- maximum dose 1mg.

Instruct patient to swallow or spit out tablet once pain relief obtained.

Repeat p.r.n. when spasm/colic is transient and intermittent. For persistent spasm consider:

- glyceryl trinitrate skin patches
- orally active nitrates, e.g. **isosorbide mononitrate**
- ointment 0.2% for pain due to anal fissure; a pea-sized quantitiy applied to the anal rim b.d. for a least 6 weeks.[2,7]

Supply

Glyceryl trinitrate (non-proprietary)

Tablets SL 500microgram, 100 = £1.06; because of degradation, unused tablets should be discarded after 8 weeks.

Aerosol spray SL 400microgram/metered dose, 200 dose unit = £3.13.

Transdermal preparations

Nitro-Dur® (Schering Plough 01707 363636)

Transdermal patch 200microgram/h (approx 5mg/24h), 400microgram/h (approx 10mg/24h), 600microgram/h (approx 15mg/24h), 28 days @ 1 patch o.d. = £11.84, £13.10 and £14.42 respectively.

Ointment 0.2% (Unlicensed, available as a special order from Queens Medical Centre Pharmacy, Nottingham 0115 924 9924; see Special orders and named patient supplies, p.349.) Can be made extemporaneously by diluting 2% glyceryl trinitrate ointment (Percutol® Dominion 01428 661078) 1:10 with white soft paraffin.[7]

This is not a complete list; see BNF for full details.

1 McDonnell F and Walsh D (1999) Treatment of odynophagia and dysphagia in advanced cancer with sublingual glyceryl trinitrate. *Palliative Medicine.* **13**: 251–252.
2 Lund J and Scholefield J (1997) A randomised, prospective, double-blind, placebo-controlled trial of glyceryl trinitrate ointment in treatment of anal fissure. *Lancet.* **349**: 11–14.
3 Elliott K *et al.* (1994) The NMDA receptor antagonists, LY274614 and MK-801, and the nitric oxide synthase inhibitor, NG-nitro-L-arginine, attenuate analgesic tolerance to the mu-opioid morphine but not to kappa opioids. *Pain.* **56**: 69–75.
4 Ferreira S *et al.* (1992) Blockade of hyperalgesia and neurogenic oedema by topical application of nitroglycerin. *European Journal of Pharmacology.* **217**: 207–209.
5 Berrazueta J *et al.* (1994) Local transdermal glyceryl trinitrate has an antiinflammatory action on thrombophlebitis induced by sclerosis of leg varicose veins. *Angiology.* **5**: 347–351.
6 Lauretti G *et al.* (1999) Oral ketamine and transdermal nitroglycerin as analgesic adjuvants to oral morphine therapy and amitriptyline for cancer pain management. *Anesthesiology.* **90**: 1528–1533.
7 Anonymous (1998) Glyceryl trinitrate for anal fissure? *Drug and Therapeutics Bulletin.* **36**: 55–56.

NIFEDIPINE — BNF 2.6

Class: Calcium-channel blocker.

Indications: Angina, hypertension, Raynaud's phenomenon, †severe smooth muscle spasm pain (particularly of the oesophagus, rectum and anus[1–4]), †intractable hiccup.[5,6]

Contra-indications: Cardiogenic shock, severe aortic stenosis.

Pharmacology

Calcium-channel blockers inhibit the influx of calcium into cells, thereby modifying cell function e.g. smooth muscle contraction, nerve cell transmission of messages.[7] They have an anti-nociceptive effect and augment opioid antinociception. Nifedipine may help hiccup by relieving oesophageal spasm or by interference with neural pathways involved in hiccup.[5,6]

Nifedipine exhibits most of its effects on blood vessels, less on the myocardium and has no anti-arrhythmic activity. It rarely precipitates heart failure as any negative inotropic effect is offset by a reduction in left ventricular work. Nifedipine undergoes extensive first-pass metabolism in the liver to inactive metabolites that are excreted in the urine. Higher plasma concentrations are seen in 'slow' metabolisers, which are more prevalent in South American, South Asian and African populations.[8,9] Hepatic impairment increases bio-availability and halflife.

Bio-availability 45–68% PO.
Onset of action 15min (normal release); 1.5h (Adalat® Retard).
Time to peak plasma concentration 30min PO (capsules).
Plasma halflife 2–3.4h (normal release); 6–11h (Adalat® Retard).
Duration of action 8h (normal release); 12h (Adalat® Retard).

Cautions

Serious drug interactions: augments the hypotensive and negative inotropic effects of other drugs.

Initial exacerbation of angina. Hepatic impairment, may impair glucose tolerance. Plasma concentration increased by grapefruit juice and **cimetidine**; reduced by **rifampicin**, **carbamazepine**,

phenytoin and **phenobarbital**. Nifedipine increases plasma concentrations of **cyclosporin**, **digoxin**, **phenytoin** and **theophylline**; reduces plasma concentrations of **quinidine**; inhibits the inotropic effect of **theophylline** on muscle (see Cytochrome P450, p.331).

Undesirable effects

For full list, see manufacturer's SPC.

Common: headache, vasodilation, nausea, dizziness, peripheral oedema (*not* associated with heart failure or weight gain).

Uncommon: agitation, nervousness, sleep disorder, tremor, vertigo, hypertension, palpitations, postural hypotension, tachycardia, dyspnoea, abdominal pain, lethargy, chest pain, oedema, rash, sweating, abnormal vision.

Dose and use

- starting dose 10mg PO/SL stat
- followed by 10–20mg t.d.s. with or after food, or m/r 20mg b.d.
- in achalasia use 10–20mg SL 30min a.c.
- usual maximum dose 60–80mg/day.

Up to 160mg/day has been used for intractable hiccup with concurrent **fludrocortisone** 0.5–1mg to overcome associated orthostatic hypotension.[6]

Supply

Adalat® (Bayer 01635 563000)
Capsules 5mg, 10mg, 28 days @ 10mg t.d.s. = £7.22.

Adalat® Retard (Bayer 01635 563000)
Tablets m/r 20mg, 28 days @ 20mg b.d. = £10.20.

This is not a complete list; see BNF for full details.

1 Cargill G *et al.* (1982) Nifedipine for relief of esophageal chest pain. *New England Journal of Medicine.* **307**: 187–188.
2 McLoughlin R and McQuillan R (1997) Using nifedipine to treat tenesmus. *Palliative Medicine.* **11**: 419–420.
3 Celik A *et al.* (1995) Hereditary proctalgia fugax and constipation: report of a second family. *Gut.* **36**: 581–584.
4 Al-Waili N (1990) Nifedipine for intestinal colic. *Journal of the American Medical Association.* **263**: 3258.
5 Lipps DC *et al.* (1990) Nifedipine for intractable hiccups. *Neurology.* **40**: 531–532.
6 Brigham B and Bolin T (1992) High dose nifedipine and fludrocortisone for intractable hiccups. *Medical Journal of Australia.* **157**: 70.
7 Castell DO (1985) Calcium-channel blocking agents for gastrointestinal disorders. *American Journal of Cardiology.* **55**: 210B–213B.
8 Sowunmi A *et al.* (1995) Ethnic differences in nifedipine kinetics: comparisons between Nigerians, Caucasians and South Asians. *British Journal of Clinical Pharmacology.* **40**: 489–493.
9 Castaneda-Hernandez G *et al.* (1996) Interethnic variability in nifedipine disposition: reduced systemic plasma clearance in Mexican subjects. *British Journal of Clinical Pharmacology.* **41**: 433–434.

DALTEPARIN BNF 2.8

Class: Low molecular weight heparin (LMWH).

Indications: Prevention and treatment of deep vein thrombosis, pulmonary embolism, †thrombophlebitis migrans, †disseminated intravascular coagulation (DIC).

Contra-indications: Patients at risk of haemorrhage (e.g. bleeding diathesis, thrombocytopenia *except disseminated intravascular coagulation*), peptic ulcer, recent cerebral haemorrhage and severe liver disease, subacute bacterial endocarditis.

Pharmacology

Dalteparin acts within minutes by potentiating the inhibitory effect of antithrombin III on Factor Xa and thrombin. It has a relatively higher ability to potentiate Factor Xa inhibition than to prolong plasma clotting time (APTT) which cannot be used to guide dosage. Anti-factor Xa levels can be measured if necessary but routine monitoring is not required because the dose is determined by the patient's weight. LMWH is now the initial treatment of choice for deep vein thrombosis. It is as effective and cheaper than standard heparin.[1] Other advantages include a better safety profile (it has less of an effect on platelet function and thus primary haemostasis) and a longer duration of action which allows administration o.d. Heparin is the treatment of choice for chronic DIC; this commonly presents as recurrent thromboses in both superficial and deep veins which do not respond to **warfarin**. Even when haemorrhagic manifestations (e.g. ecchymoses and haematomas) are the predominant manifestations, the correct treatment is still heparin because the original trigger for DIC is clot formation. **Tranexamic acid** (an antifibrinolytic drug) should not be used in DIC because it would increase the risk of end-organ damage from microvascular thromboses.
Bio-availability 87% SC.
Onset of action 3min IV; 2–4h SC.
Time to peak plasma concentration 3–4h SC.
Plasma halflife 2h IV; 3–5h SC.
Duration of action 10–24h SC.

Cautions

Serious drug interactions: enhanced anticoagulant effect with anticoagulant/antiplatelet drugs e.g. NSAIDS; reduced anticoagulant effect with antihistamines, cardiac glycosides, **tetracycline** and **ascorbic acid**.

Renal failure, uncontrolled hypertension, retinopathy.

Undesirable effects

For full list, see manufacturer's SPC.
Local skin reactions at the injection site (erythema, induration, pruritus) and, rarely, systemic reactions (urticaria, angioedema, anaphylaxis). Abnormal liver function tests have been reported. Osteoporosis (long-term use).

Both standard heparin and LMWH can cause thrombocytopenia (platelet count $<100 \times 10^9$/L). An early (<4 days) mild fall in platelet count is often seen after starting heparin therapy, particularly after surgery. This corrects spontaneously despite the continued use of heparin and is asymptomatic.[2] However, occasionally, an immune heparin-induced thrombocytopenia (HIT) develops associated with heparin-dependent IgG antibodies. The antibodies form a complex with platelet factor 4 and bind to the platelet surface, *causing disruption of the platelets and a release of procoagulant material*. It can occur up to 4 weeks after starting heparin and manifests as venous or arterial thrombo-embolism which may be fatal. Heparin should be stopped immediately if there is a dramatic fall in the platelet count. If continued anticoagulation is desirable, a heparinoid, e.g. **danaparoid** or **hirudin** should be used. Cross-reactivity is rare. HIT is less common with prophylactic regimens (low doses) than with therapeutic ones (higher doses). The risk is further reduced by using LMWH rather than unfractionated heparin. HIT typically develops 5–8 days after starting heparin and, for this reason, some centres check the platelet count at this time (Box 2.A). HIT is more common in the USA (where more bovine heparin is used) than in the UK (where more porcine heparin is used). The risk in the USA has been put at 3% for unfractionated heparin.[2]

Dose and use

Inject SC, preferably into the abdomen or lateral thigh; introduce the total length of the needle vertically into the thickest part of a skin fold produced by squeezing the skin between the thumb and forefinger.
Surgical thromboprophylaxis
- give 2500units 1–2h before and 8–12h after the operation, then 2500units daily until mobile
- use 5000units daily in high-risk patients.

Box 2.A Diagnosis and management of HIT[2]

High clinical suspicion for HIT
Platelet count fall generally of 50% or more, or to below 100×10^9/L, beginning after 5 days of heparin use.
New thrombotic or thrombo-embolic event.

Laboratory confirmation
Do one of the following tests but if negative or borderline, do both.
Functional assay for antibodies using washed platelets or citrated platelet-rich plasmas.
Antigen assay (platelet factor 4/heparin ELISA).

Therapeutic approach
Stop heparin.
Start treatment with danaparoid or hirudin.
Unless already fully anticoagulated with warfarin, do not start warfarin until the thrombocytopenia has resolved and the patient is satisfactorily anticoagulated with danaparoid or hirudin.

Thrombophlebitis migrans
- generally responds rapidly to a small dose, i.e. 2500–5000units SC daily
- titrate dose if necessary to maximum allowed according to weight i.e. 200units/kg.

Deep vein thrombosis and pulmonary embolism
- confirm diagnosis radiologically (ultrasound, venogram, V/Q scan)
- give 200units/kg SC o.d., up to a maximum of 18 000units
- use 100units/kg SC b.d. if patients are considered to be at a greater risk of bleeding
- in patients whose cancer is relatively stable, **warfarin** should be commenced at the same time and LMWH continued for 2 days after achieving a therapeutic INR.

In patients with advanced cancer, because haemorrhagic complications with **warfarin** occur in nearly 50% (possibly related to drug interactions and hepatic dysfunction), dalteparin can be used alone for 4–8 weeks or indefinitely if risk of recurrence is high.[3,4]

Disseminated intravascular coagulation (DIC)
- confirm the diagnosis
  thrombocytopenia (platelet count $<150\,000 \times 10^9$/L in 95% of cases)
  decreased plasma fibrinogen concentration
  elevated plasma D-dimer concentration, a fibrin degradation product (85% of cases)
  prolonged prothrombin time and/or partial thromboplastin time.[5]

A normal plasma fibrinogen concentration (200–250mg/100ml) is also suspicious because fibrinogen levels are generally raised in cancer (e.g. 450–500mg/100ml) unless there is extensive hepatic disease. Infection and cancer both may be associated with an increased platelet count which likewise may mask an evolving thrombocytopenia.
- give dalteparin o.d. as for deep vein thrombosis
- *do not use **warfarin** because it is ineffective.*

Overdose
- In emergencies, 1mg of **protamine sulphate** inhibits 100units of dalteparin; maximum dose 50mg by slow IV injection.

Supply

Fragmin® (Pharmacia 01908 661101)
Injection (single dose syringe for subcutaneous injection)
12 500units/ml, 0.2ml (2500units) = £1.86.
25 000units/ml, 0.2ml (5000units) = £2.82, 0.3ml (7500units) = £4.23, 0.4ml (10 000units) = £5.65, 0.5ml (12 500units) = £7.06, 0.6ml (15 000units) = £8.47, 0.72ml (18 000units) = £10.16.
Injection (vial; for subcutaneous injection)
25 000units/ml, 4ml (100 000units) = £48.66.

This is not a complete list; see BNF for full details.

1 Hull R *et al.* (1997) Treatment of proximal vein thrombosis with subcutaneous low molecular-weight heparin vs intravenous heparin. An economic perspective. *Archives of Internal Medicine.* **157**: 289–294.
2 Warkentin T *et al.* (1995) Heparin-induced thrombocytopenia in patients treated with low molecular weight heparin or unfractionated heparin. *New England Journal of Medicine.* **332**: 1330–1335.
3 Johnson M (1997) Problems of anticoagulation within a palliative care setting: an audit of hospice patients taking warfarin. *Palliative Medicine.* **11**: 306–312.
4 Johnson M and Sherry K (1997) How do palliative physicians manage venous thromboembolism? *Palliative Medicine.* **11**: 462–468.
5 Spero J *et al.* (1980) Disseminated intravascular coagulation: findings in 346 patients. *Thrombosis and Haemostasis.* **43**: 28–33.

ETAMSYLATE — BNF 2.11

Class: Haemostatic agent.

Indications: Menorrhagia, periventricular haemorrhage in neonates, †surface bleeding from ulcerating tumours, nasal cavity and other organs (bladder, uterus, rectum, stomach and lungs).

Contra-indication: Porphyria.

Pharmacology

Etamsylate is thought to act by increasing capillary vascular wall resistance and platelet adhesiveness in the presence of a vascular lesion, by inhibiting the biosynthesis and actions of those PGs which cause platelet disaggregation, vasodilation and increased capillary permeability; it does not have a vasoconstricting action. Etamsylate does not affect normal coagulation; administration is without effect on prothrombin time, fibrinolysis, platelet count or function. It can be used in conjunction with **tranexamic acid** (see p.44). Rarely, parenteral use may be necessary, e.g. in patients with bleeding and complete dysphagia due to oesophageal cancer. Etamsylate is excreted in the urine mainly unchanged.
Bio-availability no data.
Onset of action 30min IV.
Time to peak plasma concentration 4h PO; 1h IV.
Plasma halflife 5–17h PO; 1.7–2.5h IM; 1.8–2h IV.
Duration of action no data.

Undesirable effects

For full list, see manufacturer's SPC.
Headaches, rash, nausea (when taken on an empty stomach).

Dose and use

- 500mg q.d.s. either indefinitely or until 1 week after cessation of bleeding
- if causes nausea, take p.c.

Supply

Dicynene® (Sanofi-Synthelabo 01483 505515)
Tablets 500mg, 28 days @ 500mg q.d.s. = £23.67.
Injection 125mg/ml, 2ml amp = £0.78.

TRANEXAMIC ACID BNF 2.11

Class: Antifibrinolytic agent.

Indications: Prevention of postoperative bleeding in haemophilia, menorrhagia, hereditary angioedema, epistaxis, †surface bleeding from ulcerating tumours, nasal cavity and other organs (bladder, uterus, rectum, stomach and lungs).

Contra-indications: Thrombo-embolic disease, DIC.

Pharmacology

Tranexamic acid, like **aminocaproic acid**, inhibits the breakdown of fibrin clots. It acts primarily by competitively blocking the binding of plasminogen and plasmin; direct inhibition of plasmin occurs to a limited extent. Tranexamic acid has greater potency, efficacy and is more convenient to give than **aminocaproic acid**.[1] In DIC, even when haemorrhagic manifestations (e.g. ecchymoses and haematomas) are the predominant manifestations, tranexamic acid should not be used because clot formation is the trigger for further intravascular coagulation and platelet consumption, and an increased risk of end-organ damage from microvascular thromboses. It can be used in conjunction with **etamsylate** (see p.43). Solutions of tranexamic acid have been applied topically for surface bleeding from fungating cancer in the skin or body cavities, e.g. as a mouth wash, bladder irrigation, rectal instillation and intrapleurally.[2–4] Rarely, parenteral use may be necessary, e.g. in patients with bleeding and complete dysphagia due to oesophageal cancer. Tranexamic acid is excreted in the urine mainly as unchanged drug and will cumulate in renal failure.

Bio-availability 30–50% PO; topical mouth rinse minimal.
Onset of action no data.
Time to peak plasma concentration 3h PO; 1h IM.
Plasma halflife 2h.
Duration of action 24h.

Cautions

Serious drug interactions: increased risk of thrombosis with other thrombogenic drugs.

Renal failure. In patients with haematuria there is risk of ureteric obstruction and retention.

Undesirable effects

For full list, see manufacturer's SPC.

Nausea, vomiting, diarrhoea, disturbance of colour vision (withdraw treatment), hypotension (IV), thrombo-embolism (rare).

Dose and use

- 1.5g PO stat and 1g t.d.s.
- usual maximum dose 2g q.d.s.[5]
- discontinue 1 week after cessation of bleeding or reduce to 500mg t.d.s.
- restart if bleeding occurs.[6]

Topical solution for surface bleeding from fungating cancer in the skin

- 500mg in 5ml soaked into gauze and apply with pressure for 10min.[4]

Topical solution for surface bleeding from fungating cancer in a body cavity

Generally used only if PO tranexamic acid has failed:

- 5g o.d.–b.d. diluted with a suitable volume of water i.e. 50ml (at body temperature for bladder/rectal instillation).[3]

Supply

Cyklokapron® (Pharmacia 01908 661101)
Tablets 500mg, 28 days @ 500mg t.d.s. = £20.02.
Injection 100mg/ml, 5ml amp = £1.29.

Tranexamic acid (Pharmaceutical Unit, St Mary's Hospital, Penarth 02920 705545).
Oral solution 500mg/5ml (Unlicensed, available as a special order from Pharmaceutical Unit, St Mary's Hospital, Penarth 02920 705545; see Special orders and named patient supplies, p.349.)

1 Okamoto S *et al.* (1964) An active stereoisomer (trans form) of AMCHA and its antifibrinolytic (antiplasminic) action in vitro and in vivo. *Keio Journal of Medicine.* **13**: 177–185.
2 deBoer W *et al.* (1991) Tranexamic acid treatment of haemothorax in two patients with malignant mesothelioma. *Chest.* **100**: 847–848.
3 McElligott E *et al.* (1991) Tranexamic acid and rectal bleeding. *Lancet.* **337**: 431.
4 Twycross R and Wilcock A (2001) *Symptom Management in Advanced Cancer* (3e). Radcliffe Medical Press, Oxford, pp.237–244.
5 Anonymous (1996) Tranexamic acid in oncology. *Annals of Pharmacology.* **30**: 868–870.
6 Dean A and Tuffin P (1997) Fibrinolytic inhibitors for cancer-associated bleeding problems. *Journal of Pain and Symptom Management.* **13**: 20–24.

3: RESPIRATORY SYSTEM

BRONCHODILATORS BNF 3.1

Selective β_2-adrenoceptor stimulants (e.g. **salbutamol**, **terbutaline**) are the safest and most effective bronchodilators for patients with airflow obstruction. British Thoracic Society guidelines for their use in patients with asthma and COPD are available (Boxes 3.A–3.C).[1,2] Ideally, a patient should be evaluated before and after a test dose of a bronchodilator or a corticosteroid to confirm benefit, and the results documented in the patient's notes (Box 3.D). Patients with mild-to-moderate asthma should use the minimum dose of short-acting β_2-stimulants to control their symptoms, e.g. **salbutamol** p.r.n. In more severe asthma a long-acting β_2-stimulant, e.g. **salmeterol**, is prescribed in addition to inhaled corticosteroid (step 3 and above). Inhalation delivers the drug directly to the bronchi and enables a smaller dose to work more quickly and with fewer undesirable systemic effects. Inhaler technique should be carefully explained and checked periodically. The patient should be instructed to inhale slowly and then to hold their breath for 10sec if possible. Even with a good technique, 80% of a dose is deposited in the mouth and oropharynx. If inhaler technique does not improve with training, consider using a large-volume (650–850ml) spacer device to deliver single-dose actuations. Build up of static on the spacer attracts drug particles and reduces drug delivery. To reduce static, spacers should be washed weekly with washing-up liquid, rinsed and left to dry *without wiping*. Spacers should be replaced every 6–12 months.[3] Turbohalers and breath-actuated aerosol inhalers are other options. Turbohalers are not suited to patients with poor inspiratory effort. Breath-actuated ones are triggered at low inspiratory flow rates and are the most popular device with patients.[4]

Hydrofluoroalkane (HFA) is replacing chlorofluorocarbons (CFC) as the propellant in pressurised metered-dose inhalers, and the aerosol may differ in feel and taste. Because of a reduced exit velocity, 'clogging' is more likely and frequent cleaning of the nozzle is recommended, particularly with drugs suspended rather than dissolved in the propellant, e.g. **salbutamol**. HFA and CFC inhalers are generally equivalent, although differences can arise with the use of spacer devices. Only spacers specified in the SPC for a particular HFA inhaler should be used. To avoid confusion, prescriptions should state either the brand or state clearly whether a CFC or a HFA (i.e. CFC-free) inhaler is intended.[3]

In patients with lung cancer, concurrent COPD can be a major cause of breathlessness but may be unrecognised and so go untreated. Breathlessness can be improved in most patients with lung cancer and COPD by a combination of a β_2-stimulant and an antimuscarinic.[5] Administration by aerosol inhaler through a spacer is as effective as a nebuliser.[5] Also see Nebulised drugs, p.351.

1 British Thoracic Society (1997) BTS guidelines on asthma management. *Thorax.* **52**: S1–S21.
2 British Thoracic Society (1997) BTS guidelines for the management of chronic obstructive pulmonary disease. *Thorax.* **52**: S1–S28.
3 Anonymous (2000) Inhaler devices for asthma. *Drug and Therapeutics Bulletin.* **38**: 9–14.

Box 3.A Management of chronic asthma in adults[1]

Start at the step most appropriate to the initial severity. *A corticosteroid should be prescribed for a non-responsive acute exacerbation, e.g. prednisolone 30–60mg o.m.*

Step 1: occasional relief bronchodilators
Inhaled short-acting β_2-stimulant p.r.n.
Move to step 2 if needed more than o.d. or if symptoms at night.

Step 2: regular inhaled preventer therapy
Regular standard-dose of inhaled corticosteroid (beclometasone dipropionate or budesonide 100–400microgram b.d. *or* fluticasone propionate 50–200microgram b.d.)
+ inhaled short-acting β_2-stimulant p.r.n.
High-dose inhaled corticosteroid may be required to gain initial relief; some people benefit from doubling the dose for a short period during an exacerbation.

Step 3: high-dose inhaled corticosteroids *or* standard-dose inhaled corticosteroids + long-acting inhaled β_2-stimulant
Regular high-dose inhaled corticosteroids (beclometasone dipropionate or budesonide 800–2000microgram daily *or* fluticasone 400–1000microgram daily; given in 2–4 doses via a large-volume spacer), *or*
Regular standard-dose inhaled corticosteroids + regular long-acting inhaled β_2-stimulant (salmeterol 50microgram b.d., formoterol (eformoterol) 12microgram b.d.)
+ inhaled short-acting β_2-stimulant p.r.n.
The few who have problems (i.e. sore throat, hoarse voice) with high-dose inhaled corticosteroids should change to standard-dose inhaled corticosteroid with long-acting β_2-stimulant (as above) or regular oral m/r theophylline or try regular cromoglicate or nedocromil.

Step 4: high-dose inhaled corticosteroids + regular bronchodilators
Regular high-dose inhaled corticosteroids
+ sequential therapeutic trial of one or more of:
  inhaled long-acting β_2-stimulant
  oral m/r theophylline
  inhaled antimuscarinic
  oral m/r β_2-stimulant
  high-dose inhaled bronchodilators
  inhaled sodium cromoglicate or nedocromil
+ inhaled short-acting β_2-stimulant p.r.n.

Step 5: regular corticosteroid tablets
Regular prednisolone tablets (the minimum dose that controls symptoms o.m.)
+ regular high-dose inhaled corticosteroid
+ one or more long-acting bronchodilators (see Step 4)
+ inhaled short-acting β_2-stimulant p.r.n.
Refer to asthma clinic.

Stepping down
Review treatment every 3–6 months; if good control has been achieved for 1–3 months, it may be possible to go down one or more steps. If treatment started recently at Step 4 or 5 (or contains corticosteroid tablets) reduction should be considered after a shorter interval.

Box 3.B Severe acute asthma

Characterised by persistent breathlessness despite usual bronchodilators, exhaustion, tachycardia (>110/min) and a low peak expiratory flow rate (<50% of best). It requires urgent treatment by experienced physicians with:

- oxygen
- corticosteroids (hydrocortisone 200mg IV *or* prednisolone 30–60mg PO)
- salbutamol 5mg or terbutaline 10mg by nebuliser (repeat as necessary).

If little response, consider:

- ipratropium bromide 500microgram by nebuliser
- aminophylline 250mg by slow IV injection *but not if the patient is already taking oral theophylline*
- change route of administration of β_2-stimulant to SC/IV.

If continued decline, consider:

- intermittent positive pressure ventilation.

Box 3.C Bronchodilator therapy in COPD[2]

At all stages patients must be taught how and when to use their treatments. The use of medication which may cause bronchoconstriction (e.g. β-blockers) should be avoided.

Mild COPD

FEV_1 60–79% of predicted value; FEV_1/FVC and other indices of expiratory flow mildly reduced:

- asymptomatic → no drug treatment
- symptomatic → a trial of an inhaled β_2-stimulant *or* an antimuscarinic taken p.r.n. using an appropriate inhaler device, stop if ineffective.

Moderate COPD

FEV_1 40–59% of predicted value, often with increased FRC and reduced Tlco.
Some patients are hypoxaemic but not hypercapnic:

- regular inhaled bronchodilators as above.

Treatment depends on the severity of symptoms and their effect on lifestyle; most patients need only a single drug but a few require combined treatment.
Oral bronchodilators are generally not necessary.

Severe COPD

FEV_1 <40% of predicted value with marked overinflation; Tlco variable but often low. Hypoxaemia usual, hypercapnia in some:

- combined treatment with a β_2-stimulant and an antimuscarinic bronchodilator
- theophyllines can be tried but must be monitored for adverse effects.

Some patients request 'stronger' therapy. However, the dose-response curve is limited by the maximum bronchodilation possible. High-dose treatment including nebulised drugs should be prescribed only after a formal assessment.

Box 3.D Bronchodilator and reversibility testing[2]

These tests are done when a patient is clinically stable in order to:

- detect patients whose FEV_1 increases substantially, i.e. are asthmatic
- establish the post-bronchodilator FEV_1 (the best predictor of long-term outcome).

The patient should not have taken inhaled short-acting bronchodilators in the previous 6h, long-acting ones in the previous 12h, or m/r theophylline in the preceding 24h.

Response

Measure FEV_1

- before and 15min after 2.5–5mg nebulised salbutamol *or* 5–10mg terbutaline
- before and after 500microgram nebulised ipratropium bromide
- before and after both in combination

or

- before and after a course of oral prednisolone (e.g. 30mg o.m. for 2 weeks) or inhaled corticosteroid (e.g. beclometasone 500microgram b.d. for 6 weeks).

Interpretation

- an increase in FEV_1 that is both greater than 200ml and a 15% increase over the pre-bronchodilator value is the definition of reversibility
- a negative FEV_1 response does not preclude benefit from bronchodilators in terms of improved walking distance or a reduction in the perception of breathlessness.

4 Lenney J *et al.* (2000) Inappropriate inhaler use: assessment of use and patient preference of seven inhalation devices. *Respiratory Medicine.* **94**: 496–500.

5 Congelton J and Meurs M (1995) The incidence of airflow obstruction in bronchial carcinoma, its relation to breathlessness and response to bronchodilator therapy. *Respiratory Medicine.* **89**: 291–296.

IPRATROPIUM — BNF 3.1.2

Class: Quarternary ammonium antimuscarinic bronchodilator.

Indications: Reversible airways obstruction, particularly in COPD.

Pharmacology

Antimuscarinic bronchodilators are as effective as β_2-stimulants in patients with COPD with some studies suggesting a greater and more prolonged bronchodilator response.[1,2] The combination of an antimuscarinic with a β_2-stimulant provides a greater degree of bronchodilation than either alone but no greater symptom relief.[3] The combination should be tried only when ipratropium or a β_2-stimulant individually have failed to give adequate relief.

Bio-availability 10–20% of the dose reaches the lower airways.

Onset of action 3–30min asthma; 15min COPD.

Peak response 1.5–3h asthma; 1–2h COPD.

Plasma halflife 2.3–3.8h.

Duration of action 4–8h.

Cautions

Glaucoma, prostatic hypertrophy.

Undesirable effects

For full list, see manufacturer's SPC.

Acute-angle closure glaucoma (nebulised), dry mouth. Rarely urinary retention, constipation and paradoxical bronchoconstriction.

Dose and use

In most patients, bronchodilation can be maintained with administration t.d.s.

Aerosol inhalation

- 20–40microgram t.d.s.–q.d.s. p.r.n.
- 20–40microgram before exercise in exercise-induced bronchoconstriction.

Nebuliser solution

- 250–500microgram q.d.s. p.r.n.

Supply

Ipratropium bromide (non-proprietary)
Nebuliser solution 250microgram/ml, 1ml (250microgram) and 2ml (500microgram) dose vials, 28 days @ 500microgram q.d.s. = £36.34.

Atrovent® (Boehringer Ingelheim 01344 424600)
Aerosol inhalation 20microgram/metered inhalation, 28 days @ 40microgram (2 puffs) q.d.s. = £4.72 (*includes CFC propellant*).
Forte aerosol inhalation 40microgram/metered inhalation, 28 days @ 40microgram (1 puff) q.d.s. = £3.48 (*includes CFC propellant*).
Nebuliser solution 250microgram/ml, 1ml (250microgram) and 2ml (500microgram) dose vials, 28 days @ 500microgram q.d.s. = £42.56.

Ipratropium Steri-Neb® (IVAX 08705 020304)
Nebuliser solution 250microgram/ml, 1ml (250microgram) and 2ml (500microgram) dose vials, 28 days @ 500microgram q.d.s. = £30.52.

Respontin® (GSK 0800 221441)
Nebuliser solution 250microgram/ml, 1ml (250microgram) and 2ml (500microgram) dose vials, 28 days @ 500microgram q.d.s. = £35.84.

1 Tashkin D *et al.* (1986) Comparison of the anticholinergic bronchodilator ipratropium bromide with metaproterenol in chronic obstructive pulmonary disease. A 90-day multi-center study. *American Journal of Medicine.* **81**: 81–90.
2 Combivent Inhalation Aerosol Study Group (1994) In chronic obstructive pulmonary disease a combination of ipratropium and albuterol is more effective than either agent alone. *Chest.* **105**: 1411–1419.
3 Combivent Inhalation Study Group (1997) Routine nebulized ipratropium and albuterol together are better than either alone in COPD. *Chest.* **112**: 1514–1521.

SALBUTAMOL — BNF 3.1.1

Class: β_2-adrenoceptor agonist (sympathomimetic).

Indications: Asthma and other conditions associated with reversible airways obstruction.

Pharmacology

In patients with asthma, short-acting β_2-adrenoceptor agonists should generally only be used for symptom relief p.r.n. Use more than o.d. indicates the need for prophylactic therapy with an inhaled corticosteroid (see p.55). If insufficient, a *long-acting* (i.e. 12h) β_2-adrenoceptor agonist, e.g. **salmeterol**, should be added b.d. (see Box 3.A, p.48). These improve symptoms and lung function and decrease the frequency of exacerbations without the safety concerns associated with the regular use of short-acting β_2-adrenoceptor agonists.[1] In patients with COPD, regular *short-acting* or *long-acting* β_2-adrenoceptor agonists can be used.[2–4] Salbutamol has predominantly a β_2-stimulant bronchodilator effect, i.e. does not have a major impact on the heart. It is safer than less selective β-adrenoceptor agonists, e.g. **orciprenaline** and **adrenaline** (epinephrine) although some patients develop prolongation of the QT interval that may predispose to the ventricular tachyarrhythmia, *torsade de pointes* (see Prolongation of QT interval in palliative care, p.327).

Serum potassium should be monitored in severe asthma as β_2-adrenoceptor agonists, particularly in combination with other asthma therapies, e.g. **theophylline** and inhaled corticosteroids, can cause hypokalaemia which further increases the QT interval and risk of arrhythmia. Conversely, nebulised salbutamol has surpassed **insulin** and **dextrose** as a more convenient and equally effective method of treating hyperkalaemia in uraemic patients.

Bio-availability 10–20% of the dose reaches the lower airways.
Onset of action 5min inhaled; 3–5min nebulised.
Peak response 0.5–2h inhaled; 1.2h nebulised.
Plasma halflife 4–6h inhaled and nebulised.
Duration of action 4–6h inhaled and nebulised.

Cautions

Serious drug interaction: increased risk of hypokalaemia with corticosteroids, diuretics, theophylline.

Hyperthyroidism, myocardial insufficiency, hypertension, diabetes mellitus (risk of keto-acidosis if given by CIVI).

Undesirable effects

For full list, see manufacturer's SPC.
Tremor, palpitations, muscle cramps. In higher doses: tachycardia (occasionally arrhythmias), tenseness, headaches, peripheral vasodilation, hypokalaemia, allergic reactions.

Dose and use

Aerosol inhalation

- 100–200microgram (1–2 puffs) t.d.s.–q.d.s. p.r.n.
- 200microgram (2 puffs) before exercise in exercise-induced bronchoconstriction.

Nebuliser solution

- 2.5–5mg up to q.d.s., occasionally q4h.

Supply

Salbutamol (non-proprietary)
Aerosol inhalation 100microgram/metered inhalation, 28 days @ 200microgram (2 puffs) q.d.s. = £2.14 (*includes CFC propellant*).
Aerosol inhalation (*CFC-free*) 100microgram/metered inhalation, 28 days @ 200 microgram (2 puffs) q.d.s. = £2.14.
Nebuliser solution 1mg/ml, 2.5ml (2.5mg) and 2mg/ml, 2.5ml (5mg) dose vials, 28 days @ 5mg q.d.s. = £27.89.

Airomir® (3M 01509 611611)
Aerosol inhalation (*CFC-free*) 100microgram/metered inhalation, 28 days @ 200microgram (2 puffs) q.d.s. = £2.21.

Ventolin® (GSK 0800 221441)
Aerosol inhalation (*CFC-free*) Evohaler® 100microgram/metered inhalation, 28 days @ 200microgram (2 puffs) q.d.s. = £2.58.
Nebuliser solution 1mg/ml, 2.5ml (2.5mg) and 2mg/ml, 2.5ml (5mg) dose Nebules®, 28 days @ 5mg q.d.s. = £38.64.

Inhaler and spacer devices
Haleraid® (GSK 0800 221441) to aid operation by patients with impaired strength in hands, available for 120 and 200 dose inhalers = £0.80.

Nebuhaler® (AstraZeneca 0800 783 0033) large-volume spacer device, for **terbutaline** and **budesonide** = £4.28.
Volumatic® (Allen & Hanburys 020 8990 9888) large-volume spacer device, for salbutamol, **salmeterol**, **ipratropium**, **beclometasone**, **fluticasone** = £2.75.

1 Sears M (2000) Short-acting inhaled B-agonists: to be taken regularly or as needed? *Lancet*. **355**: 1658–1659.
2 British Thoracic Society (1997) BTS guidelines for the management of chronic obstructive pulmonary disease. *Thorax*. **52**: S1–S28.
3 Jones P and Bosh T (1997) Quality of life changes in COPD patients treated with salmeterol. *American Journal of Respiratory and Critical Care Medicine*. **155**: 1283–1289.
4 Rennard S *et al.* (2001) Use of a long-acting inhaled beta$_2$-adrenergic agonist, salmeterol xinafoate, in patients with chronic obstructive pulmonary disease. *American Journal of Respiratory and Critical Care Medicine*. **163**: 1087–1092.

THEOPHYLLINE BNF 3.1.3

Class: Methylxanthine.

Indications: Reversible airways obstruction, severe acute asthma (see Box 3.B, p.49).

Pharmacology

In patients with asthma, a *long-acting* β_2-adrenoceptor agonist, e.g. **salmeterol,** is generally used before theophylline because of its superior safety and efficacy (see Box 3.A, p.48).[1] This is probably also true for patients with COPD. Theophylline shares the actions of the other xanthine alkaloids (e.g. caffeine) on the CNS, myocardium, kidney and smooth muscle. It has a relatively weak CNS effect but a more powerful relaxant effect on bronchial smooth muscle. It probably acts by inhibiting cyclic nucleotide phosphodiesterase. This leads to an accumulation of cyclic AMP/GMP which prevents the use of intracellular calcium for muscle contraction. In addition, an immunomodulator effect on cells important in airway inflammation has been shown at plasma concentrations as low as 5microgram/ml.[2,3] Other effects include an improvement in respiratory muscle strength, the release of catecholamines from the adrenal medulla, inhibition of catechol-O-methyl transferase and blockade of adenosine receptors – all of which may play a part in the beneficial effect of theophylline.

Theophylline is given by injection as **aminophylline**, a mixture of theophylline with **ethylenediamine**; it is 20 times more soluble than theophylline alone. **Aminophylline** must be given by *very slow* IV injection; it is too irritant for IM use and is a potent gastric irritant PO. Theophylline is metabolised by the liver. Its therapeutic index is narrow and some patients experience undesirable effects even in the therapeutic range. Plasma concentrations of theophylline are influenced by infection, hypoxia, smoking, various drugs, hepatic impairment and heart failure; all these can make the use of theophylline difficult.

Steady-state theophylline levels are attained within 3–4 days of adjusting the dose of a m/r preparation. Blood for theophylline levels should be taken 6–8h after the last dose or immediately before the next dose. *Because it is not possible to ensure bio-equivalence between different m/r theophylline products, they should not be interchanged.* The Royal Pharmaceutical Society requires a prescription to specify the brand name of the product.
Bio-availability ≥90%; 80% m/r.
Onset of action 40–60min PO; immunomodulation ≤3 weeks.
Peak response up to 24h.
Plasma halflife 6–12h.
Duration of action 6–12h aminophylline IV; 12h m/r theophylline PO; immunomodulation several days.

Cautions

Serious drug interactions: plasma concentrations of theophylline are increased by **allopurinol, cimetidine, ciprofloxacin, clarithromycin, diltiazem, erythromycin, fluconazole, fluvoxamine, norfloxacin, thiabendazole, verapamil, viloxazine** and oral contraceptives. Plasma concentrations are decreased in smokers, heavy drinkers and by barbiturates, **carbamazepine, isoprenaline, phenytoin, rifampicin** and **sulphinpyrazone**. May potentiate hypokalaemia associated with β_2-adrenoceptor agonists, corticosteroids, diuretics and hypoxia. Also see Cytochrome P450, p.331.

Elderly, cardiac disease, hypertension, hyperthyroidism, peptic ulcer, liver failure, pyrexia.

Undesirable effects

For full list, see manufacturer's SPC.

Dyspepsia, nausea, headache, CNS stimulation (less with m/r preparations). Arrhythmias and seizures (IV use).

Dose and use

Generally, a m/r preparation is preferable, e.g. Uniphyllin-Continus®:

- usual starting dose 200mg b.d.; increase after one week
- in the elderly or patients weighing <70kg, the usual maintenance dose is 300mg b.d.
- in younger heavier patients, the usual maintenance dose is 400mg b.d.
- in patients whose symptoms manifest diurnal fluctuation, a larger evening or morning dose is appropriate to ensure maximum therapeutic benefit when symptoms are most severe
- the recommended therapeutic range is 10–20microgram/ml.

In view of the beneficial immunomodulator effect of theophylline in patients with asthma at relatively low plasma concentrations,[3,4] dose adjustments should be made according to clinical response rather than necessarily trying to achieve the recommended therapeutic range.

Give by injection in acute severe asthma if patient not already taking oral theophylline:

- **aminophylline** 250–500mg (maximum 5mg/kg) IV *over 20min*
- continue as 500microgram/kg/h CIVI; adjust dose according to theophylline levels.

Patients already receiving theophylline PO should not receive **aminophylline** IV unless plasma theophylline concentrations can be monitored to guide dosing.

Supply

Uniphyllin Continus® (Napp 01223 424444)

Tablets m/r theophylline 200mg, 300mg, 400mg, 28 days @ 200mg, 300mg, 400mg b.d. = £4.12, £6.27 and £7.44 respectively.

Aminophylline (non-proprietary)

Injection aminophylline 25mg/ml, 10ml amp = £0.67.

This is not a complete list; see BNF for full details.

1 Davies B et *al.* (1998) The efficacy and safety of salmeterol compared to theophylline: meta-analysis of nine controlled studies. *Respiratory Medicine.* **92**: 256–263.

2 Sullivan P et *al.* (1994) Anti-inflammatory effects of low-dose oral theophylline in atopic asthma. *Lancet.* **343**: 1006–1008.

3 Kidney J et *al.* (1995) Immunomodulation by theophylline in asthma. Demonstration by withdrawal of therapy. *American Journal of Respiratory and Critical Care Medicine.* **151**: 1907–1914.

4 Evans D et *al.* (1997) A comparison of low-dose inhaled budesonide plus theophylline and high-dose inhaled budesonide for moderate asthma. *New England Journal of Medicine.* **337**: 1412–1418.

INHALED CORTICOSTEROIDS BNF 3.2

Indications: Reversible airways obstruction, †stridor, †lymphangitis carcinomatosa, †radiation pneumonitis, †cough after insertion of a bronchial stent (see Nebulised drugs, p.351).

Pharmacology

Corticosteroids reduce the inflammatory response by lowering peripheral lymphocyte levels and inhibiting phospholipase A_2, the enzyme which releases arachidonic acid (the precursor of PGs and leukotrienes) from cell membrane phospholipid. Inhaled corticosteroids reduce bronchial mucosa inflammation and are indicated in asthma (see Box 3.A, p.48 and Box 3.B, p.49). Symptoms may take 3–7 days to improve. For most formulations, **fluticasone** is at least twice as potent as **beclometasone** and **budesonide** and only half the dose is required for an equivalent effect. Improvement in symptoms may take 7 days, but maximal improvement in airway inflammation may take 3 months. At the lower dose range (e.g. **budesonide** 200–400microgram/day), o.d. administration is as effective as b.d.[1] If moderate doses fail to improve symptoms, consider using a higher dose (e.g. **budesonide** 800–2000microgram) or add a *long-acting* β_2-adrenoceptor agonist, e.g. **salmeterol**. The anti-inflammatory effect of inhaled corticosteroids is complemented by the leukotriene-receptor antagonists given PO. These block the effects of cysteinyl-leukotrienes on bronchial smooth muscle and other airway tissue, improving asthma control and protecting against exercise-induced bronchoconstriction.

In patients with COPD, although systemic corticosteroids (e.g. **prednisolone** 30–60mg PO for 2 weeks) are of benefit in treating exacerbations,[2] the role of long-term inhaled corticosteroids is less well defined. Generally, they should be used in those 10–15% of patients who show objective improvement after a trial of corticosteroid therapy (see Box 3.D, p.50). In patients with moderate-to-severe COPD, **fluticasone** 500microgram b.d. has recently been shown to reduce exacerbations and rate of decline in health and increase FEV_1 compared to placebo.[3] The only evidence to support the other uses of inhaled or nebulised corticosteroids listed above is clinical experience. Inhaled corticosteroids can reach the systemic circulation via the pulmonary circulation or via the gastro-intestinal tract if swallowed. Daily doses of **budesonide** $\leq$1500microgram or equivalent do not generally lead to adrenal suppression. The systemic bio-availability of the swallowed fraction is less with corticosteroids with high first-pass clearance by the liver, e.g. **budesonide** (11%) and **fluticasone** (1%), and there may be less risk of adrenal suppression than with **beclometasone** (20%).[4] However, there is significant variation amongst individuals and formulation and duration of treatment are also important. Systemic corticosteroids (see p.219) should therefore be considered to cover stressful periods (e.g. infection, surgery) in patients receiving moderate-to-large doses of inhaled corticosteroids long-term.[5]

For pharmacokinetic details, see Table 3.1.

Table 3.1 Pharmacokinetics of inhaled corticosteroids[a]

	Beclometasone	*Budesonide*	*Fluticasone*
Bio-availability	No data	39% Turbohaler® 6% Respules®	30% aerosol inhaler 13.5% powder inhaler
Onset of action	1–4 weeks inhaler	24h inhaler 2–8 days Respules®	24h
Time to peak plasma concentration	1–1.5h	20min Turbohaler® 10–30min Respules®	No data
Peak response	No data	1–2 weeks inhaler 4–6 weeks Respules®	1–2 weeks
Plasma halflife	3h	2–3h	8h
Duration of action	No data	12–24h inhaler	No data

a. data from Micromedex, relating to use in asthma.

Cautions

Active or quiescent tuberculosis.

Undesirable effects

For full list, see manufacturer's SPC.
Oropharyngeal candidiasis, sore throat, hoarse voice, paradoxical bronchospasm, hypersensitivity reactions (e.g. rashes). At higher doses (e.g. **beclometasone** >1000microgram/day), adrenal suppression and osteoporosis. Prolonged use of inhaled corticosteroids is associated with an increased risk of cataract.[6,7]

Dose and use

Aerosol inhalation

- check the patient's inhaler technique
- use a large-volume spacer device if
  poor inhaler technique
  patient is on a high dose (e.g. **beclometasone** >1000microgram/day)
  patient develops a hoarse voice or sore throat
- take the corticosteroid 5min *after* a β_2-stimulant if being used concurrently
- instruct patient to rinse mouth after use to reduce systemic availability
- usual starting dose to gain control quickly is **beclometasone** 400microgram b.d. or equivalent; dose can be reduced in steps of 25–50% every 1–3months, until minimum effective dose for maintenance is found
- titrate dose against symptoms; usual maximum dose is **beclometasone** 2000microgram/day (or equivalent) in divided doses.

Nebuliser solution

- **budesonide** 1–2mg b.d.; occasionally more.

Patients should be given a *Steroid Card* with doses associated with adrenal suppression (see Box 7.G, p.223).

Supply

Beclometasone (non-proprietary)
Aerosol inhalation 50microgram, 100microgram, 200microgram/metered inhalation, 28 days @ 200microgram (1 puff) b.d. = £5.49 (*includes CFC propellant*).
Aerosol inhalation 250microgram/metered inhalation, 28 days @ 500microgram (2 puff) b.d. = £9.95 (*includes CFC propellant*).

Becotide® (GSK 0800 221441)
Aerosol inhalation 50microgram, 100microgram, 200microgram/metered inhalation, 28 days @ 200microgram (1 puff) b.d. = £5.49 (*includes CFC propellant*).
Becloforte® (GSK 0800 221441)
Aerosol inhalation 250microgram/metered inhalation, 28 days @ 500microgram (2 puff) b.d. = £12.94 (*includes CFC propellant*).

Qvar® (3M 01509 611611)
Aerosol inhalation (*CFC-free*) 50microgram, 100microgram/metered inhalation, 28 days @ 100microgram (1 puff) b.d. = £4.82.

Budesonide
Pulmicort® (AstraZeneca 0800 783 0033)
Aerosol inhalation 50microgram, 200microgram/metered inhalation, 28 days @ 200microgram (1 puff) b.d. = £5.32 (*includes CFC propellant*).
Dry powder inhalation Turbohaler® 100microgram, 200microgram, 400microgram/inhalation, 28 days @ 200microgram (1 puff) b.d. = £10.36.
Nebuliser solution 250microgram/ml, 2ml (500microgram) and 500microgram/ml, 2ml (1mg) Respules®, 28 days @ 1mg b.d. = £124.99.

Fluticasone
Flixotide® (GSK 0800 221441)
Aerosol inhalation 25microgram, 50microgram, 125microgram, 250microgram/metered inhalation, 28 days @ 100microgram (2 puff) b.d. = £5.46 (*includes CFC propellant*).

Aerosol inhalation (*CFC-free*) Evohaler® 50microgram, 125microgram, 250microgram/metered inhalation, 28 days @ 100microgram (2 puff) b.d. = £5.46.
Nebuliser solution 250microgram/ml, 2ml (500microgram) and 1mg/ml, 2ml (2mg) Nebules®, 28 days @ 1mg b.d. = £112.45.

This is not a complete list; see BNF for full details.

1 Chisholm S *et al.* (1998) Once-daily budesonide in mild asthma. *Respiratory Medicine.* **92**: 421–425.
2 Niewoehner D *et al.* (1999) Effect of systemic glucocorticoids on exacerbations of chronic obstructive pulmonary disease. *New England Journal of Medicine.* **340**: 1941–1947.
3 Burge P *et al.* (2000) Randomised, double blind, placebo controlled study of fluticasone propionate in patients with moderate to severe chronic obstructive pulmonary disease: the ISOLDE trial. *British Medical Journal.* **320**: 1297–1303.
4 Dekhuijzen P and Honour J (2000) Inhaled corticosteroids and the hypothalamic-pituitary-adrenal (HPA) axis: do we understand their interaction? *Respiratory Medicine.* **94**: 627–631.
5 Anonymous (2000) The use of inhaled corticosteroids in adults with asthma. *Drug and Therapeutics Bulletin.* **38**: 5–8.
6 Cumming R and Mitchell P (1999) Inhaled corticosteroids and cataract. Prevalence, prevention and management. *Drug Safety.* **20**: 77–84.
7 Carnahan M and Goldstein D (2000) Ocular complications of topical, peri-ocular, and systemic corticosteroids. *Current Opinion in Ophthalmology.* **11**: 478–483.

OXYGEN — BNF 3.6

Indications: Breathlessness on exertion (intermittent use); breathlessness at rest (continuous use).

Pharmacology

Oxygen is prescribed for breathless patients to increase alveolar oxygen tension and decrease the work of breathing necessary to maintain a given arterial tension. The concentration given varies with the underlying condition. Inappropriate prescription can have serious or fatal effects. Ideally, domiciliary oxygen should be prescribed only after careful evaluation, preferably by a respiratory specialist. Some patients obtain as much benefit from piped air delivered by nasal prongs.[1] This suggests that a sensation of airflow is an important determinant of benefit.[2–5] Patients should be encouraged to test the benefit of a cool draught (open window or fan) before being offered oxygen. In mildly hypoxic patients, the benefit from oxygen is independent of the degree of arterial oxygen desaturation.[1] In severely hypoxic patients (oxygen saturation $<90\%$), oxygen is generally better than air.[6]
Helium 79%-oxygen 21% mixture is less dense and viscous than room air.[7] Its use helps to reduce the respiratory work required to overcome upper airway obstruction.[8–10] It can be used as a temporary measure while more definitive therapy is arranged.

Cautions

Patients with hypercapnic ventilatory failure who are dependent upon hypoxia for their respiratory drive. Patients should be advised of the fire risks of oxygen therapy:

- no smoking in the vicinity of the cylinder
- no naked flames, including candles, matches and gas cookers
- keep away from sources of heat, e.g. radiators and direct sunlight.

Undesirable effects

An oxygen mask may be claustrophobic for some; use of nasal prongs can cause dryness and soreness of the nasal mucosa.

Dose and use

Oxygen therapy should be available for severely hypoxic patients, most of whom will be breathless at rest and/or on minimal exertion. In those less hypoxic the role of oxygen is more difficult to determine because there is great variation in response to oxygen. This cannot be predicted by the level of oxygen saturation at rest or the degree of desaturation on exercise. A trial of oxygen therapy can be given via nasal prongs for 10–15min. Although initial oxygen saturation is a poor predictor of who will benefit subjectively, a pulse oximeter will help identify those patients whose oxygen saturation is objectively improved by oxygen therapy. If on review the patient has persisted in using the oxygen and has found it useful, it can be continued; if the patient has any doubts about its efficacy it should be discontinued.

Short-term/intermittent

High concentration oxygen (60%) is given for pneumonia, pulmonary embolism and fibrosing alveolitis. In these situations a low arterial oxygen (PaO_2) is usually associated with normal or low levels of carbon dioxide ($PaCO_2$). High concentrations of oxygen are also given in acute asthma; $PaCO_2$ levels are generally subnormal but can rise rapidly with deterioration. If patients fail to improve with treatment, ventilation needs to be considered urgently.

Low concentration oxygen (≤28%) is reserved for patients with ventilatory failure related to COPD and other causes. The aim is to improve breathlessness caused by hypoxaemia without worsening pre-existing CO_2 retention. Intermittent (short-burst) oxygen can be considered for episodic breathlessness not relieved by other treatments in patients with advanced cancer, COPD, interstitial lung disease and heart failure. For exercise-induced breathlessness some patients prefer to use oxygen before the exercise and others afterwards to aid recovery.[11]

Long-term/continuous

Long-term oxygen (≥15h/day) can be considered for use in patients with severe disabling breathlessness due to cancer and other progressive life-threatening diseases. More specifically in patients with:

- COPD or cystic fibrosis with PaO_2 <7.3kPa *or* ≤8kPa with either secondary polycythaemia or nocturnal hypoxaemia (SaO_2 below 90% for at least 30% of night) or peripheral oedema or evidence of pulmonary hypertension
- interstitial lung disease and PaO_2 ≤8kPa
- pulmonary hypertension, without parenchymal lung involvement and PaO_2 ≤8kPa
- obstructive sleep apnoea who remain hypoxic during sleep despite nasal continuous positive airway pressure (CPAP)
- heart failure and PaO_2 <7.3kPa or nocturnal hypoxaemia
- neuromuscular or skeletal disorders, either alone or in combination with ventilatory support.[12]

Long-term oxygen therapy prolongs survival only in patients with severe COPD.[13] Ideally, in COPD, blood gas tensions should be measured before treatment when the patient's condition is stable (e.g. not less than 4 weeks after an exacerbation) on two occasions at least 3 weeks apart to ensure the criteria are met (see bullet 1 above). When treatment is commenced, blood gas tensions should be measured to ensure that the set flow is achieving a PaO_2 of >8kPa without an unacceptable rise in $PaCO_2$. It is more economical to use a concentrator if oxygen is given >8h/day (equivalent to 21 cylinders per month).

Supply

Oxygen cylinders

1360L (domiciliary use) and 3400L (hospital use) supplied by pharmacy contractors; flow settings medium (2L/min) or high (4L/min). Patients are supplied with either constant or variable performance masks. Constant supply masks such as the Intersurgical 010 28% (£0.97) or Ventimask MK IV 28% (£1.36) provide an almost constant supply of 28% oxygen over a wide range of oxygen supply (generally 4L/min) irrespective of the patient's breathing pattern. The flow rate should be adjusted for optimal patient comfort and symptom relief. *Constant supply masks should be used when an accurate delivery of oxygen is necessary, i.e. in patients at risk of hypercapnic respiratory failure.* The variable performance masks include the Intersurgical 005 mask (£0.78) and the Venticaire masks (£0.65); the concentration of oxygen supplied to the patient varies with the rate of flow of oxygen (2L/min is recommended and provides 24% oxygen) and with the patient's breathing pattern. Nasal cannulae are best suited for chronic usage but they are the least accurate. The concentration of oxygen delivered is dependent on factors other than flow rate and at 2L/min, oxygen concentrations can vary 24–35%.[14] Health authorities have lists of pharmacy contractors who provide domiciliary oxygen services.

Portable oxygen cylinders

'PD oxygen cylinder' (300L capacity) allows 2h of use at 2L/min, supplied by Medigas or BOC. Other portable oxygen cylinders are not prescribable on the NHS as the fittings are not compatible with the Drug Tariff oxygen equipment.

Oxygen concentrators
Concentrators and accessories (face mask, nasal cannula and humidifier) are prescribed by GPs specifying the flow rate (2–4L/min) and h/day. If necessary, two concentrators can be linked by a tubing and T-piece to deliver higher flow rates (4–8L/min). The GP should contact the supplier who will arrange to deliver the concentrator and collect the FP10 from the patient. Suppliers are specified by health authorities, on a regional tendering basis (see BNF 3.6 for list). An installation fee is charged to the health authority (about £90) plus a monthly rental and service charge (about £35) and an additional fee if a back-up cylinder is required (about £4). The price for private purchase is about £1000 (+ VAT). Patients may be re-imbursed for the electricity costs.
Helium 79%-oxygen 21%
Lindy Gas (0800 056 7345) supplies 1200ml cylinder, contract price.
BOC (0800 111333) supplies 1200ml cylinder, £31.47.

1 Booth S *et al.* (1996) Does oxygen help dyspnea in patients with cancer? *American Journal of Respiratory and Critical Care Medicine.* **153**: 1515–1518.
2 Schwartzstein R *et al.* (1987) Cold facial stimulation reduces breathlessness induced in normal subjects. *American Review of Respiratory Disease.* **136**: 58–61.
3 Burgess K and Whitelaw W (1988) Effects of nasal cold receptors on pattern of breathing. *Journal of Applied Physiology.* **64**: 371–376.
4 Freedman S (1988) Cold facial stimulation reduces breathlessness induced in normal subjects. *American Review of Respiratory Diseases.* **137**: 492–493.
5 Kerr D (1989) A bedside fan for terminal dyspnea. *American Journal of Hospice Care.* **89**: 22.
6 Bruera E *et al.* (1993) Effects of oxygen on dyspnoea in hypoxaemic terminal cancer patients. *Lancet.* **342**: 13–14.
7 Boorstein J *et al.* (1989) Using helium-oxygen mixtures in the emergency management of acute upper airway obstruction. *Annals of Emergency Medicine.* **18**: 688–690.
8 Lu T-S *et al.* (1976) Helium-oxygen in treatment of upper airway obstruction. *Anesthesiology.* **45**: 678–680.
9 Rudow M *et al.* (1986) Helium-oxygen mixtures in airway obstruction due to thyroid carcinoma. *Canadian Anaesthesiology Society Journal.* **33**: 498–501.
10 Khanlou H and Eiger G (2001) Safety and efficacy of heliox as a treatment for upper airway obstruction due to radiation-induced laryngeal dysfunction. *Heart and Lung.* **30**: 146–147.
11 Killen JW and Corris PA (2000) a pragmatic assessment of the placement of oxygen when given for exercise induced dyspnoea. *Thorax.* **55**: 544–546.
12 Royal College of Physicians of London (1999) *Domiciliary oxygen therapy services: clinical guidelines and advice for prescribers.* Royal College of Physicians, London.
13 Crockett A *et al.* (2001) A review of long-term oxygen therapy for chronic obstructive pulmonary disease. *Respiratory Medicine.* **95**: 437–443.
14 Bazuaye E *et al.* (1992) Variability of inspired oxygen concentration with nasal cannulas. *Thorax.* **47**: 609–611.

COUGH SUPPRESSANTS — BNF 3.9

Indications: Dry cough which is distressing to the patient, nocturnal wet cough which is disturbing sleep, wet cough in a patient too weak to expectorate properly.

Management strategy
Coughing helps clear the central airways of foreign matter, secretions or pus and should generally be encouraged. It is pathological when ineffective and when it adversely affects sleep, rest, eating or social activity. It may cause embarrassment, exhaustion, muscle strain, rib or vertebral fracture, vomiting, syncope, headache, urinary incontinence or retinal haemorrhage. The primary aim is to identify and treat the cause of the distressing cough but, when this is not possible or is inappropriate, a cough suppressant should be used (Figure 3.1).[1]

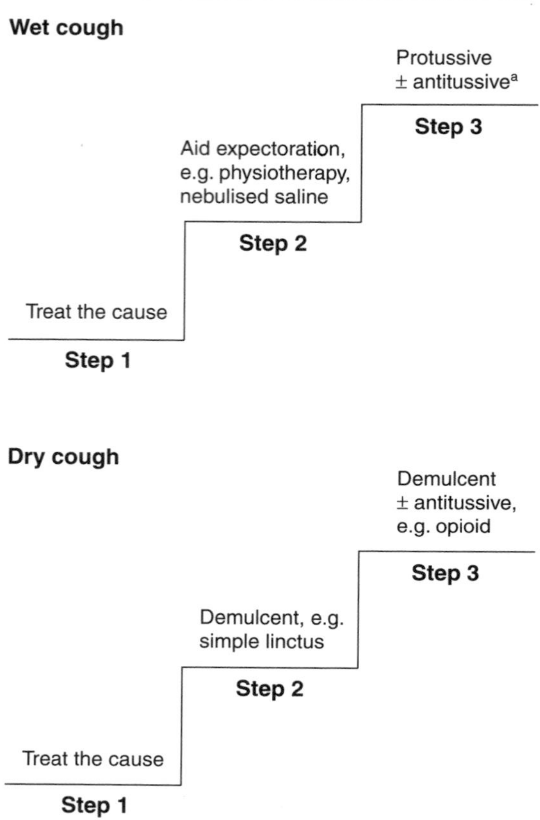

Figure 3.1 Treatment ladders for cough.

a. an antitussive reduces the frequency of coughing; a protussive makes coughing more effective and less distressing.

Dose and use

Demulcents: contain soothing substances such as syrup or glycerol. The high sugar content stimulates the production of saliva and soothes the oropharynx. The associated swallowing may also interfere with the cough reflex. The effect is short-lived and there is no evidence that compound preparations are better than **Simple Linctus** BP (5ml t.d.s.–q.d.s.). Thus, if simple linctus is ineffective, there is little point in trying compound preparations.

Opioids: act primarily by suppressing the cough reflex centre in the brain stem. **Codeine, pholcodine** and **dextromethorphan** are common ingredients in compound cough preparations. **Dextromethorphan** is a synthetic opioid derivative but does not act through opioid receptors. The effective dose of **codeine** or **dextromethorphan** is greater than the dose typically recommended by manufacturers of compound preparations.[2] The benefit of compound preparations may reside mainly in the sugar content. If **codeine** linctus 5–10ml (15–30mg) t.d.s.–q.d.s. is ineffective, a strong opioid such as **morphine** should be used. If a patient is already receiving a strong opioid for pain relief it is nonsense to prescribe **codeine** as well. **Morphine** solution can be used instead of **codeine** linctus, initially 2.5–5mg q.d.s.–q4h, or when **codeine** linctus fails to relieve, 5–10mg q.d.s.–q4h. The dose is titrated up as necessary or until undesirable effects occur. For patients already receiving strong opioids, if an 'as needed' dose relieves the cough, continue to use in this way or increase the regular **morphine** dose. If no benefit is obtained from a p.r.n. dose of **morphine**, there is little point in further regular dose increments. Some patients with cough but no pain benefit from a bedtime dose of **morphine** to prevent cough disturbing sleep.

Nebulised local anaesthetics: of limited value because of the unpleasant taste, oropharyngeal numbness, risk of bronchoconstriction and short duration of action (10–30min). The use of nebulised local anaesthetics in patients with cough caused by cancer has not been evaluated and cannot be routinely recommended. However, there are case reports of patients with chronic lung disease, sarcoid or cancer, in whom a single treatment with nebulised **lidocaine** (lignocaine) 400mg relieved cough for 1–8 weeks.[3–5] They should be considered only when other avenues have failed, including nebulised saline. Suggested doses are 2% **lidocaine** (5ml) or 0.25% **bupivacaine** (5ml) q8h–q6h.

Other drugs: used in patients with lung cancer include:

- **sodium cromoglicate** 10mg inhaled q.d.s. improves cough within 36–48h[6]
- **levodropropizine** 75mg PO t.d.s. is as effective as **dihydrocodeine** 10mg t.d.s. and causes less drowsiness (not UK)[7]
- **benzonatate** 100–200mg PO t.d.s. is a cough suppressant with a local anaesthetic effect (not UK).[8]

Supply

Simple Linctus BP

Oral syrup 28 days @ 5ml q.d.s. = £0.90.

Codeine Linctus BP

Oral syrup 15mg/5ml, 28 days @ 15mg q.d.s. = £2.24.
Diabetic oral syrup 15mg/5ml, 28 days @ 15mg q.d.s. = £4.09.
All of the above preparations are available OTC.

Morphine

Sevredol® (Napp 01223 424444)
Oral solution 10mg/5ml, 28 days @ 5mg q.d.s. = £5.57.
Also see **morphine**, p.173 for other preparations.

1 Wilcock A (1998) The management of respiratory symptoms. In: C Faull *et al.* (eds) *The Handbook of Palliative Care*. Blackwell Scientific, London, pp.157–176.
2 Fuller R and Jackson D (1990) Physiology and treatment of cough. *Thorax*. **45**: 425–430.
3 Howard P *et al.* (1977) Lignocaine aerosol and persistent cough. *British Journal of Diseases of the Chest*. **71**: 19–24.
4 Stewart C and Coady T (1977) Suppression of intractable cough. *British Medical Journal*. **1**: 1660–1661.
5 Saunders R and Kirkpatrick M (1984) Prolonged suppression of cough after inhalation of lidocaine in a patient with sarcoid. *Journal of the American Medical Association*. **252**: 2452–2457.
6 Moroni M *et al.* (1996) Inhaled sodium cromoglycate to treat cough in advanced lung cancer patients. *British Journal of Cancer*. **74**: 309–311.
7 Luporini G *et al.* (1998) Efficacy and safety of levodropropizine and dihydrocodeine on non-productive cough in primary and metastatic lung cancer. *European Respiratory Journal*. **12**: 97–101.
8 Doona M and Walsh D (1997) Benzonatate for opioid-resistant cough in advanced cancer. *Palliative Medicine*. **16**: 212–219.

AROMATIC INHALATIONS — BNF 3.8

Class of drug: Demulcent.

Indications: Wet cough (to aid expectoration).

Dose and use

Add 5ml to 500ml ('one teaspoon to a pint') of hot (not boiling) water and inhale vapour.

Supply

Benzoin Tincture Compound BP
Tincture (Friars' Balsam) balsamic acids 4.5%, 100ml = £0.88.

Menthol and Eucalyptus Inhalation BP 1980
Inhalation 100ml = £0.59.
These preparations are available OTC.

CARBOCISTEINE BNF 3.7

Class: Mucolytic.

Indications: Reduction of sputum viscosity.

Contra-indications: Active peptic ulceration.

Pharmacology

Carbocisteine reduces the viscosity of bronchial secretions and facilitates expectoration. It alters the physical and chemical characteristics of the mucin components of sputum to a more 'normal' pattern (by reducing fructose and sulphate content and increasing the proportion of sialomucins). In patients with COPD, mucolytics reduce the number of exacerbations and days of illness but the benefit appears small and their routine use remains debatable.[1,2] However, some individual patients benefit from their use and a therapeutic trial may be justified if all other approaches have failed, particularly in patients with more severe COPD and frequent or prolonged exacerbations.

Cautions

Rare reports of rashes and gastro-intestinal bleeding.

Undesirable effects

For full list, see manufacturer's SPC.
Occasional gastro-intestinal irritation.

Dose and use

- starting dose 750mg t.d.s.
- reduce to 750mg b.d. once satisfactory response obtained.

Supply

Mucodyne® (Aventis Pharma 01732 584000)
Capsules 375mg, 28 days @ 750mg t.d.s. = £25.09 (~~NHS~~).
Oral solution 250mg/5ml, 28 days @ 750mg t.d.s. = £26.38 (~~NHS~~).
Both preparations are available on NHS prescription for children in specific circumstances (see BNF 3.7).

1 Stey C *et al.* (2000) The effect of oral N-acetylcysteine in chronic bronchitis: quantitative systematic review. *European Respiratory Journal.* **16**: 253–262.
2 Poole P and Black P (2001) Oral mucolytic drugs for exacerbations of chronic obstructive pulmonary disease: systematic review. *British Medical Journal.* **322**: 1271–1274.

4: CENTRAL NERVOUS SYSTEM

Psychotropics

Benzodiazepines
Clonazepam
Diazepam
Lorazepam
Midazolam

Typical antipsychotics
Haloperidol
Levomepromazine (methotrimeprazine)
Thioridazine

Atypical antipsychotics
Olanzapine
Risperidone

Antidepressants
Amitriptyline
Mirtazapine
Sertraline
Venlafaxine

Psychostimulants
*Methylphenidate

Cannabinoids
*Nabilone

Anti-emetics
Metoclopramide
Domperidone
Cyclizine
$5HT_3$-receptor antagonists

Hyoscine hydrobromide

Anti-epileptics
Gabapentin

Orphenadrine

PSYCHOTROPICS — BNF 4.2

Psychotropic drugs are primarily used to alter a patient's psychological state.[1] They can be classified as:

- anxiolytic sedatives
- antipsychotics (neuroleptics)
- antidepressants
- psychostimulants
- psychodysleptics.

Generally, smaller doses should be used in debilitated patients with advanced cancer than in physically fit patients, particularly if they are already receiving **morphine** or another psychotropic drug. Close supervision is essential, particularly during the first few days. There may be a need for either a reduction in dose because of drug cumulation or a further increase because of a lack of response. A few patients respond paradoxically when prescribed psychotropic drugs, e.g. **diazepam** (become more distressed) or **amitriptyline** (become wakeful and restless at night). Other patients derive little benefit from a benzodiazepine, e.g. **diazepam**, but are helped by an antipsychotic, e.g. **haloperidol**.

Antidepressants are widely used to relieve neuropathic pain; dose escalation is often limited by undesirable effects.

1 Stahl S (2000) *Essential Psychopharmacology: neuroscientific basis and practical applications* (2e). Cambridge University Press, Cambridge.

BENZODIAZEPINES BNF 4.1, 4.8.3, 10.2.2 & 15.1.4.1

Benzodiazepines are a group of drugs which:
- reduce anxiety and aggression
- sedate and improve sleep
- relax muscles
- suppress seizures.

Benzodiazepines bind to a specific site on the $GABA_A$-receptor and enhance the inhibitory effect of GABA. Subtypes of the $GABA_A$-receptor exist in different regions of the brain, and differ in their sensitivity to benzodiazepines. Anxiolytic benzodiazepines are agonists at this regulatory site. Other benzodiazepines (e.g. **flumazenil**) are antagonists, and prevent the actions of the anxiolytic benzodiazepines. There is also a class of inverse agonists. These reduce the effectiveness of GABA and are anxiogenic; they are not used clinically. Endogenous ligands for the benzodiazepine binding site include peptide and steroid molecules, but their physiological function is not yet understood.

Although the relationship is non-linear, the plasma halflife of a benzodiazepine and its pharmacologically active metabolites reflect its duration of action (Figure 4.1); those with long halflives can be taken o.d., generally o.n. Short-acting agents (e.g. **oxazepam** and **temazepam**) are metabolised to inactive compounds, and are used mainly as sleeping pills. Some long-acting agents (e.g. **diazepam** and **chlordiazepoxide**) are converted to a long-lasting active metabolite (nordiazepam). **Zolpidem** is a short-acting drug which is not a benzodiazepine but acts similarly. Differences in the pharmacological profile of different benzodiazepines are relatively minor (Table 4.1). **Clonazepam** appears to have more anti-epileptic action in relation to its other effects. Potency varies considerably (Table 4.2).

The main undesirable effects of benzodiazepines are dose-dependent drowsiness, impaired psychomotor skills and hypotonia (manifesting as unsteadiness/ataxia), with an increased risk (× 1.7) of femoral fracture in the elderly.[1] Their effects are exacerbated by alcohol. They are relatively safe in overdose. Benzodiazepines with long halflives cumulate when given repeatedly and undesirable effects may manifest after several days or weeks. Because benzodiazepines can cause physical and psychological dependence, the CSM discourages use in the general population (Box 4.A). However, benzodiazepines are essential drugs in palliative care (Box 4.B).

Table 4.1 Pharmacological properties of selected benzodiazepines[2]

Drug name	*Anxiolytic*	*Night sedative*	*Muscle relaxant*	*Anti-epileptic*
Diazepam	+++	++	+++	+++
Lorazepam	+++	++	+	+[a]
Clonazepam	+	+++	+	+++
Nitrazepam	++	+++	+	++
Oxazepam	+++	+	0	0
Temazepam	+	0[a]	0	0

Pharmacological activity: 0 = minimal effect; + = slight; ++ = moderate; +++ = marked.

a. the failure to demonstrate a major anti-epileptic effect with lorazepam or a significant night sedative effect with temazepam emphasises a limitation of a single dose study in volunteers.

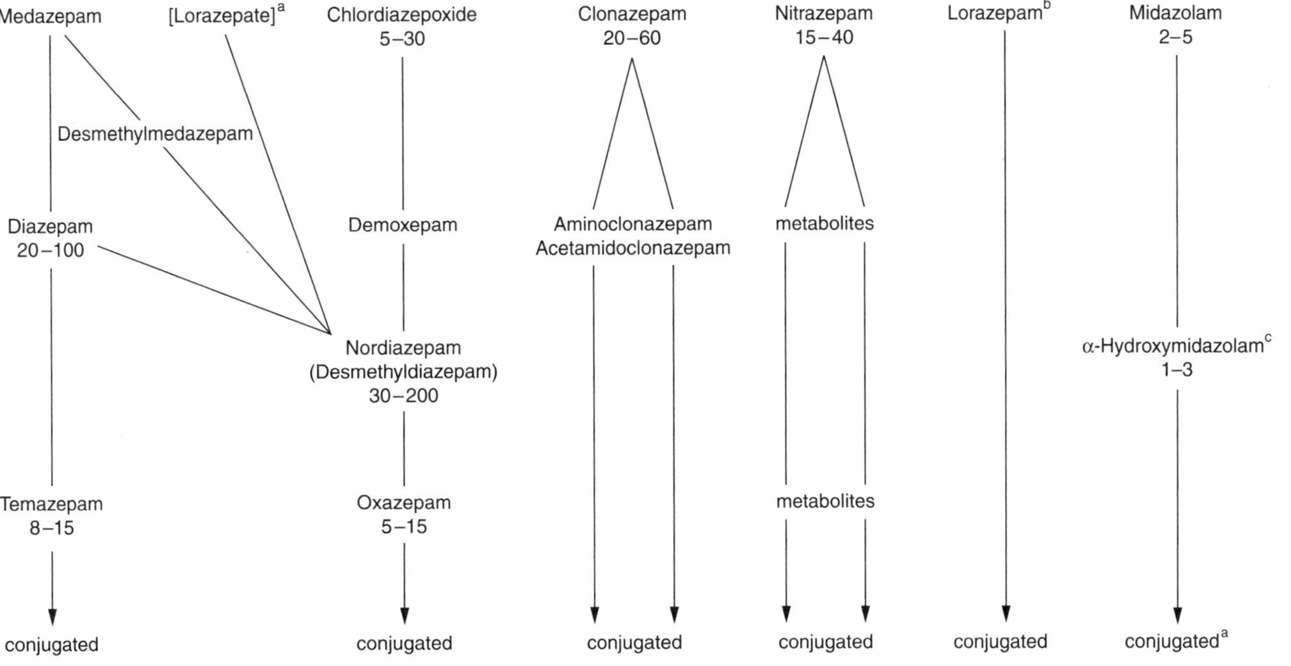

Figure 4.1 Metabolic pathways for selected benzodiazepines. Figures refer to plasma elimination halflives in hours of pharmacologically active substances.

a. lorazepate is a pro-drug

b. lorazepam does not use the P450 hepatic metabolic pathway and avoids interactions relating to competitive inhibition of metabolism

c. α-hydroxymidazolam glucuronide is an active substance, about 10 times less potent than both the unconjugated form and midazolam; cumulation in severe renal failure may lead to prolonged sedation.

Table 4.2 Approximate equivalent anxiolytic-sedative doses[3]

Drug	*Dose*
Lorazepam	500mg
Diazepam	5mg
Nitrazepam	5mg
Temazepam	10mg
Chlordiazepoxide	15mg
Oxazepam	15mg

Box 4.A CSM advice

1 Benzodiazepines are indicated for the short-term relief (2–4 weeks only) of anxiety that is severe, disabling or subjecting the individual to unacceptable distress, occurring alone or in association with insomnia or short-term psychosomatic, organic or psychotic illness.

2 The use of benzodiazepines to treat short-term mild anxiety is inappropriate and unsuitable.

3 Benzodiazepines should be used to treat insomnia only when it is severe, disabling, or subjecting the individual to extreme distress.

Box 4.B Benzodiazepines in palliative care

Night sedation

Short-acting drugs

- midazolam is not available in tablet form in the UK (halflife = 2–5h)
- zopiclone and zolpidem are alternatives available in the UK (halflives = 2–5h); they are not benzodiazepines, but act on the same receptors.

Intermediate-acting drug

- temazepam 10–40mg PO o.n., occasionally 60mg, is widely used (halflife = 8–15h).

Long-acting drug

- flunitrazepam, although marketed as a night sedative (0.5–2mg), has a plasma halflife of 16–35h; it is therefore *not* recommended as a night sedative in palliative care.

Some patients with insomnia respond better to an antipsychotic drug or a tricyclic antidepressant.

Anxiety and panic disorder

Intermediate-acting drugs

- oxazepam 10–15mg PO b.d.–t.d.s. (halflife = 5–15h)
- lorazepam 1–2mg PO b.d.–t.d.s. (halflife = 10–20h).

Lorazepam tablets are used SL at some centres for episodes of acute severe distress (e.g. respiratory panic attacks). For regular use, given its halflife, o.n. or b.d. administration should suffice.

Long-acting drug

- diazepam 2–20mg PO o.n. (halflife = 20–100h).

The BNF recommends t.d.s. administration but the long halflife means that o.n. will generally be as effective, and easier for the patient.

continued

Box 4.B Continued

Acute psychotic agitation
In acute psychotic agitation, lorazepam 2mg PO/IM every 30min until settled is as effective as haloperidol 5mg every 30min.[4]

Muscle relaxant
- diazepam 2–10mg PO o.n., occasionally more
- baclofen is a useful non-benzodiazepine alternative, particularly if diazepam is too sedative and anxiety is not an associated problem.

Anti-epileptic
Acute treatment[5]
- clonazepam 1mg IV, injected over 30sec; repeat after 15min × 2 p.r.n.[6]
- diazepam 10mg IV, injected over 2–4min; repeat after 15min × 2 p.r.n.
- lorazepam 100microgram/kg IV, injected at 2mg/min.[6,7]
- midazolam 10mg IV, injected over 2min; repeat after 15min × 2 p.r.n.

Chronic treatment
- clonazepam 500microgram–1mg PO o.n., rising by 500microgram every 3–5 days up to 2–4mg, occasionally more; doses above 2mg can be divided, e.g. 2mg o.n. and the rest o.m.

Myoclonus
Same choice as for seizures but lower doses:
- diazepam 5mg PO o.n.
- midazolam 5mg SC stat and 10mg/24h CSCI in moribund patients.

Alcohol withdrawal
Same choice as for seizure with dose and route dependent on severity of withdrawal syndrome.[8,9]

1 Grad R (1995) Benzodiazepines for insomnia in community-dwelling elderly: a review of benefit and risk. *Journal of Family Practice*. **41**: 473–481.
2 Ansseau M *et al.* (1984) Methodology required to show clinical differences between benzodiazepines. *Current Medical Research and Opinion*. **8**: 108–113.
3 Anonymous (1998) Hypnotics and anxiolytics. In: *British National Formulary* No. 41. British Medical Association and Royal Pharmaceutical Society of Great Britain, London, p.154.
4 Foster S *et al.* (1997) Efficacy of lorazepam and haloperidol for rapid tranquilization in the psychiatric emergency room setting. *International Clinical Psychopharmacology*. **12**: 175–179.
5 Rey E *et al.* (1999) Pharmacokinetic optimization of benzodiazepines therapy for acute seizures. Focus on delivery routes. *Clinical Pharmacokinetics*. **36**: 409–424.
6 British National Formulary (2001) Drugs used in status epilepticus. In: *British National Formulary* No. 41. British Medical Association and Royal Pharmaceutical Society of Great Britain, London, p.234.
7 Treiman D *et al.* (1998) A comparison of four treatments for generalized convulsive status epilepticus. *New England Journal of Medicine*. **339**: 792–798.
8 Peppers M (1996) Benzodiazepines for alcohol withdrawal in the elderly and in patients with liver disease. *Pharmacotherapy*. **16**: 49–57.
9 Chick J (1998) Review: benzodiazepines are more effective than neuroleptics in reducing delirium and seizures in alcohol withdrawal. *Evidence-Based Medicine*. **3**: 11.

CLONAZEPAM BNF 4.8.1

Class: Benzodiazepine.

Indications: Epilepsy, myoclonus, †anxiety, †panic disorder,[1,2] †restless legs syndrome,[3] †neuropathic pain,[4–6] †terminal agitation.

Contra-indications: Respiratory depression; acute pulmonary insufficiency, severe hepatic disease, sleep apnoea syndrome, myasthenia gravis.

Pharmacology

Clonazepam is a typical benzodiazepine with GABA-potentiating actions in the CNS, notably spinal cord, hippocampus, cerebellum and cerebrum. At all these sites, clonazepam reduces neuronal activity. It can be administered via CSCI (see Syringe Drivers, p.297) or, because of its long halflife, may be administered as a SC injection o.n. Clonazepam is extensively metabolised to inactive metabolites and the cytochrome CYP3A pathway may be important (see Cytochrome P450, p.331).
Bio-availability 100% PO.
Onset of action 5–10min SC; 20–60min PO.
Time to peak plasma concentration 1–4h.
Halflife 20–60h (mean 30h).
Duration of action 12h.

Cautions

Respiratory disease, hepatic and renal impairment.

Undesirable effects

For full list, see manufacturer's SPC.

Fatigue, drowsiness, muscular hypotonia and inco-ordination. These effects are generally transitory and can be minimised by starting with low doses at bedtime. In children, clonazepam has been associated with salivary hypersecretion and drooling.

Dose and use

Due to the development of tolerance to the anti-epileptic effect, clonazepam is generally reserved for the treatment of refractory tonic-clonic or partial seizures.[1-3] Although there is no controlled data to support its use, clonazepam is the first-line treatment in several centres for neuropathic pain in cancer. Like **midazolam** (see p.73), clonazepam can be administered by CSCI for the treatment of terminal agitation (Table 4.3).

Table 4.3 Dose recommendations for clonazepam

Indication	*Stat & p.r.n. doses*	*Initial dose*	*Common range*
Epilepsy	n/a[a]	500microgram–1mg o.n. PO 500microgram–1mg/24h CSCI[b]	4–8mg daily PO 2–8mg/24h CSCI[b]
Panic disorder	n/a	250microgram b.d. *or* 500microgram o.n. PO	1–4mg daily PO
Restless legs	n/a	500microgram o.n. PO	1–2mg o.n. PO
Neuropathic pain	500microgram PO	500microgram o.n. PO	2–8mg daily PO
Terminal sedation	500microgram SC	2mg/24h CSCI[a]	2–8mg/24h CSCI[a]

a. for acute use in status epilepticus (see Box 4.B, p.66)
b. clonazepam adsorbs to PVC in giving sets; clinical significance unknown.

Supply

Rivotril® (Roche 01707 366000)
Tablets 500microgram, 2mg, 28 days @ 2mg o.d. = £1.57.
Injection 1mg/ml, 1ml amp (with 1ml diluent) = £0. 68.

1 Davidson J and Moroz G (1998) Pivotal studies of clonazepam in panic disorder. *Psychopharmacology Bulletin.* **34**: 169–174.
2 Wulsin L *et al.* (1999) Clonazepam treatment of panic disorder in patients with recurrent chest pain and normal coronary arteries. *International Journal of Psychiatry and Medicine.* **29**: 97–105.
3 Joy M (1997) Clonazepam: benzodiazepine therapy for the restless legs syndrome. *ANNA Journal.* **24**: 686–689.
4 Reddy S and Patt R (1994) The benzodiazepines as adjuvant analgesics. *Journal of Pain and Symptom Management.* **9**: 510–514.
5 McQuay H *et al.* (1995) Anticonvulsant drugs for the management of pain: a systematic review. *British Medical Journal.* **311**: 1047–1052.
6 Bartusch S *et al.* (1996) Clonazepam for the treatment of lancinating phantom limb pain. *Clinical Journal of Pain.* **12**: 59–62.

DIAZEPAM BNF 4.1.2, 4.8.2, 10.2.2 & 15.1.4.1

Class: Benzodiazepine.

Indications: Anxiety, insomnia, muscle spasm, myoclonus, epilepsy, alcohol withdrawal (delirium tremens).

Pharmacology

Diazepam is a typical benzodiazepine with GABA-potentiating actions in the CNS, notably spinal cord, hippocampus, cerebellum and cerebrum. At all these sites, diazepam reduces neuronal activity. Diazepam is relatively devoid of autonomic effects and does not significantly reduce locomotor activity at low doses, or depress **amfetamine**-induced excitation. In high doses, it activates the drug metabolising enzymes in the liver. Diazepam also possesses dependence liability and may produce withdrawal symptoms, but has a wide margin of safety against poisoning. Standard parenteral preparations are oil-based and absorption from muscle after IM injection is slower and more variable than after PO and PR administration. Diazepam has a long plasma half-life and several active metabolites, one of which has a plasma halflife of up to 200h in the elderly. Because of marked interindividual variation, the effects of a constant dose will vary greatly. Doses for individual patients are determined empirically.
Bio-availability 100% PO.
Onset of action 15min PO.
Time to peak plasma concentration 30–90min PO.
Plasma halflife 20–100h; active metabolite nordiazepam 30–200h.
Duration of action 3–30h, situation dependent.

Cautions

Concurrent administration with other sedative drugs, including strong opioids, old age, debilitation, hepatic impairment. If given IV can cause hypotension and transient apnoea. Cumulation of active metabolites may necessitate a dose reduction after several days.

Diazepam is metabolised via the cytochrome P450 group of hepatic enzymes which gives rise to several potentially important drug interactions (see Cytochrome P450, p.331); **amiodarone, cimetidine, fluconazole, metronidazole, omeprazole, sodium valproate** all inhibit the clearance of diazepam, resulting in an enhanced and more prolonged effect.[1,2] Genetic polymorphism occurs and some people are slow metabolisers (whites 3–5%, Asians 20%); this also results in an enhanced and more prolonged effect (see Cytochrome P450, p.331).

Undesirable effects

For full list, see manufacturer's SPC.

Drowsiness, muscle flaccidity, unsteadiness (ataxia). When given IV, the oil-based solution may cause painful thrombophlebitis. Paradoxical reactions have been reported: insomnia, anxiety, excitement, rage, hallucinations, increased muscle spasticity.

Dose and use

Typical doses for diazepam are shown in Table 4.4. The initial dose will depend on the patient's age, general condition, previous use of diazepam and other benzodiazepines, the intensity of distress, and the urgency of relief. Generally, elderly and debilitated patients should be started on low doses.

Table 4.4 Dose recommendations for diazepam

Indication	*Stat dose*	*Initial daily dose*	*Common range*
Anxiety[a]	2–10mg PO	2–10mg PO o.n.	2–20mg PO
Muscle spasm[b] Multifocal myoclonus	5mg PO	5mg PO o.n.	2–10mg PO
Anti-epileptic[c]	10mg PR/IV	10–20mg	10–30mg

a. given as an adjunct to non-drug approaches, e.g. relaxation therapy and massage
b. if localised, consider injection of a trigger point with local anaesthetic or acupuncture
c. acute use but in the moribund can be used as a convenient substitute for long-term oral anti-epileptic therapy (also see midazolam, p.73).

In an agitated moribund patient, b.d.–t.d.s. dosing is sometimes indicated so as to reduce the number of hours awake. Rectal diazepam is useful in a crisis or if the patient is moribund:

- suppositories 10mg
- rectal solution 5–10mg in 2.5ml
- parenteral formulation adminstered with a cannula.

If IV administration is necessary, use diazepam oil-in-water emulsion (Diazemuls®) if possible or substitute **midazolam** (see p.73). Patients occasionally react paradoxically, i.e. become more distressed; if this happens, **haloperidol** or **levomepromazine** (methotrimeprazine) should be given instead.

Supply

Diazepam (non-proprietary)
Tablets 2mg, 5mg, 10mg, 28 days @ 5mg o.n. = £0.57.
Oral solution 2mg/5ml, 28 days @ 5mg o.n. = £7.81.
Suppositories 10mg, 1 = £1.09.
Rectal tubes (rectal solution) 5mg and 10mg/2.5ml tube = £1.34 and £1.73 respectively.
Injection (oil-based solution) 5mg/ml, 2ml amp = £0.25.
Injection (oil-in-water emulsion) 5mg/ml, 2ml amp = £0.73.

1 Klotz U and Reimann I (1980) Delayed clearance of diazepam due to cimetidine. *New England Journal of Medicine*. **302**: 1012–1014.
2 Wagner B and O'Hara D (1997) Pharmacokinetics and pharmacodynamics of sedatives and analgesics in the treatment of agitated critically ill patients. *Clinical Pharmacokinetics*. **33**: 426–453.

LORAZEPAM BNF 4.1.2, 4.8.2 & 15.1.4.1

Class: Benzodiazepine.

Indications: Anxiety, insomnia, status epilepticus, peri-operative sedation, †acute agitation, †terminal agitation, †alcohol withdrawal (delirium tremens),[1] †serotonin syndrome.[2]

Contra-indications: Do not use alone in delirium unless alcohol withdrawal.[3]

Pharmacology

Lorazepam is a typical benzodiazepine with GABA-potentiating actions in the CNS, notably spinal cord, hippocampus, cerebellum and cerebrum. At all these sites, lorazepam reduces neuronal activity.[4] Like other benzodiazepines, lorazepam can cause amnesia. Lorazepam is rapidly absorbed SL and PO. Despite being 85% protein-bound, it quickly reaches its sites of action in the CNS.[5] Lorazepam is glucuronidated in the liver to an inactive compound and is excreted both by the kidneys and in the bile. The conjugated metabolite undergoes enterohepatic circulation. Duration of action does not correlate with plasma concentrations and can be up to 3 days. Lorazepam can be given SL, PO, PR, IM, IV but is not recommended for SC use in its present formulation because of the risk of precipitation.[6] Intra-arterial administration has been associated with vascular compromise and gangrene. Lorazepam is now regarded as the benzodiazepine of choice in the control of status epilepticus.[7] Most commonly, lorazepam is used as an anxiolytic.[8] IV lorazepam is an alternative to SC **midazolam** for sedation in the imminently dying.[6,9] It is used with **haloperidol** or **risperidone** to control manic agitation,[10] although at some centres it is used as the sole medication in this circumstance.[11,12] IV lorazepam is cheaper than SC/IV **midazolam** for sedation and seizure therapy.[6,13]

Bio-availability 93% PO.
Onset of action 5min SL; 10–15min PO.
Time to peak plasma concentration 1h SL; 1–1.5h IM; 1–6h PO.
Plasma halflife 12–15h.
Duration of action 6–72h.

Cautions

Although it can be used alone in mania,[11,12] lorazepam should not be used alone in an agitated delirium because it is likely to exacerbate the condition.[3,14] Cumulation can occur, particularly in the elderly and debilitated. Concurrent administration with alcohol and/or other centrally-acting drugs, e.g. tricyclic antidepressants, H_1-antihistamines, antipsychotics and opioids, may result in excessive sedation and/or delirium. The metabolism of lorazepam is impeded by **valproic acid.**[15] Lorazepam interacts with oral anticoagulants at the protein-binding site. It has less interaction with **dextropropoxyphene** than other benzodiazepines.[16] It may increase **digoxin** levels. **Carbamazepine** and **rifampicin** decrease benzodiazepine levels.

Undesirable effects

For full list, see manufacturer's SPC.

Drowsiness, fatigue, impaired co-ordination, blurred vision, lightheadedness, memory impairment, insomnia, dysarthria, anxiety, decreased libido, depression, headaches, tachycardia, chest pain, dry mouth, constipation, diarrhoea, nausea, vomiting, increased or decreased appetite, sweating, rash.

Dose and use

Insomnia

- 2–4mg PO o.n.

Anxiety

- 1mg SL/PO stat and b.d.
- if necessary, increase to 2–6mg/24h.

Agitation

- give 2mg PO every 30min until the patient is settled.[11]

Sedation in the imminently dying

- use in conjunction with an antipsychotic
- 2–4mg IV stat
- 4–20mg/24h CIVI.

Status epilepticus

- lorazepam 0.5–20mg/h IV titrated to sedation (Figure 4.2).

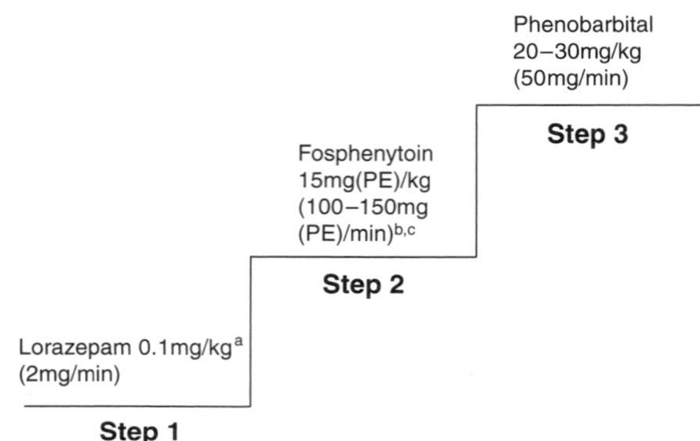

Figure 4.2 IV treatment for status epilepticus. Some centres reverse step 2 and step 3. If all else fails, proceed to general anaesthesia with thiopental, propofol, etc.

a. BNF recommendations; clonazepam, diazepam or midazolam can be used instead
b. fosphenytoin is a pro-drug of phenytoin and can be given more rapidly; fosphenytoin sodium 1.5mg = phenytoin sodium 1mg. Dose is expressed as *phenytoin sodium equivalent (PE)*
c. IV phenytoin 20–30mg/kg (50mg/min) can be used instead with ECG monitoring.

Supply

Lorazepam (non-proprietary)
Tablets 1mg, 2.5mg, 28 days @ 2mg b.d. = £4.93.
Injection 4mg/ml, 1ml amp = £0.51. For IM injection, dilute with equal volume WFI or saline 0.9%.

1 Peppers M (1996) Benzodiazepines for alcohol withdrawal in the elderly and in patients with liver disease. *Pharmacotherapy*. **16**: 49–57.
2 Brown T *et al.* (1996) Pathophysiology and management of the serotonin syndrome. *Annals of Pharmacotherapy*. **30**: 527–533.
3 Breitbart W *et al.* (1996) A double-blind trial of haloperidol, chlorpromazine, and lorazepam in the treatment of delirium in hospitalized AIDS patients. *American Journal of Psychiatry*. **153**: 231–237.
4 Ziemann U *et al.* (1996) The effect of lorazepam on the motor cortical excitability in man. *Experimental Brain Research*. **109**: 127–135.
5 Wagner B and O'Hara D (1997) Pharmacokinetics and pharmacodynamics of sedatives and analgesics in the treatment of agitated critically ill patients. *Clinical Pharmacokinetics*. **33**: 426–453.
6 McCollam J *et al.* (1999) Continuous infusions of lorazepam, midazolam and propofol for sedation of the critically ill surgery trauma patient: a prospective, randomized comparison. *Critical Care Medicine*. **27**: 2454–2458.
7 Rey E *et al.* (1999) Pharmacokinetic optimization of benzodiazepines therapy for acute seizures. Focus on delivery routes. *Clinical Pharmacokinetics*. **36**: 409–424.
8 MacLaren R *et al.* (2000) A prospective evaluation of empiric versus protocol-based sedation and analgesia. *Pharmacotherapy*. **20**: 662–672.

9 Fainsinger R *et al.* (2000) Sedation for delirium and other symptoms in terminally ill patients in Edmonton. *Journal of Palliative Care.* **16(2)**: 5–10.
10 Currier G and Simpson G (2001) Risperidone liquid concentrate and oral lorazepam versus intramuscular haloperidol and intramuscular lorazepam for treatment of psychotic agitation. *Journal of Clinical Psychiatry.* **62**: 153–157.
11 Foster S *et al.* (1997) Efficacy of lorazepam and haloperidol for rapid tranquilization in the psychiatric emergency room setting. *International Clinical Psychopharmacology.* **12**: 175–179.
12 Lenox R *et al.* (1992) Adjunctive treatment of manic agitation with lorazepam versus haloperidol: a double-blind study. *Journal of Clinical Psychiatry.* **53**: 47–52.
13 Swart E *et al.* (1999) Continuous infusion of lorazepam versus midazolam in patients in the intensive care unit: sedation with lorazepam is easier to manage and is more cost-effective. *Critical Care Medicine.* **27**: 1461–1465.
14 Salzman C *et al.* (1991) Parenteral lorazepam versus parenteral haloperidol for the control of psychotic disruptive behavior. *Journal of Clinical Psychiatry.* **52**: 177–180.
15 Samara E *et al.* (1997) Effect of valproate on the pharmacokinetics and pharmacodynamics of lorazepam. *Journal of Clinical Pharmacology.* **37**: 442–450.
16 Abernethy D *et al.* (1985) Interaction of propoxyphene with diazepam, alprazolam and lorazepam. *British Journal of Clinical Pharmacology.* **19**: 51–57.

MIDAZOLAM — BNF 15.1.4.1

Class: Benzodiazepine.

Indications: Anaesthetic induction agent, sedative for minor procedures, myoclonus, epilepsy, terminal agitation,[1,2] †intractable hiccup.[3]

Pharmacology

Midazolam is a short-acting, water-soluble benzodiazepine with GABA-potentiating actions in the CNS, notably spinal cord, hippocampus, cerebellum and cerebrum. At all these sites, midazolam reduces neuronal activity. In single doses for sedation, midazolam is 3 times more potent than **diazepam**; as an anti-epileptic, it is twice as potent. With multiple doses, **diazepam** will gain in potency because of its prolonged plasma halflife, i.e. 20–100h versus 2–5h for midazolam. In adults >60 years, the plasma halflife of midazolam is prolonged up to 3 times and in some intensive care patients having CIVI for sedation, the plasma halflife may be prolonged up to 6 times. It also may be prolonged in hepatic impairment and cardiac failure. Cumulation of hydroxymidazolam glucuronide occurs in renal impairment. There is an active metabolite with a receptor affinity of about 1/10 that of midazolam. In severe renal impairment (creatinine clearance <10ml/min) massive cumulation can result in prolonged sedation.[4] The main advantage of midazolam is that it is water-soluble and is miscible with most of the drugs commonly given by CSCI. It is also better for IV injection because it does not cause thrombophlebitis. Also see Benzodiazepines, p.64.
Bio-availability >90% IM; 75% buccal; 35–44% PO.
Onset of action 5–10min SC; 2–3min IV; 15min buccal.
Time to peak plasma concentration 30min IM; 30min buccal; 60min PO.
Plasma halflife 2–5h; increased to about 10h by CSCI.
Duration of action 5mg = 240min (*max*) depending on the individual.[5]

Cautions

If given IV can cause hypotension and transient apnoea. Enhanced effect if given concurrently with **diltiazem**, **erythromycin**, **fluconazole** (possibly), **itraconazole**, **ketoconazole** (see Cytochrome P450, p.331).

Undesirable effects

For full list, see manufacturer's SPC.
Drowsiness.

Dose and use

Typical doses for midazolam are shown in Table 4.5. In terminal agitation, if the patient does not settle on 30mg/24h, an antipsychotic (e.g. **haloperidol**) is best introduced before further increasing the dose of midazolam. Its use for intractable hiccup is limited to patients in whom persistent distressing hiccup is contributing to terminal restlessness at a time when sedation is acceptable to aid symptom relief.

Table 4.5 Dose recommendations for SC midazolam

Indication	*Stat and p.r.n. doses*	*Initial infusion rate/24h*	*Common range*
Muscle tension/spasm Multifocal myoclonus	5mg	10mg	10–30mg
Terminal agitation Intractable hiccup	5–10mg[a]	30mg	30–60mg[b]
Anti-epileptic	10mg	30mg	30–60mg

a. for hiccup, give initial stat dose IV
b. reported upper dose range 120mg for hiccup; 240mg for agitation.

Supply

Midazolam (non-proprietary)
Injection 1mg/ml, 50ml vial = £6.00; 5mg/ml, 2ml, 5ml 10ml, 18ml amp = £0.78, £2.50, £4.86, £6.80 respectively.

Hypnovel® (Roche 01707 366000)
Injection 2mg/ml, 5ml amp = £0.96; 5mg/ml, 2ml amp = £0.81.

1 Bottomley DM and Hanks GW (1990) Subcutaneous midazolam infusion in palliative care. *Journal of Pain and Symptom Management.* **5**: 259–261.
2 McNamara P *et al.* (1991) Use of midazolam in palliative care. *Palliative Medicine.* **5**: 244–249.
3 Wilcock A and Twycross R (1996) Case report: midazolam for intractable hiccup. *Journal of Pain and Symptom Management.* **12**: 59–61.
4 Bauer TM *et al.* (1995) Prolonged sedation due to accumulation of conjugated metabolites of midazolam. *Lancet.* **346**: 145–147.
5 Schwagmeier R *et al.* (1998) Midazolam pharmacokinetics following intravenous and buccal administration. *British Journal of Clinical Pharmacology.* **46:** 203–206.

TYPICAL ANTIPSYCHOTICS BNF 4.2.1

Antipsychotic drugs are now conventionally divided into two categories, *typical* and *atypical*. The distinction between the two categories is not clearly defined but is based on:

- incidence of extrapyramidal effects (less in atypicals)
- efficacy in treatment-resistant schizophrenics (greater in atypicals)
- efficacy against negative symptoms in schizophrenia (greater in atypicals).

Phenothiazines and butyrophenones are the main typical antipsychotics. They are principally D_2 antagonists; phenothiazines also antagonise muscarinic, α-adrenergic and H_1-receptors. All antipsychotics can cause extrapyramidal reactions (see Drug-induced movement disorders, p.339). **Haloperidol** is the typical antipsychotic of choice in palliative care. It is used as an anti-emetic as well as an antipsychotic.

In the past, antipsychotics were used as part of an analgesic 'cocktail'. However, in chronic pain, the combination of an antipsychotic with an antidepressant is no more effective than treatment with an antidepressant alone,[1] and in combination with **morphine** causes more sedation without more pain relief. [2] However, antipsychotics are of benefit in selected highly anxious patients overwhelmed by persisting pain and insomnia.[3] Benefit may also be seen in patients whose pain escalates with the onset of delirium (acute confusion) and who derive no benefit from increased doses of opioids.[4] **Levomepromazine** (methotrimeprazine) is the only phenothiazine with specific analgesic properties.[5]

The pharmacology of phenothiazines is complex because they interact with numerous transmitter systems in both the CNS and the periphery. The antipsychotic effect is mediated through D_2-receptor blockade in the mesolimbic and cortical areas. D_2-receptor blockade also has an inhibitory effect on the area postrema (chemoreceptor trigger zone), stimulates prolactin release, and reduces growth hormone levels. Extrapyramidal effects may occur as a result of D_2-receptor blockade in the basal ganglia (globus pallidus and corpus striatum). Phenothiazines bind to α-adrenoceptors to varying extents and cause postural hypotension; they also bind to H_1-receptors and cause sedation. Some phenothiazines are less sedative than others, and **trifluoperazine** may be stimulating. Akathisia, an extrapyramidal effect, may be misinterpreted as cerebral stimulation or deterioration of an underlying psychosis. Phenothiazines have differing antimuscarinic activity, which may be marked, e.g. **thioridazine**. Antiparkinsonian drugs with antimuscarinic properties, e.g. **orphenadrine**, **procyclidine**, are used to treat extrapyramidal effects but their antimuscarinic effects will be additive to those of the antipsychotic drug itself. In these circumstances, the antiparkinsonian drug could precipitate a toxic confusional psychosis and so complicate the underlying psychosis.

Given their respective plasma halflives, most phenothiazines need to be given b.d.–t.d.s. at most; sometimes just o.n. (Table 4.6). Apart from **levomepromazine** (methotrimeprazine), phenothiazines are generally too irritant to be given SC, and are given IM instead. **Prochlorperazine** is sometimes given by intermittent SC injection.

Table 4.6 Comparative features of selected antipsychotic drugs[6–14]

Drug	*Oral bio-availability (%)*	*Plasma halflife (h)*	*Equivalent oral dose (mg)*
Haloperidol	60	12–36	2–3
Fluphenazine	3	15	1–2
Trifluoperazine	?	8–12	5
Prochlorperazine	15	8[18[a]]	?
Thioridazine	60	6–40	100
Chlorpromazine	10–25	7–15	100
Levomepromazine	40	16–30	25–50

a. chronic administration.

1 Getto C *et al.* (1987) Antidepressants and chronic nonmalignant pain: a review. *Journal of Pain and Symptom Management.* **2**: 9–18.
2 Houde RW (1966) On assaying analgesics in man. In: RS Knighton and PR Dumke (eds) *Pain.* Little Brown, Boston, pp.183–196.
3 Maltebie A and Cavenar J (1977) Haloperidol and analgesia: case reports. *Military Medicine.* **142**: 946–948.
4 Coyle N *et al.* (1994) Delirium as a contributing factor to 'crescendo' pain: three case reports. *Journal of Pain and Symptom Management.* **9**: 44–47.
5 Bonica JJ and Halpern LM (1972) Analgesics. In: W Modell (ed) *Drugs of Choice 1972–1973.* CV Mosby, St Louis, pp.185–217.
6 Foster P (1989) Neuroleptic equivalence. *Pharmaceutical Journal.* **September 30**: 431–432.
7 Data Sheet (1996) Haloperidol. In: *ABPI Compendium of Data Sheet and Summaries of Product Characteristics 1996-1997.* Datapharm Publications, London, pp.449–450.
8 Koytchev R *et al.* (1996) Absolute bioavailability of oral immediate and slow release fluphenazine in healthy volunteers. *European Journal of Clinical Pharmacology.* **51**: 183–187.
9 Smith Kline Beecham Pharmaceuticals (1997) Personal communication.
10 Dahl S and Strandjord R (1977) Pharmacokinetics of chlorpromazine after single and chronic dosage. *Clinical Pharmacology and Therapeutics.* **21**: 437–448.

11 Reynolds J (1996) Thioridazine. In: *Martindale. The Extra Pharmacopoeia* (31e). Royal Pharmaceutical Society, London, pp.738–739.
12 Yeung P *et al.* (1993) Pharmacokinetics of chlorpromazine and key metabolites. *European Journal of Clinical Pharmacology.* **45**: 563–569.
13 Dahl SG (1975) Pharmacokinetics of methotrimeprazine after single and multiple doses. *Clinical Pharmacology and Therapeutics.* **19**: 435–442.
14 Koytchev R *et al.* (1994) Absolute bioavailability of chlorpromazine, promazine and promethazine. *Arzneimittel-Forschung.* **44**: 121–125.

HALOPERIDOL — BNF 4.2.1

Class: Butyrophenone.

Indications: Nausea and vomiting, psychotic symptoms, agitated delirium (including disturbed nights in the elderly), intractable hiccup.

Haloperidol tablets and oral solution are not licensed for anti-emetic use (but are for intractable hiccup). In contrast, the injectable formulation is licensed for use as an IM anti-emetic (but not for intractable hiccup). The routes and doses recommended here are often outside the terms of the licence.

Phamacology

Haloperidol is a typical antipsychotic which is a specific D_2-receptor antagonist. Steady-state plasma concentrations do not vary greatly between patients after injection but they vary considerably after PO administration. The metabolism of haloperidol is not as complex as that of the phenothiazines but, even so, there are many metabolites. It is not possible to relate clinical response to plasma haloperidol concentrations. Haloperidol in solution is odourless, colourless and tasteless and can be administered clandestinely in extreme situations.[1] Haloperidol is widely used in palliative care in delirium and as an anti-emetic. By virtue of its D_2-receptor antagonism, it has a profound inhibitory effect on the area postrema (chemoreceptor trigger zone). Clinical experience over several decades has shown haloperidol to be an excellent anti-emetic for most chemical causes of vomiting, e.g. **morphine**, **digoxin**, renal failure, hypercalcaemia; and also after radiotherapy.[2] However, no formal clinical trials have been conducted to date.[3] Haloperidol has also been used for obstructive vomiting in relatively small doses, e.g. 2–5mg SC.[4,5] Its benefit in these circumstances is more difficult to understand. It may relate to blocking the emetogenic impact of 'toxins' absorbed from the obstructed bowel or could represent a prokinetic effect, similar to that of **domperidone**. If that is the case, it would be expected that haloperidol would correct gastric stasis induced by stress, anxiety or nausea from any cause. Haloperidol demonstrates 10-fold greater affinity at dopamine receptors than **domperidone**.[6]

Compared with **chlorpromazine**, haloperidol has less effect on the cardiovascular system and is less sedative. It has no antimuscarinic properties. However, it causes more extrapyramidal reactions, which are more likely at daily doses of >5mg (see Drug-induced movement disorders, p.339). In a study of schizophrenia, haloperidol caused akathisia in >50%.[7] The incidence in palliative care, where lower doses are the norm, will be lower. Because these are unpredictable, an antiparkinsonian drug should not be prescribed prophylactically.

Bio-availability 60–70% PO.
Onset of action 10–15min SC; >1h PO.
Time to peak plasma concentration 30–40min PO; 10–20min SC.
Plasma halflife 13–35h.
Duration of action up to 24h, sometimes longer.

Cautions

Parkinson's disease. Potentiation of CNS depression caused by other CNS depressants, e.g. anxiolytics, alcohol. Increased risk of extrapyramidal effects and possible neurotoxicity with **lithium**. Plasma concentration of haloperidol is approximately halved by concurrent use of **carbamazepine**.

Undesirable effects

For full list, see manufacturer's SPC.

Extrapyramidal effects (including tardive dyskinesia), hypothermia, sedation, hypotension, endocrine effects, blood disorders, alteration in liver function, neuroleptic (antipsychotic) malignant syndrome (see p.342).

Dose and use

Anti-emetic (for chemical/toxic causes of vomiting)

- starting dose 1.5mg stat & o.n. (standard anti-emetic for morphine-induced vomiting at many centres)
- usual dose 3–5mg o.n.; maximum dose 10–20mg o.n. or in divided dosage.

If 10mg o.n. or 5mg b.d. is ineffective, it is generally advisable to substitute **levomepromazine** (methotrimeprazine) for haloperidol.

Antipsychotic-anxiolytic

- 1.5–3mg stat & o.n. in the elderly
- 5mg stat & o.n. in the younger patients or if poor response in the elderly
- 10–30mg o.n. (or in divided dosage) if poor response.

Although haloperidol exacerbates Parkinson's disease, a small daily dose, i.e. 1–1.5mg, may not cause noticeable deterioration.

Intractable hiccup

- if severe and no response with IV **metoclopramide**, give 5–10mg PO/IV[8]
- maintenance dose 1.5–3mg o.n.[9,10]

Supply

Haloperidol (non-proprietary)
Tablets 1.5mg, 5mg, 10mg, 20mg, 28 days @ 5mg o.n. = £3.57.

Serenace® (IVAX 08705 020304)
Capsules 0.5mg, 28 days @ 5mg o.n. = £9.15.
Tablets 1.5mg, 5mg, 10mg, 28 days @ 5mg o.n. = £4.57.
Oral solution 2mg/ml, 28 days @ 5mg o.n. = £6.14.
Injection 5mg/ml, 1ml amp = £0.59.

Haldol® (Janssen-Cilag 01494 567567)
Tablets 5mg, 10mg, 28 days @ 5mg o.n. = £2.31.
Oral solution 2mg/ml, 28 days @ 5mg o.n. = £3.56.
Injection 5mg/ml, 1ml amp = £0.33.

Dozic® (Rosemont 0113 244 1999)
Oral solution 1mg/ml, 28 days @ 5mg o.n. = £10.22.

---

1 UKCC (2001) *UKCC position statement on the covert administration of medicines* (September).
2 Stoll BA (1962) Radiation sickness. *British Medical Journal.* **2**: 507–510.
3 Critchley P *et al.* (2001) Efficacy of haloperidol in the treatment of nausea and vomiting in the palliative patient: a systematic review. *Journal of Pain and Symptom Management.* **22**: 631–634.
4 Ventafridda V *et al.* (1990) The management of inoperable gastrointestinal obstruction in terminal cancer patients. *Tumori.* **76**: 389–393.
5 Mercadante S (1995) Bowel obstruction in home-care cancer patients: 4 years experience. *Support Care Cancer.* **3**: 190–193.
6 Sanger G (1993) The pharmacology of anti-emetic agents. In: P Andrews and G Sanger (eds) *Emesis in Anti-cancer Therapy: mechanisms and treatment.* Chapman & Hall, London, pp.179–210.
7 Wirshing D *et al.* (1999) Novel antipsychotics: comparison of weight gain liabilities. *Journal of Clinical Psychiatry.* **60**: 358–363.
8 Twycross R and Wilcock A (2001) *Symptom Management in Advanced Cancer* (3e). Radcliffe Medical Press, Oxford, p.174.
9 Ives TJ *et al.* (1985) Treatment of intractable hiccups with intramuscular haloperidol. *American Journal of Psychiatry.* **142**: 1368–1369.
10 Scarnati RA (1979) Intractable hiccup (singultus): report of case. *Journal of the American Osteopathic Association.* **79**: 127–129.

LEVOMEPROMAZINE (METHOTRIMEPRAZINE) BNF 4.2.1

Class: Anti-emetic, phenothiazine antipsychotic.

Indications: Nausea and vomiting, terminal agitation, intractable pain.

Pharmacology

Levomepromazine is a broad-spectrum anti-emetic which is widely used as a second- or third-line agent in patients who fail to respond to more specific drugs (see Anti-emetics, p.106). Like **chlorpromazine**, it is a potent D_2- and α_1-receptor antagonist; unlike **chlorpromazine**, levomepromazine also manifests potent $5HT_2$-receptor antagonism. This probably accounts for both its greater anti-emetic efficacy and its analgesic effect.[1] However, levomepromazine is more sedative and more likely to cause postural hypotension.
Bio-availability 40% PO.
Onset of action 30min.
Time to peak plasma concentration 1–3h PO; 30–90min SC.
Plasma halflife 15–30h.
Duration of action 12–24h.

Cautions

Parkinsonism, postural hypotension, antihypertensive medication, epilepsy, hypothyroidism, myasthenia gravis.

Undesirable effects

For full list, see manufacturer's SPC.
Sedation (particularly with SC dose of ≥25mg/24h), dose-dependent postural hypotension, antimuscarinic effects (see p.4).

Dose and use

Anti-emetic
Generally used as a second- or third-line anti-emetic:
- typical starting dose 6–12.5mg PO/SC stat, o.n. & p.r.n.
- larger doses are often associated with sedation.

If used as a first-line anti-emetic, a smaller dose may be adequate.
Terminal agitation +/– delirium
- stat dose 25mg SC and 50–75mg/24h CSCI
- titrate dose according to response; maximum 300mg/24h, occasionally more.[2,3]

Analgesic
May be of benefit in a very distressed patient with severe pain unresponsive to other measures:
- stat dose 25mg PO/SC and o.n.
- titrate dose according to response; usual maximum daily dose 100mg SC/200mg PO.

Supply

Nozinan® (Link 01403 272451)
Tablets 25mg, 28 days @ 12.5mg o.n. = £1.74.
Tablets 6mg, 28 days @ 6mg o.n. = £3.08. (Unlicensed, available as a named patient supply from Link; see Special orders and named patient supplies, p.349.) Cost of a 6mg tablet is £0.11, the equivalent cost of one quarter of a 25mg tablet is £0.06.
Injection 25mg/ml, 1ml amp = £1.85.

---

1 Twycross R *et al.* (1997) The use of low dose levomepromazine (methotrimeprazine) in the management of nausea and vomiting. *Progress in Palliative Care.* **5**: 49–53.

2 Johnson I and Patterson S (1992) Drugs used in combination in the syringe driver: a survey of hospice practice. *Palliative Medicine.* **6**: 125–130.

3 Regnard C and Tempest S (1998) *A Guide to Symptom Relief in Advanced Disease* (4e). Hochland and Hochland, Manchester.

THIORIDAZINE BNF 4.2.1

Class: Phenothiazine antipsychotic.

Indications: Need for a sedative antipsychotic, †cancer-related sweating.[1]

Contra-indications: Patients with reduced levels of CYP2D6. Concurrent use of drugs which inhibit or are metabolised by cytochrome CYP2D6 can increase plasma levels of thioridazine. Patients with prolonged QTc, a family history of prolonged QTc or those with a clinically significant cardiac disorder. Concurrent use of drugs which prolong the QTc interval. Parkinson's disease.

Pharmacology

Thioridazine is equipotent with **chlorpromazine** as an antipsychotic.[2] Compared with **chlorpromazine**, thioridazine is less anti-emetic, causes less postural hypotension and extrapyramidal effects, but has more antimuscarinic effects.[3] In 2000, the licence for thioridazine was restricted to a second-line treatment of schizophrenia in adults because of concerns about cardiotoxicity (QTc prolongation and life-threatening ventricular arrhythmias). New warnings and precautions in the SPC for the safe use of thioridazine include:

- a slow titration, maximum 100mg/week
- a maximum daily dose of 600mg
- ECG monitoring at baseline, after each dose increase and at 6-monthly intervals
- periodic checking of plasma electrolyte concentrations.

It is recommended that for patients currently receiving thioridazine the need to continue should be reviewed, and an informed decision regarding discontinuation of treatment made. Withdrawal should be gradual over a period of 1–2 weeks. Further information and a copy of the newly revised SPC can be obtained from the MCA website, www.mca.gov.uk, from the electronic compendium website, www.emc.vhn.net or by contacting the manufacturer. Also see Prolongation of QT interval in palliative care (p.327).

Bio-availability 60% PO.

Onset of action 30–60min.

Time to peak plasma concentration 2–4h PO.

Plasma halflife 6–40h; active metabolite mesoridazine 10h.

Duration of action 12–24h.

Cautions

Parkinsonism. Potentiation of CNS depression when taken with other CNS depressants, e.g. anxiolytics, alcohol. Increased risk of extrapyramidal effects and possible neurotoxicity with **lithium** (see Cytochrome P450, p.331).

Undesirable effects

For full list, see manufacturer's SPC.

See antimuscarinic effects, p.4. Electrolyte disturbance (e.g. as a result of severe diarrhoea) makes thioridazine more cardiotoxic.[4]

Dose and use

Antipsychotic

- usual starting dose 25mg stat & b.d.
- titrate according to response; usual maximum dose 100–200mg o.n. (or in divided dosage).

Night sedative

- usual starting dose 25–50mg o.n.
- titrate according to response; usual maximum dose 100–200mg o.n.

Sweating

Thioridazine is used at some centres to treat paraneoplastic sweating (Figure 4.3):

- usual starting dose 10mg o.n.
- usual effective dose 10–25mg o.n.; usual maximum dose 50mg o.n.

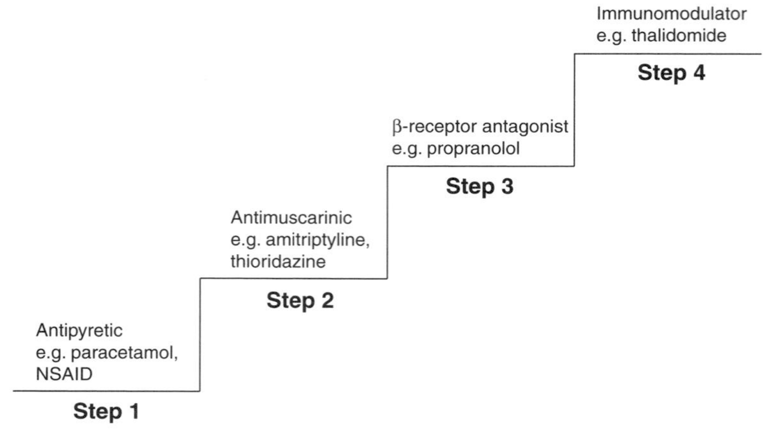

Figure 4.3 Treatment ladder for paraneoplastic sweating.[5–7]

Supply

Thioridazine (non-proprietary)
Tablets 25mg, 50mg, 100mg, 28 days @ 25mg o.n. = £0.49.
Oral solution 25mg (of thioridazine base)/5ml, 28 days @ 25mg o.n. = £0.75.

Melleril® (Novartis 01276 698370)
Tablets 10mg, 25mg, 50mg, 100mg, 28 days @ 25mg o.n. = £0.55.
Oral suspension 25mg/5ml, 100mg/5ml, 28 days @ 25mg o.n. = £0.91.
Oral syrup 25mg (of thioridazine base)/5ml, 28 days @ 25mg o.n. = £0.92.

1 Regnard C (1996) Use of low dose thioridazine to control sweating in advanced cancer. *Palliative Medicine*. **10**: 78–79.
2 Foster P (1989) Neuroleptic equivalence. *Pharmaceutical Journal*. **September 30**: 431–432.
3 Axelsson R and Martensson E (1976) Serum concentration and elimination from serum of thioridazine in psychiatric patients. *Current Therapeutic Research*. **19**: 242–265.
4 Denvir M *et al.* (1998) Thioridazine, diarrhoea and torsades de pointe. *Journal of the Royal Society of Medicine*. **91**: 145–147.
5 Tsavaris N *et al.* (1990) A randomized trial of the effect of three nonsteroidal anti-inflammatory agents in ameliorating cancer-induced fever. *Journal of Internal Medicine*. **228**: 451–455.
6 Johnson M (1996) Neoplastic fever. *Palliative Medicine*. **10**: 217–224.
7 Deaner P (1998) Thalidomide for distressing night sweats in advanced malignant disease. *Palliative Medicine*. **12**: 208–209.

ATYPICAL ANTIPSYCHOTICS BNF 4.2.1

The relatively new atypical antipsychotics include **amisulpride**, **clozapine**, **olanzapine**, **quetiapine**, **risperidone** and **zotepine**.[1] (**Sertindole** has been suspended following reports of arrhythmias and sudden cardiac death.) They have a lower propensity than typical antipsychotics for causing drug-induced movement disorders (see p.339), probably because of a balanced central antagonism of serotonin (5HT) and D_2-receptors.[2]

Clozapine is not recommended because it can cause neutropenia, and the WBC needs to be checked monthly for several months. In palliative care, the choice lies between **olanzapine** and

risperidone. These differ in their receptor site affinities; **olanzapine** has antimuscarinic properties whereas **risperidone** does not.

Although drug-induced movement disorders are less common than with typical antipsychotics, they still occur. In a retrospective review of 42 patients with bipolar disorder who had received **clozapine**, **olanzapine** or **risperidone**, >25% developed either parkinsonism or akathisia.[3] In a study comparing **risperidone** and **haloperidol** in schizophrenics, the incidence of akathisia was 24% with **risperidone** but 53% with **haloperidol**.[4] However, a postmarketing survey comparing **risperidone** with typical antipsychotics extending over 4 years and embracing 1.2 million patient-years gave 0.2% (1 in 500) as the annual reporting rate for extrapyramidal symptoms and 0.0006% (6 in 100 000) for tardive dyskinesia.[5]

Because of the lower incidence of drug-induced movement disorders and patient preference, an atypical antipsychotic is the drug of choice for chronic psychoses.[6] **Olanzapine** probably is safer than **risperidone** in this respect.[7] However, because **olanzapine** and **risperidone** are available only in oral formulations, **haloperidol** remains the most versatile choice for delirium and acute psychoses in palliative care. As with all antipsychotics, hallucinations in delirium resolve in hours-to-days whereas seemingly identical phenomena in a psychosis may not resolve for 1–2 weeks.

Given their receptor site affinities, atypical antipsychotics are likely to be potent anti-emetics, particularly **olanzapine**. Anecdotal reports support this contention but so far there has been no formal evaluation in this respect. Acquisition costs for atypical antipsychotics are higher than for typical antipsychotics. However, they cause less harm (particularly in relation to tardive dyskinesia) and long-term healthcare costs have been calculated to be significantly less.[8]

1 Hoes M (1998) Recent developments in the management of psychosis. *Pharmacy and World Science*. **20**: 101–106.
2 Geddes J *et al.* (2000) Atypical antipsychotics in the treatment of schizophrenia: systematic overview and meta-regression analysis. *British Medical Journal*. **321**: 1371–1376.
3 Guille C *et al.* (2000) A naturalistic comparison of clozapine, risperidone and olanzapine in the treatment of bipolar disorder. *Journal of Clinical Psychiatry*. **61**: 638–642.
4 Wirshing D *et al.* (1999) Risperidone in treatment-refractory schizophrenia. *American Journal of Psychiatry*. **156**: 1374–1379.
5 Tooley P and Zuiderwijk P (1997) Drug safety: experience with risperidone. *Advances in Therapy*. **14**: 262–266.
6 Kapur S and Remington G (2000) Atypical antipsychotics. Patients value the lower incidence of extrapyramidal side effects. *British Medical Journal*. **321**: 1360–1361.
7 Gilbody S *et al.* (2000) Risperidone versus other atypical antipsychotic medication for schizophrenia. *Cochrane Database Systems Review*. **3**: CD002306.
8 Davies A *et al.* (1998) Risperidone versus haloperidol: II. cost-effectiveness. *Clinical Therapeutics*. **20**: 196–213.

OLANZAPINE — BNF 4.2.1

Class: Atypical antipsychotic.

Indications: Schizophrenia; †agitation, †delirium; †anti-emetic; drug-induced movement disorders with **haloperidol**.

Contra-indications: Narrow-angle glaucoma; breast-feeding.

Pharmacology

Olanzapine is a potent D_1, D_2, D_4-receptor and $5HT_{2A}$, $5HT_{2C}$-receptor antagonist.[1,2] It also binds to other receptors, including α_1-adrenergic, H_1 and muscarinic receptors.[3] Olanzapine is used primarily in schizophrenia and other psychoses.[4] In a non-randomised comparison of olanzapine with **haloperidol** in the treatment of delirium, once daily doses o.n. adjusted according

to response were equally effective, with maximum benefit seen after 1 week.[5] Compared with **haloperidol**, olanzapine causes fewer drug-induced movement disorders, including tardive dyskinesia,[6] but dose-related weight gain is more common (40% vs 12%).[7] Weight gain is greater than with **risperidone**.[8] Given its receptor site affinities, olanzapine is likely to be a potent anti-emetic. Anecdotal reports support this contention but so far there has been no formal evaluation.[9] It is metabolised in the liver by glucuronidation and, to a lesser extent, oxidation via the cytochrome P450 system (see p.331), primarily via CYP1A2 with a minor contribution via CYP2D6. The major metabolite is the 10-N-glucuronide which does not pass the blood-brain barrier. Elimination of metabolites is both renal (60%) and faecal (30%).[10] Clearance varies 4-fold among patients.[2,6]
Bio-availability 60%, sometimes >80% PO.
Onset of action hours-to-days in delirium; days-to-weeks in psychoses.
Time to peak plasma concentration 5–8h, not affected by food.
Plasma halflife 34h; 52h in the elderly; *shorter* in smokers and in hepatic impairment; unchanged in renal impairment.
Duration of action 12–48h, situation dependent.

Cautions

Parkinson's disease (potentially can cause a deterioration). Possibly epilepsy (*typical* antipsychotics and *atypical* **clozapine** lower seizure threshold). Elderly patients and those with renal or hepatic impairment. May cause or adversely affect diabetes mellitus; rare reports of keto-acidosis.

Omeprazole, **carbamazepine**, **rifampicin** and tobacco exposure stimulate CYP1A2 and decrease olanzapine plasma concentrations; **fluvoxamine**, an inhibitor of CYP1A2, increases plasma concentrations. Olanzapine potentiates the sedative effects of alcohol and other CNS depressants.

Undesirable effects

For full list, see manufacturer's SPC.
Common: drowsiness, weight gain.
Less common: dry mouth, constipation, orthostatic hypotension,[11–13] agitation, nervousness, dizziness, peripheral oedema.
The incidence and severity of drug-induced movement disorders are significantly less than with **haloperidol**.[6,14] Acute disorders are generally mild and are reversible if the dose is reduced and/or an antimuscarinic antiparkinsonian drug prescribed.

Dose and use

Schizophrenia

An atypical antipsychotic should be used preferentially:
- starting dose 5–10mg o.n.
- increase if necessary to 20mg o.n.

Agitation and/or delirium

Used as an alternative to **haloperidol**:
- starting dose 2.5mg stat, p.r.n. & o.n.
- increase if necessary to 5–10mg o.n.[15,16]

Anti-emetic

Used as an alternative to **levomepromazine** (methotrimeprazine):
- starting dose 1.25–2.5mg stat, q2h p.r.n. & o.n.
- increase if necessary to 5mg o.n.

The higher dose may be necessary in patients receiving highly emetogenic chemotherapy, e.g. **cisplatin**.

Oral dispersible tablets are placed on the tongue and allowed to dissolve or dispersed in water, orange juice, apple juice, milk or coffee immediately before administration.

Supply

Zyprexa® (Lilly 01256 315000)
Tablets 2.5mg, 5mg, 7.5mg, 10mg, 28 days @ 5mg o.n. = £48.78.
Dispersible tablets (Velotab®) 5mg, 10mg, 28 days @ 5mg o.n. = £56.10.

Injections of olanzapine are not available.

1 Hale A (1996) Olanzapine. *British Journal of Hospital Medicine.* **58**: 442–445.
2 Stephenson C and Pilowsky L (1999) Psychopharmacology of olanzapine. A review. *British Journal of Psychiatry Supplement.* **38**: 52–58.
3 Raedler T *et al.* (2000) In vivo olanzapine occupancy of muscarinic acetylcholine receptors in patients with schizophrenia. *Neuropsychopharmacology.* **23**: 56–68.
4 Fulton B and Goa K (1997) Olanzapine. A review of phamarcological properties and therapeutic efficacy in the management of schizophrenia and related psychoses. *Drugs.* **53**: 281–297.
5 Sipahimalani A and Masand P (1998) Olanzapine in the treatment of delirium. *Psychosomatics.* **39**: 422–430.
6 Beasley C *et al.* (1997) Efficacy of olanzapine: an overview of pivotal clinical trials. *Journal of Clinical Psychiatry.* **58 (suppl 10)**: 7–12.
7 Eli Lilly Company (2001) *Olanzapine. Clinical and laboratory experience. A comprehensive monograph.* Dextra Court, Chapel Hill, Basingstoke RG21 5SY.
8 Wirshing D *et al.* (1999) Novel antipsychotics: comparison of weight gain liabilities. *Journal of Clinical Psychiatry.* **60**: 358–363.
9 Pirl W and Roth A (2000) Remission of chemotherapy-induced emesis with concurrent olanzapine treatment: a case report. *Psycho-Oncology.* **9**: 84–87.
10 Callaghan J *et al.* (1999) Olanzapine. Pharmacokinetic and pharmacodynamic profile. *Clinical Pharmacokinetics.* **37**: 177–193.
11 Tollefson G *et al.* (1997) Olanzapine versus haloperidol in the treatment of schizophrenia and schizoaffective and schizophreniform disorders: results of an international collaborative trial. *American Journal of Psychiatry.* **154**: 457–465.
12 Conley R and Meltzer H (2000) Adverse events related to olanzapine. *Journal of Clinical Psychiatry.* **61**: 26–29.
13 Worrel J *et al.* (2000) Atypical antipsychotic agents: a critical review. *American Journal of Health-System Pharmacy.* **57**: 238–358.
14 Geddes J *et al.* (2000) Atypical antipsychotics in the treatment of schizophrenia: systematic overview and meta-regression analysis. *British Medical Journal.* **321**: 1371–1376.
15 Passik S and Cooper M (1999) Complicated delirium in a cancer patient successfully treated with olanzapine. *Journal of Pain and Symptom Management.* **17**: 191–223.
16 Meehan K *et al.* (2002) Comparison of rapidly acting IM olanzapine, lorazepam, and placebo: a double-blind, randomized study in acutely agitated patients with dementia. *Neuropsychopharmacology.* **26**: 494–504.

RISPERIDONE — BNF 4.2.1

Class: Atypical antipsychotic.

Indications: Acute and chronic psychoses; †delirium; †behavioural and psychological symptoms in dementia;[1] poor response to or drug-induced movement disorders with **haloperidol**.

Pharmacology

Risperidone is a potent D_2-receptor and $5HT_{2A}$-receptor antagonist.[2] It also binds to α_1-adrenergic receptors and with lower affinity to H_1- and α_2-receptors. Unlike **olanzapine**, risperidone does *not* bind to muscarinic receptors. Compared with typical antipsychotics, the incidence of drug-induced movement disorders is less.[3,4] This is probably because of balanced central serotonin (5HT) and dopamine antagonism. Even so, a retrospective survey reported that $>$25% of patients developed akathisia or parkinsonism.[5]

Although in animal studies risperidone is 4–10 times less potent than **haloperidol** as a central D_2-receptor antagonist, [2] it is several times more potent as an antipsychotic, presumably because of the dual impact on both D_2- and $5HT_2$-receptors. In schizophrenia, risperidone has an earlier onset of action than **haloperidol**,[4,6,7] and is associated with fewer relapses.[8] In delirium, hallucinations respond to risperidone within hours but generally only after 1–2 weeks in a psychotic illness; this is true of all antipsychotics.

The major metabolite of risperidone is 9-hydroxyrisperidone. This hydroxylation is subject to debrisoquine-type genetic CYP2D6-related polymorphism but, because both risperidone and its major metabolite are equally active, the efficacy of risperidone is unaffected.[9] Risperidone is more slowly eliminated in the elderly and in patients with renal impairment. Plasma concentrations are not affected in hepatic impairment.[10]

Risperidone is as effective as **haloperidol** in treating delirium[11] and behavioural disturbances in dementia.[1] Its efficacy as an anti-emetic is unknown but it could be more effective than **haloperidol** because of its antagonism of $5HT_2$-receptors (see **levomepromazine** (methotrimeprazine), p.78). Risperidone can cause a weight gain of several kg particularly over the first 2 months; this is generally less than with other atypical antipsychotics but may be more marked if it is given together with **sodium valproate** or **lithium**.[4,5]

Bio-availability 99%.

Time to peak plasma concentration 1–2h, not affected by food.

Onset of action hours-to-days in delirium; days-to-weeks in psychoses.

Plasma halflife of active fraction (risperidone + 9-hydroxyrisperidone) 24h.

Duration of action 12–48h, situation dependent.

Cautions

Because of its α-adrenergic receptor antagonism, risperidone can cause orthostatic hypotension, particularly initially. Parkinson's disease (potentially could cause deterioration). Epilepsy (no direct evidence of a deleterious effect but typical antipsychotics and **clozapine**, an atypical antipsychotic, lower seizure threshold). Elderly patients and those with renal impairment.

Carbamazepine has been shown to decrease the combined plasma concentration of risperidone and 9-hydroxyrisperidone. A similar effect might be anticipated with other drugs which stimulate metabolising enzymes in the liver. On initiation of **carbamazepine** or other hepatic enzyme-inducing drugs, the dosage of risperidone should be re-evaluated and increased if necessary. Conversely, on discontinuation of such drugs, the dosage of risperidone should be re-evaluated and decreased if necessary.

Phenothiazines, tricyclic antidepressants and some beta-blockers may increase the plasma concentrations of risperidone but not the combined concentration of risperidone and its active metabolite. **Fluoxetine** may increase the plasma concentration of risperidone but the impact on the combined concentration is less. A dose reduction of risperidone should be considered when **fluoxetine** is added to risperidone therapy. Based on *in vitro* studies, the same interaction may occur with **haloperidol**.

Undesirable effects

For full list, see manufacturer's SPC.

Common: insomnia, agitation, anxiety, headache, movement disorders (see below).

Less common: drowsiness, fatigue, dizziness, impaired concentration, blurred vision, dyspepsia, nausea and vomiting, constipation, sexual dysfunction (including priapism and erectile dysfunction), urinary incontinence, rhinitis.

The incidence and severity of drug-induced movement disorders are significantly less than with **haloperidol**.[12–14] Acute disorders are generally mild and are reversible if the dose is reduced and/or an antimuscarinic antiparkinsonian drug prescribed.

Dose and use

Psychosis

An atypical antipsychotic should be used preferentially in chronic psychoses:

- normal starting dose 1mg b.d.
- increase to 2mg b.d. and 3mg b.d. on successive days
- in elderly patients or with renal impairment, the starting dose should be halved to 500microgram b.d. (or 1mg o.d.) and titration extended over 6 days.[15]

Delirium

- begin with 500microgram b.d. & p.r.n.
- increase if necessary by 500microgram b.d. every other day
- median maintenance dose is 1mg/day
- uncommon to need >3mg/day.[11]

Dementia

In dementia, a dose of 1mg o.d. is generally adequate.[16] The manufacturer also recommends a lower starting dose if there is hepatic impairment, although in a single-dose study plasma concentrations were not affected.[10] Despite being commonly given b.d. there is no advantage in dividing the daily dose, which can conveniently be given at bedtime.[17] Doses above 10mg/day generally do not provide added benefit and may increase the risk of drug-induced movement disorders.

Supply

Risperdal® (Janssen-Cilag 01494 567567)

Tablets 500microgram, 1mg, 2mg, 3mg, 4mg, 6mg, 28 days @ 500microgram b.d. = £21.48.

Oral solution 1mg/1ml (with dosing pipette), 28 days @ 500microgram b.d. = £18.20.

1 Zaudig M (2000) A risk-benefit assessment of risperidone for the treatment of behavioural and psychological symptoms in dementia. *Drug Safety.* **23**: 183–195.

2 Green B (2000) Focus on risperidone. *Current Medical Research and Opinion.* **16**: 57–65.

3 Tooley P and Zuiderwijk P (1997) Drug safety: experience with risperidone. *Advances in Therapy.* **14**: 262–266.

4 Wirshing D *et al.* (1999) Risperidone in treatment-refractory schizophrenia. *American Journal of Psychiatry.* **156**: 1374–1379.

5 Guille C *et al.* (2000) A naturalistic comparison of clozapine, risperidone and olanzapine in the treatment of bipolar disorder. *Journal of Clinical Psychiatry.* **61**: 638–642.

6 Couinard G (1993) A Canadian multicenter placebo-controlled study of fixed doses of risperidone and haloperidol in the treatment of chronic schizophrenic patients. *Journal of Clinical Psychopharmacology.* **13**: 25–40.

7 Rabinowitz J *et al.* (2001) Rapid onset of therapeutic effect of risperidone versus haloperidol in a double-blind randomized trial. *Journal of Clinical Psychiatry.* **62**: 343–346.

8 Csernanksy JG *et al.* (2002) A comparison of risperidone and haloperidol for the prevention of relapse in patients with schizophrenia. *New England Journal of Medicine.* **346**: 16–22.

9 Bork J *et al.* (1999) A pilot study on risperidone metabolism: the role of cytochromes P450 2D6 and 3A. *Journal of Clinical Psychiatry.* **60**: 469–476.

10 Snoecke E *et al.* (1995) Influence of age, renal and liver impairment on the pharmacokinetics of risperidone in man. *Psychopharmacology (Berl).* **122**: 223–229.

11 Sipahimalani A *et al.* (1997) Treatment of delirium with risperidone. *International Journal of Geriatric Psychopharmacology.* **1**: 24–26.

12 Umbricht D and Kane J (1995) Risperidone: efficacy and safety. *Schizophrenia Bulletin.* **21**: 593–606.

13 Jeste D *et al.* (1999) Lower incidence of tardive dyskinesia with risperidone compared with haloperidol in older patients. *Journal of the American Geriatric Society.* **47**: 716–719.

14 Geddes J *et al.* (2000) Atypical antipsychotics in the treatment of schizophrenia: systematic overview and meta-regression analysis. *British Medical Journal.* **321**: 1371–1376.

15 Luchins D *et al.* (1998) Alteration in the recommended dosing schedule for risperidone. *American Journal of Psychiatry.* **155**: 365–366.

16 Bhana N and Spencer C (2000) Risperidone: a review of its use in the management of the behavioural and psychological symptoms of dementia. *Drugs Aging.* **16**: 451–471.

17 Nair N (1998) Therapeutic equivalence of risperidone given once daily and twice daily in patients with schizophrenia. The Risperidone Study. *Journal of Clinical Psychopharmacology.* **18**: 10–110.

ANTIDEPRESSANTS BNF 4.3

The range of antidepressants has increased considerably in recent years (Box 4.C). Choice is dictated partly by cost, availability and fashion but also by a desire to keep undesirable effects to a minimum. Thus, although **amitriptyline** is cheap and widely available with equal or better efficacy than other antidepressants,[1,2] it causes more undesirable effects.[3] As a result, **amitriptyline** is now seldom used as the first-line antidepressant in the UK. However, undesirable effects may still be troublesome with other antidepressants; for example, nausea and anxiety are common reasons for discontinuing an SSRI.[4] For patients with epilepsy, an SSRI or **venlafaxine** are good choices because they are less likely to cause seizures.[5]

Antidepressants which inhibit presynaptic serotonin re-uptake, particularly SSRIs, **clomipramine**, **amitriptyline**, **venlafaxine**, decrease serotonin uptake from the blood by platelets. Because platelets do not synthesise serotonin, the amount of serotonin in platelets is reduced.[6] This may have an adverse effect on platelet aggregation.[7] Serotonin re-uptake inhibitors have been shown to increase the risk of gastro-intestinal bleeding in the elderly, even after confounding factors have been controlled for.[8] For patients with a history of active peptic ulcer disease, bleeding rates in octogenarians increased by about 1/3 (number needed to harm = 85).[8] Awareness that serotonin re-uptake inhibitors are an additional risk factor is important in high-risk patients.

Box 4.C Classification of antidepressants according to principal actions

Enzyme inhibitors (mono-amine oxidase inhibitors, MAOIs)
Phenelzine, moclobemide (reversible inhibitor of mono-oxidase, RIMA)

Re-uptake inhibitors (mono-amine *re-uptake* inhibitors, MARIs)
Serotonin and noradrenaline (norepinephrine)
Amitriptyline, imipramine, dosulepin (dothiepin), venlafaxine
Serotonin (selective serotonin re-uptake inhibitors, SSRIs)
Fluoxetine, paroxetine, sertraline, citalopram
Noradrenaline (norepinephrine)
Desipramine[a], lofepramine[a], maprotiline, reboxetine

Receptor antagonists[b]
Trazodone (α_1, $5HT_2$)
Nefazodone ($5HT_2$); also a MARI
Mirtazapine (central α_2, $5HT_2$, $5HT_3$)[c]

a. also has a clinically unimportant effect on serotonin re-uptake
b. antagonism of $5HT_2$- and $5HT_3$-receptors facilitates increased $5HT_{1a}$ binding; this enhances the antidepressant effect
c. mirtazapine is described as a noradrenergic and specific serotoninergic antidepressant (NaSSA).

Each palliative care service needs to choose its own preferred antidepressants and become familiar with their use (Box 4.D). Antidepressants take time to work, particularly when slow dose escalation is necessary. With the older antidepressants, the *median* response time for depression in older patients is 2–3 months.[9] However, **mirtazapine** and **venlafaxine** are faster-acting.[10,11] The British Association for Psychopharmacology have produced evidence-based guidelines for the treatment of depression.[12]

Prescribing more than one antidepressant at the same time is *not* recommended. Compound preparations of an antidepressant and an anxiolytic are also *not* recommended because the dose of the individual components cannot be adjusted separately. Further, whereas antidepressants are generally given continuously over several months, anxiolytics are prescribed on a short-term basis. Although anxiety is often present in depressive illness and may be the presenting symptom, the use of antipsychotics or anxiolytics (benzodiazepines) may mask the true diagnosis. They should therefore be used with caution, although they are useful adjuncts in agitated depression. Maintenance treatment helps to prevent a recurrence of depression and is recommended for patients who have had $\geqslant$3 depressive episodes in the preceding 5 years.[13]

Tricyclic antidepressants
Tricyclic drugs have a range of actions, including:
- blockade of re-uptake by presynaptic terminals of
  - serotonin (5-hydroxytryptamine, 5HT) } responsible for antidepressant
  - noradrenaline (norepinephrine) } and analgesic effects
- receptor blockade
  - muscarinic, responsible for benefit in urgency and bladder spasms
  - H_1-histaminergic, responsible for sedation } tend to be
  - α_1-adrenergic, responsible for postural hypotension } correlated.

Sedative effects are more common in physically ill patients, particularly if receiving other psychoactive drugs, including opioids. Tricyclic antidepressants are also used for pain relief (particularly neuropathic pain) and for bladder spasms. A meta-analysis concluded that mixed serotonin and noradrenaline (norepinephrine) re-uptake inhibitors are more effective analgesics than placebo.[14]

Box 4.D Preferred antidepressants at Sir Michael Sobell House

If there is no response after 4 weeks, consider changing from TCA → SSRI or vice versa, or switch to a second-line antidepressant.

First-line antidepressants
Tricyclic antidepressant (TCA)
Amitriptyline (mixed noradrenaline and serotonin re-uptake inhibitor)

- universally available and minimal cost
- 10–25mg o.n. initially, increasing to 25–50mg o.n.
- if no benefit after 2 weeks, increase to 75–150mg o.n. in steps
- dose escalation often limited by undesirable effects, e.g. dry mouth and sedation.

Selective serotonin re-uptake inhibitor (SSRI)
Sertraline

- no antimuscarinic effects; may cause an initial increase in anxiety; low likelihood of a withdrawal (discontinuation) syndrome
- usual dose 50mg o.m., preferably after food
- occasionally necessary to increase the dose to 100–200mg o.m.

Second-line antidepressants
Venlafaxine (mixed noradrenaline and serotonin re-uptake inhibitor)

- a good choice for patients with psychomotor retardation
- 37.5mg b.d., increasing to 75mg b.d. after 2 weeks if necessary
- can use m/r preparations, i.e. 75mg or 150mg capsules o.m.
- fewer undesirable effects than amitriptyline but much more expensive.

Mirtazapine (noradrenergic and specific serotoninergic antidepressant, NaSSA)

- a good choice for patients with marked anxiety/agitation
- is not a mono-amine re-uptake inhibitor; acts on receptors
- 15mg o.n. initially, increasing to 30mg o.n.
- concurrent H_1-receptor antagonism leads to sedation *but this may decrease with higher dose because of noradrenergic effects*
- fewer undesirable effects than amitriptyline but much more expensive.

Selective serotonin re-uptake inhibitors (SSRIs)
SSRIs selectively block the presynaptic re-uptake of serotonin.[15,16] Compared with tricyclic antidepressants, SSRIs are unlikely to cause weight gain, sedation, delirium, cardiac arrhythmias and heart block. Apart from **paroxetine**, SSRIs do not have antimuscarinic effects but may cause extrapyramidal effects (see Drug-induced movement disorders, p.339). SSRIs often initially cause nausea as a consequence of increased serotonin activity in the gastro-intestinal tract and possibly via central $5HT_3$-receptors. $5HT_3$-receptor antagonists are effective anti-emetics in this situation,[17] as is **cisapride**, a $5HT_4$-receptor agonist.[18] Some SSRIs significantly inhibit the hepatic cytochrome P450 enzyme system, e.g. **fluvoxamine** (CYP1A2) and **paroxetine** (CYP2D6).[19]

The efficacy of SSRIs in neuropathic pain relief is not completely clear.[20] In randomised controlled trials in diabetic neuropathy and postherpetic neuralgia, **fluoxetine** and **zimelidine** were no better than placebo.[21–23] On the other hand, **paroxetine** and **sertraline** have been shown to relieve diabetic neuropathic pain.[24,25] Relief correlates with plasma drug concentrations; a **paroxetine** plasma concentration above 150nmol provides relief similar to that obtained with **imipramine** and with fewer undesirable effects.[24] **Paroxetine** is of value in some patients with pruritus.[26]

Mono-amine oxidase inhibitors (MAOIs)
There is little place for MAOIs in palliative care. In certain circumstances, excessive noradrenaline (norepinephrine) or excessive serotonin can cumulate and give rise to either a hypertensive crisis (associated with headache and potentially fatal intracranial haemorrhage) or the serotonin

syndrome (see Box 4.F, p.89). The hypertensive crisis ('noradrenergic syndrome') is associated with the consumption of tyramine-containing foods (Table 4.7) or drug interactions with indirect-acting sympathomimetic amine drugs, e.g. **ephedrine**, **pseudoephedrine**, **dexamfetamine**, tricyclic antidepressants, SSRIs. Hypertensive crises have also occurred when an MAOI and **pethidine** have been given concurrently, but not with other opioids (Box 4.E).[27–29]

Table 4.7 Tyramine-containing foods associated with MAOI-related syndrome

Alcohol	Meat (smoked or pickled)
red wine (white wine is safe)	Meat or yeast extracts
beer	Bovril
Broad bean pods	Oxo
Cheese (old)	Marmite
Fava beans	Pickled herring

Box 4.E A misleading report about morphine and MAOIs[27]

A patient who regularly took a MAOI and trifluoperazine 20mg daily was given pre-operative promethazine 50mg IM and morphine 1mg IV followed by two doses of morphine 2.5mg IV. About 3min later she became unresponsive and hypotensive (systolic pressure 40mmHg); responding within 2min to IV naloxone. Although repeatedly referenced as such, this was *not* a MAOI-related serotonin syndrome, it was a hypotensive response to IV morphine in someone chronically taking trifluoperazine, an α-adrenergic antagonist.

St. John's wort

St. John's wort (hypericum extract) is a popular OTC antidepressant. It is as effective as **imipramine** and **amitriptyline** in treating mild-to-moderate depression and causes fewer undesirable effects.[30–34] However, if OTC hypericum is combined with prescription antidepressants, there is a risk of developing a central serotonin syndrome (see Cautions).[35,36]

Cautions

CSM advice (hyponatraemia). Hyponatraemia (usually in the elderly and possibly due to inappropriate secretion of antidiuretic hormone) has been associated with all types of antidepressants and should be considered in all patients who develop drowsiness, confusion or seizures while taking an antidepressant.

Serotonin syndrome is a potential hazard with most antidepressants (Box 4.F). **Mirtazapine** appears to be safe in this respect; indeed, it has been used successfully to treat serotonin syndrome.[37]

Box 4.F Serotonin syndrome[38,39]

Highest risk	Significant risk	Dubious association
MAOI +	SSRI +	Carbamazepine
dextromethorphan	dextromethorphan	Fentanyl
levodopa	lithium	
lithium	moclobemide	
pethidine	pentazocine	
SSRI	tramadol	
tricyclic	trazodone	
tryptophan	tryptophan	
	Buspirone (5HT agonist)	
	Bromocriptine	
	'Ecstasy' (methylene dioxymethamfetamine)	

Can also be caused by a single drug,[40] or in overdose.[41]

Clinical features

Restlessness, agitation, delirium, tachycardia, myoclonus, hyperreflexia, tremor, shivering and hyperthermia (>40.5°C). Hyperthermia is a bad prognostic sign. Onset generally within a few hours of drug/dose changes and most resolve in 24h. Recurrent mild symptoms may occur for weeks before a full-blown syndrome. Hypertension (and headache), convulsions and death have been reported.

Clinical features overlap with those of neuroleptic (antipsychotic) malignant syndrome (see p.342), suggesting a common pathophysiology.[42]

Treatment

Discontinue serotoninergic medication.

Symptomatic measures (based on animal studies and clinical reports):

- paracetamol as an antipyretic
- external cooling if hyperthermia
- propranolol 20mg q8h[43] *or* } have antiserotonin properties
- cyproheptadine 4–8mg PO q2h–q4h p.r.n. }
- midazolam 5–10mg SC p.r.n. for myoclonus and convulsions
- mirtazapine 15–30mg PO o.d.[37]

Undesirable effects

These vary from antidepressant to antidepressant (see individual drug monographs). A synopsis is contained in Table 4.8.

Stopping antidepressants

Abrupt cessation of antidepressant therapy (particularly a MAOI) after regular administration for ⩾8 weeks may result in withdrawal phenomena.[44] Discontinuation reactions are distinct from recurrence of the primary psychiatric disorder. They generally start abruptly within a few days of stopping the antidepressant (or of reducing its dose) and may last up to 3 weeks. In contrast, a depressive relapse is uncommon in the first week after stopping an antidepressant, and symptoms tend to build up gradually and persist. Discontinuation symptoms are varied and differ depending on the class of antidepressant. Common symptoms include:

- gastro-intestinal disturbance (nausea, abdominal pain, diarrhoea)
- sleep disturbance (insomnia, vivid dreams, nightmares)
- general somatic distress (sweating, lethargy, headaches)
- affective symptoms (low mood, anxiety, irritability).

Table 4.8 Undesirable effects of antidepressant drugs[12]

Drug	*Action*	*Anti-muscarinic*	*Sedation*	*Insomnia/ agitation*	*Postural hypotension*	*Nausea/ gastro-intestinal*	*Sexual dysfunction*	*Weight gain*	*Specific effects*	*Inhibition of hepatic enzymes*	*Lethality in overdose*
Tricyclic antidepressants											
Amitriptyline, dosulepin[a]	NRI > SRI	++	++	–	++	–	+	++		++	High
Clomipramine	SRI + NRI	++	++	+	++	+	++	+		++	Moderate
Imipramine	NRI > SRI	++	+	+	++	–	+	+		++	High
Desipramine, nortriptyline	NRI	+	+	+	+	–	+	–		++	High
Lofepramine	NRI	+	–	+	+	–	?	–		+	Low
SSRIs											
Citalopram, sertraline	SRI	–	–	+	–	++	++	–	Initial nausea and vomiting	–	Low
Fluoxetine, fluvoxamine	SRI	–	–	+	–	++	++	–	Serotonin syndrome (see Box 4.F)	++	Low
Paroxetine	SRI	+	–	+	–	++	++	–		++	Low
Other re-uptake inhibitors											
Maprotiline	NRI	++	++	–	–	–	+	++	Increased seizure potential	?	High
Venlafaxine	SRI > NRI	–	–	+	–	++	++	–	Hypertension	–	Low
Reboxetine	NRI	+	–	–	–	–	+	–		–	Low

continued

Table 4.8 Continued

Drug	*Action*	*Anti-muscarinic*	*Sedation*	*Insomnia/ agitation*	*Postural hypotension*	*Nausea/ gastro-intestinal*	*Sexual dysfunction*	*Weight gain*	*Specific effects*	*Inhibition of hepatic enzymes*	*Lethality in overdose*
Receptor antagonists											
Trazodone	5-HT_2 + α_1>SRI	–	++	–	++	–	–	+	Priapism	?	Low
Nefazodone	5-HT_2 > SRI	+	+	–	+	+	–	++		++	Low
Mianserin	5-HT_2 + α_1 + α_2	+	++	–	–	–	–	–	Blood dyscrasia	?	Low
Mirtazapine	5-HT_2 + 5-HT_3 + α_2	–	++	–	–	–	–	++		–	Low
MAOIs											
Phenelzine, tranylcypromine, isocarboxazid	Irreversible	+	+	++	++	+	++	++	Hypertensive crisis with sympathomimetics Serotonin syndrome (see Box 4.F)	?	High
Moclobemide	RIMA	–	–	+	–	+	–	–		–	Low

a. dothiepin.
Abbreviations: NRI = noradrenaline (norepinephrine) re-uptake inhibitor; SRI = serotonin re-uptake inhibitor; 5-HT_2 = 5-HT_2 antagonist; 5-HT_3 = 5-HT_3 antagonists; α_1/α_2 = α_1-adrenergic antagonist/α_2 antagonist; RIMA = reversible inhibitor of monoamine oxidase-A; ++ = relatively common or strong; + = may occur or moderately strong; – = absent or rare/weak; ? = unknown/insufficient information.

With SSRIs (e.g. **sertraline**) the commonest symptoms appear to be dizziness/lightheadedness and sensory abnormalities (including numbness, paraesthesia, and electric shock-like sensations). Discontinuation reactions usually resolve within 24h of re-instating antidepressant therapy, whereas with a depressive relapse the response is slower.

To reduce the likelihood of discontinuation reactions the BNF recommends that antidepressants which have been continuously prescribed for ⩾8 weeks should be gradually reduced over 4 weeks. Tapering is probably unnecessary when switching between SSRIs. If a discontinuation reaction is suspected, the antidepressant should be restarted and reduced more gradually. If mild, however, re-assurance alone may be adequate ± a benzodiazepine to overcome insomnia.

1 Barbui C and Hotopf M (2001) Amitriptyline v. the rest: still the leading antidepressant after 40 years of randomised controlled trials. *British Journal of Psychiatry.* **178**: 129–144.
2 Thompson C (2001) Amitriptyline: still efficacious, but at what cost? *British Journal of Psychiatry.* **178**: 99–100.
3 Martin R *et al.* (1997) General practitioner's perception of the tolerability of antidepressant drugs: a comparison of selective serotonin reuptake inhibitors and tricyclic antidepressants. *British Medical Journal.* **314**: 646–651.
4 Trindade E *et al.* (1998) Adverse effects associated with selective reuptake inhibitors and tricyclic antidepressants: a meta-analysis. *Canadian Medical Association Journal.* **17**: 1245–1252.
5 Curran S and dePauw K (1998) Selecting an antidepressant for use in a patient with epilepsy. Safety considerations. *Drug Safety.* **18**: 125–133.
6 Ross S *et al.* (1980) Inhibition of 5-hydroxytryptamine uptake in human platelets by antidepressant agents in vivo. *Psychopharmacology.* **67**: 1–7.
7 Li N *et al.* (1997) Effects of serotonin on platelet activation in whole blood. *Blood Coagulation Fibrinolysis.* **8**: 517–523.
8 vanWalraven C *et al.* (2001) Inhibition of serotonin reuptake by antidepressants and upper gastrointestinal bleeding in elderly patients: retrospective cohort study. *British Medical Journal.* **323**: 655–657.
9 Reynolds C *et al.* (1998) Effects of age at onset of first lifetime episode of recurrent major depression on treatment response and illness course in elderly patients. *American Journal of Psychiatry.* **155**: 795–799.
10 Burrows G and Kremer C (1997) Mirtazapine: clinical advantages in the treatment of depression. *Journal of Clinical Psychopharmacology.* **1**: 34–39.
11 Thase M *et al.* (2001) Remission rates during treatment with venlafaxine or selective serotonin reuptake inhibitors. *British Journal of Psychiatry.* **178**: 234–241.
12 Anderson I *et al.* (2000) Evidence-based guidelines for treating depressive disorders with antidepressants: a revision of the 1993 British Association for psychopharmacology guidelines. *Journal of Pyschopharmacology.* **14**: 3–20.
13 Edwards J (1998) Long term pharmacotherapy of depression. *British Medical Journal.* **316**: 1180–1181.
14 Onghena P and Houdenhove BV (1992) Antidepressant-induced analgesia in chronic nonmalignant pain: a meta-analysis of 39 placebo-controlled trials. *Pain.* **49**: 205–219.
15 Finley P (1994) Selective serotonin reuptake inhibitors: pharmacologic profiles and potential therapeutic distinctions. *Annals of Pharmacotherapy.* **28**: 1359–1369.
16 Edwards G and Anderson I (1999) Systematic review and guide to selection of selective serotonin reuptake inhibitors. *Drugs.* **57**: 507–533.
17 Bailey J *et al.* (1995) The 5HT3 antagonist ondansetron reduces gastrointestinal side effects induced by a specific serotonin re-uptake inhibitor in man. *Journal of Psychopharmacology.* **9**: 137–141.
18 Bergeron R and Blier P (1994) Cisapride for the treatment of nausea produced by selective serotonin reuptake inhibitors. *American Journal of Psychiatry.* **151**: 1084–1086.
19 Richelson E (1997) Pharmacokinetic drug interactions of new antidepressants: A review of the effects on the metabolism of other drugs. *Mayo Clinic Proceedings.* **72**: 835–847.
20 Ansari A (2000) The efficacy of newer antidepressants in the treatment of chronic pain: a review of current literature. *Harvard Review Psychiatry.* **7**: 257–277.
21 Max M *et al.* (1992) Effects of desipramine, amitriptyline, and fluoxetine on pain in diabetic neuropathy. *New England Journal of Medicine.* **326**: 1287–1288.

22 Watson C and Evans R (1985) A comparative trial of amitriptyline and zimelidine in postherpetic neuralgia. *Pain*. **23**: 387–394.
23 Lynch S *et al.* (1990) Efficacy of antidepressants in relieving diabetic neuropathy pain: amitriptyline vs. desipramine and fluoxetine vs. placebo. *Neurology*. **40**: 437.
24 Sindrup S *et al.* (1990) The selective serotonin re-uptake inhibitor paroxetine is effective in the treatment of diabetic neuropathy symptoms. *Pain*. **42**: 135–144.
25 Goodnick P *et al.* (1997) Sertraline in diabetic neuropathy: preliminary results. *Annals of Clinical Psychiatry*. **9**: 255–257.
26 Zylicz Z *et al.* (1998) Paroxetine for pruritus in advanced cancer. *Journal of Pain and Symptom Management*. **16**: 121–124.
27 Barry B (1979) Adverse effects of MAO inhibitors with narcotics reversed with naloxone. *Anaesthesia and Intensive Care*. **7**: 194.
28 Browne B and Linter S (1987) Monoamine oxidase inhibitors and narcotic analgesics. A critical review of the implications for treatment. *British Journal of Psychiatry*. **151**: 210–212.
29 Stockley I (1994) Monamine oxidase inhibitors + morphine or methadone. In: I Stockley (ed) *Drug Interactions* (3e). Blackwell Scientific, Oxford, pp.642–644.
30 Vorbach E *et al.* (1997) Efficacy and tolerability of St John's wort extract LI160 versus imipramine in patients with severe depressive episodes according to ICD10. *Pharmacopsychiatry*. **30**: 81–85.
31 Wheatley D (1997) LI160, an extract of St John's wort versus amitriptyline in mildly to moderately depressed outpatients – a controlled 6-week clinical trial. *Pharmacopsychiatry*. **30**: 77–80.
32 Gaster B and Holroyd J (2000) St John's wort for depression: a systematic review. *Archives of Internal Medicine*. **160**: 152–156.
33 Woelk H (2000) Comparison of St John's wort and imipramine for treating depression: randomised controlled trial. *British Medical Journal*. **321**: 536–539.
34 Linde K and Mulrow C (2001) St. John's wort for depression (Cochrane Review). In: *Cochrane Library*, Oxford.
35 Lantz M *et al.* (1999) St John's wort and antidepressant drug interactions in the elderly. *Journal of Geriatric Psychiatry and Neurology*. **12**: 7–10.
36 Anonymous (2000) St. John's wort (Hypericum perforatum) interactions. *Current Problems in Pharmacovigilance*. **26**: 6–7.
37 Hoes M and Zeijpveld J (1996) Mirtazapine as treatment for serotonin syndrome. *Pharmacopsychiatry*. **29**: 81.
38 Sporer K (1995) The serotonin syndrome: Implicated drugs, pathophysiology and management. *Drug Safety*. **13**: 94–104.
39 Mir S and Taylor D (1999) Serotonin syndrome. *Psychiatric Bulletin*. **23**: 742–747.
40 Lejoyeux M *et al.* (1992) The serotonin syndrome. *American Journal of Psychiatry*. **149**: 410–1411.
41 Kaminski C *et al.* (1994) Sertraline intoxication in a child. *Annals of Emergency Medicine*. **23**: 1371–1374.
42 Kontaxakis V *et al.* (2000) Olanzapine-associated neuroleptic malignant syndrome: Is there any overlap with the serotonin syndrome? *Journal of the European College of Neuropsychopharmacology*. **10 (suppl 3)**: S313.
43 Guze B and Baxter L (1986) The serotonin syndrome: case responsive to propranolol. *Journal of Clinical Psychopharmacology*. **6**: 119–120.
44 Haddad P *et al.* (1998) Antidepressant discontinuation reactions. *British Medical Journal*. **316**: 1105–1106.

AMITRIPTYLINE BNF 4.3.1

Class: Tricyclic antidepressant.

Indications: Depression, panic disorder, nocturnal enuresis in children, †neuropathic pain, †urgency of micturition, †urge incontinence, †bladder spasms.

Contra-indications: Co-administration with an MAOI, recent myocardial infarction, arrhythmias (particularly heart block of any degree), mania, severe hepatic impairment.

Pharmacology

Amitriptyline exerts its antidepressant and analgesic effects by blocking the presynaptic re-uptake of serotonin and noradrenaline (norepinephrine). It may also act as a NMDA-receptor antagonist.[1] It has a sedative effect and this manifests immediately; improved sleep is the first benefit of therapy. The analgesic effect may manifest after 3–7 days, whereas the antidepressant effect may not be apparent for 2 weeks or more. A dose-response relationship has been shown for its analgesic effect.[2,3] There appears to be a 'therapeutic window' for amitriptyline in some patients.[4] Patients with postherpetic neuralgia or painful diabetic neuropathy had good relief with amitriptyline 20–100mg (median 50mg). With this dose the pain was reduced from severe to mild. When the dose was increased, the pain became severe again and, when decreased, the pain became mild again. However, most patients do not manifest this effect. Amitriptyline frequently causes increased appetite and weight gain – a bonus in palliative care but often an undesirable effect for others. Some 20% of patients fail to respond to amitriptyline (or related antidepressant drug); some of the failures relate to the dose being inadequate. However, because of the potential for undesirable effects, low doses should be used initially in the frail elderly.

Bio-availability no data.

Onset of action up to 30 days for depression.

Time to peak plasma concentration 4h PO; 24–48h IM.

Plasma halflife 9–25h; active metabolite nortriptyline 13–93h.

Duration of action 24h, situation dependent.

Cautions

Elderly, cardiac disease (particularly if history of arrhythmia), epilepsy, hepatic impairment, history of mania, psychoses (may aggravate), closed-angle glaucoma, urinary hesitancy, history of urinary retention. Drowsiness may affect performance of skilled tasks, e.g. driving; effects of alcohol enhanced. Avoid abrupt withdrawal after prolonged use. Also see Stopping antidepressants, p.89 and Cytochrome P450, p.331.

Undesirable effects

For full list, see manufacturer's SPC.

Antimuscarinic effects, sedation, delirium, postural hypotension, hyponatraemia. The use of amitriptyline in the elderly is associated with a doubling of the incidence of femoral fractures.[5]

Dose and use

Amitriptyline, like other tricyclic drugs, can be given as a single dose o.n. for all indications. If a patient experiences early morning drowsiness, or takes a long time settling at night, advise to take 2h before bedtime. A small number of patients are stimulated by amitriptyline and experience insomnia, unpleasant vivid dreams, myoclonus and physical restlessness. In these patients, change to a SSRI or administer amitriptyline o.m. Relatively small doses are often effective in relieving depression in debilitated cancer patients, e.g. amitriptyline 25–50mg o.n.; start with a small dose in the frail elderly (Table 4.9).

Supply

Amitriptyline (non-proprietary)

Tablets 10mg, 25mg, 50mg, 28 days @ 50mg o.n. = £1.20.

Oral solution 25mg and 50mg/5ml, 28 days @ 50mg o.n. = £9.45.

Table 4.9 Dose escalation timetables for amitriptyline

Dose (o.n.)	*Elderly frail/outpatient*	*Younger patient/inpatient*
10mg	Day 1	–
25mg	Day 3	Day 1
50mg	Week 2	Day 3
75mg	Week 3–4	Week 2
100mg	Week 5–6	Week 2
150mg	Week 7–8[a]	Week 3[a]

a. not often necessary in palliative care.

Injection 10mg/ml, 10ml vial = £6.40. (Unlicensed, available as a named patient supply from IDIS 020 8410 0800; see Special orders and named patient supplies, p.349)

1 Eisenach J and Gebhart G (1995) Intrathecal amitriptyline acts as an N-Methyl-D-Aspartate receptor antagonist in the presence of inflammatory hyperalgesia in rats. *Anesthesiology.* **83**: 1046.
2 Max M *et al.* (1987) Amitriptyline relieves diabetic neuropathy pain in patients with normal or depressed mood. *Neurology (Ny).* **37**: 589–596.
3 McQuay HJ *et al.* (1993) Dose-response for analgesic effect of amitriptyline in chronic pain. *Anaesthesia.* **48**: 281–285.
4 Watson C (1984) Therapeutic window for amitriptyline analgesia. *Canadian Medical Association Journal.* **130**: 105–106.
5 Ray WA *et al.* (1987) Psychotropic drug use and the risk of hip fracture. *New England Journal of Medicine.* **316**: 363–369.

MIRTAZAPINE — BNF 4.3.4

Class: Antidepressant.

Indications: Depression, †neuropathic pain, †intractable itch, †serotonin syndrome.

Contra-indications: Should not be given with an MAOI or within 2 weeks of its cessation.

Pharmacology

Mirtazapine is a noradrenergic and specific serotoninergic antidepressant (NaSSA).[1–3] It is a centrally active presynaptic α_2-adrenergic antagonist, which increases central noradrenergic and serotoninergic neurotransmission.[4] The enhancement of serotoninergic neurotransmission is specifically mediated via 5-HT_1-receptors; 5-HT_2- and 5HT_3-receptors are blocked by mirtazapine. Thus, unlike SSRIs, mirtazapine is not associated with nausea and vomiting. Both enantiomers of mirtazapine are presumed to contribute to the antidepressant activity, the S(+) enantiomer by blocking α_2 and 5-HT_2 receptors and the R(–) enantiomer by blocking 5-HT_3 receptors. The histamine H_1-antagonistic activity of mirtazapine is responsible for its sedative properties. At lower doses, the antihistaminic effect of mirtazapine predominates, producing sedation. Mirtazapine 15mg o.n. is equivalent to 15mg of **diazepam** in terms of reducing anxiety.[1] With higher doses, sedation is reduced as noradrenergic neural transmission increases. Mirtazapine is generally well tolerated. It has no significant antimuscarinic activity. Mirtazapine is an effective antidepressant with a response rate of nearly 70%.[5,6] The antidepressant effects of mirtazapine are equivalent to **amitriptyline**, **fluoxetine**, **clomipramine** and **doxepin**[3] with a rapid onset of action, sometimes in less than a week.[7] There are fewer relapses compared to **amitriptyline**. A combination of mirtazapine and an SSRI are often effective in the treatment of refractory depression.[8] Mirtazapine is not associated with cardiovascular toxicity or sexual dysfunction.[9] A blockade of $5HT_2$ and $5HT_3$ leads to appetite stimulation and reduced nausea.[10] Some centres use mirtazapine for neuropathic pain,[11,12] and for intractable itch.[13] There is an isolated report on its use in serotonin syndrome.[14]

Mirtazapine displays linear pharmacokinetics within the recommended dose range. Food does not effect absorption. Steady state is reached after 3–4 days of o.d. administration. Binding to plasma proteins is about 85%. Mirtazapine is extensively metabolised and eliminated via the urine and faeces. Major pathways of biotransformation are demethylation and oxidation, followed by conjugation. Cytochrome P450 enzymes CYP2D6 and CYP1A2 are involved in the formation of the 8-hydroxy metabolite of mirtazapine, whereas CYP3A4 is considered to be responsible for the formation of the N-demethyl and N-oxide metabolites (see p.331). The demethyl metabolite is pharmacologically active and appears to have the same pharmacokinetic profile as the parent compound. Overdoses produce disorientation, drowsiness, memory impairment and tachycardia, but there have been no deaths with mirtazapine as a single agent. Mirtazapine has additive undesirable effects on cognition and motor performance when taken with alcohol or **diazepam**.

Bio-availability 50% PO.
Onset of action hours-to-days (unlicensed indications); 1–2 weeks (antidepressant).
Time to peak plasma concentration 2h.
Plasma halflife 20–40h; often shorter in men (26h) than women (37h) but can extend up to 65h.
Duration of action variable; up to several days.

Cautions

Hepatic or renal impairment. Can transform the depressive phase of bipolar disorder (manic depressive psychosis) into the manic phase. May accentuate the effect of alcohol and of benzodiazepines. Despite the caution in the manufacturer's SPC concerning its use in patients with epilepsy and organic brain syndrome, mirtazapine probably does not have pro-epileptic properties unlike **amitriptyline** and SSRIs.[15]

Undesirable effects

For full list, see manufacturer's SPC.
Very common (>10%): increase in appetite and weight gain;[3,16] drowsiness during the first few weeks of treatment. *Dose reduction generally does not lead to less sedation but can jeopardise antidepressant efficacy.*
Uncommon (<1%): hepatic impairment.

Dose and use

Depression

- starting dose 15mg o.n. and increase if necessary after 2 weeks
- the effective daily dose is generally 15–45mg[1,6]
- the recommended dose is the same in the elderly.

Treatment with an adequate dose should result in a positive response within 2–4 weeks. If there is no response with 45mg after 4 weeks, an alternative antidepressant should be prescribed instead. If effective, treatment should be continued until the patient has been symptom-free for 4–6 months. After this, treatment can be gradually discontinued.

Neuropathic pain and intractable itch
Use as for depression; continue indefinitely.[11–13]

Supply

Zispin® (Organon 01223 432700)
Tablets 30mg, 28 days @ 30mg o.n = £22.92.

1 Puzantian T (1998) Mirtazapine, an antidepressant. *American Journal of Health-System Pharmacy*. **55**: 44–49.

2 Anonymous (1999) Mirtazapine – another new class of antidepressant. *Drug and Therapeutics Bulletin.* **37**: 1–3.
3 Kent J (2000) SnaRIs, NaSSAs and NaRIs: new agents for the treatment of depression. *Lancet.* **355**: 911–918.
4 deBoer T (1996) The pharmacologic profile of mirtazapine. *Journal of Clinical Psychiatry.* **57**: 19–25.
5 Kasper S (1995) Clinical efficacy of mirtazapine: a review of meta-analyses of pooled data. *International Clinical Research.* **10**: 25–36.
6 Bailer U *et al.* (1998) Mirtazapine in inpatient treatment of depressed patients. *Wiener Klinische Wochenschrift.* **110**: 646–650.
7 Burrows G and Kremer C (1997) Mirtazapine: clinical advantages in the treatment of depression. *Journal of Clinical Psychopharmacology.* **1**: 34–39.
8 O'Reardon J *et al.* (2000) Treatment-resistant depression in the age of serotonin: evolving strategies. *Current Opinion in Psychiatry.* **13**: 93–98.
9 Gelenberg A *et al.* (2000) Mirtazapine substitution in SSRI-induced sexual dysfunction. *Journal of Clinical Psychiatry.* **61**: 356–360.
10 Davis M *et al.* (2001) Mirtazapine: Heir apparent to amitriptyline? *American Journal of Hospice and Palliative Care.* **18 (1)**: 42–46.
11 Brannon G and Stone K (1999) The use of mirtazapine in a patient with chronic pain. *Journal of Pain and Symptom Management.* **18**: 382–385.
12 Ritzenthaler B and Pearson D (2000) Efficacy and tolerability of mirtazapine in neuropathic pain. *Palliative Medicine.* **14**: 346.
13 Krajnik M and Zylicz Z (2001) Understanding pruritus in systemic disease. *Journal of Pain and Symptom Management.* **21**: 151–168.
14 Hoes M and Zeijpveld J (1996) Mirtazapine as treatment for serotonin syndrome. *Pharmacopsychiatry.* **29**: 81.
15 Curran S and dePauw K (1998) Selecting an antidepressant for use in a patient with epilepsy. Safety considerations. *Drug Safety.* **18**: 125–133.
16 Abed R and Cooper M (1999) Mirtazapine causing hyperphagia. *British Journal of Psychiatry.* **174**: 181–182.

SERTRALINE — BNF 4.3.1

Class: SSRI.

Indications: Depression, †neuropathic pain.

Contra-indications: Concurrent administration with an MAOI, mania.

Pharmacology

Sertraline has no affinity for muscarinic, serotoninergic, dopaminergic, adrenergic, histaminergic, GABA-ergic receptors. Unlike **amitriptyline**, sertraline does not cause weight gain. A withdrawal (discontinuation) syndrome has not been reported. Sertraline exhibits dose proportional pharmacokinetics up to 200mg. Steady-state plasma concentrations are achieved after 1 week. Food does not affect the bio-availability of sertraline. The main metabolite is inactive. Metabolites are excreted equally in faeces and urine. Sertraline is as effective as **amitriptyline** in treating depression with anxiety; its antidepressant action may be enhanced by **sodium valproate**.[1] Sertraline has been shown to relieve diabetic neuropathic pain.[2]

Bio-availability >44%.
Onset of action 1–4 weeks.
Time to peak plasma concentration 4.5–8.4h.
Plasma halflife 22–36h.
Duration of action several days, situation dependent.

Cautions

Epilepsy, hepatic impairment, renal impairment. All SSRIs increase the risk of gastro-intestinal bleeding in the elderly, particularly those over 80 years of age.[3]

Sertraline (or other SSRI) should not be started until 2 weeks after stopping a MAOI. Treatment should not be discontinued abruptly (Box 4.G). Also see Stopping antidepressants, p.89 and Cytochrome P450, p.331.

Box 4.G SSRI withdrawal syndrome[5]

Somatic symptoms	**Psychological symptoms**
Disequilibrium	*Core*
Dizziness	Anxiety/agitation
Vertigo	Crying spells
Ataxia	Irritability
Gastro-intestinal symptoms	*Other*
Nausea	Overactivity
Vomiting	Decreased concentration/slowed thinking
Flu-like symptoms	Memory problems
Fatigue	Depersonalisation
Lethargy	Lowered mood
Myalgia	Delirium
Chills	
Sensory disturbance	
Paraesthesia	
Sensations of electric shock	
Sleep disturbances	
Insomnia	
Vivid dreams	

Undesirable effects

For full list, see manufacturer's SPC.

Sexual dysfunction (diminished libido and delayed orgasm).[4] Anorexia, nausea, diarrhoea, exacerbation of anxiety (initially), restlessness, headache.

Dose and use

Sertraline is easy to use because, for most patients, the starting dose does not need to be increased:

- the standard dose is 50mg o.m. preferably p.c.
- occasionally necessary to increase the dose to 100–200mg.

Supply

Lustral® (Pfizer 01304 616161)

Tablets 50mg, 100mg, 28 days @ 50mg o.m. = £16.20.

1 Dave M (1995) Antidepressant augmentation with valproate. *Depression.* **3**: 157–158.

2 Goodnick P *et al.* (1997) Sertraline in diabetic neuropathy: preliminary results. *Annals of Clinical Psychiatry.* **9**: 255–257.

3 vanWalraven C *et al.* (2001) Inhibition of serotonin reuptake by antidepressants and upper gastrointestinal bleeding in elderly patients: retrospective cohort study. *British Medical Journal.* **323**: 655–657.

4 Modell J *et al.* (1997) Comparative sexual side effects of bupropion, fluoxetine, paroxetine, and sertraline. *Clinical Pharmacology and Therapeutics.* **61**: 476–487.

5 Schatzberg A *et al.* (1997) Serotonin reuptake inhibitor discontinuation syndrome: a hypothetical definition. *Journal of Clinical Psychiatry.* **58**: 5–10.

VENLAFAXINE BNF 4.3.4

Class: Antidepressant; serotonin and noradrenaline (norepinephrine) re-uptake inhibitor (SNRI).

Indications: Depression, generalised anxiety disorder, †neuropathic pain, †hot flushes.

Contra-indications: Concurrent use with MAOI or within 2 weeks of previous treatment with MAOI.

Pharmacology

Venlafaxine is a bicyclic phenylethylamine compound which can be thought of as 'clean' **amitriptyline**. It inhibits the presynaptic re-uptake of serotonin and noradrenaline (norepinephrine), and of dopamine to a lesser extent but, unlike **amitriptyline**, it has little or no postsynaptic antagonistic effects at muscarinic, α-adrenergic or H_1-receptors.[1,2] Venlafaxine's inhibition of presynaptic serotonin re-uptake is about 3 times greater than for noradrenaline (norepinephrine) re-uptake and at least 10 times greater than for dopamine inhibition. Significant inhibition of noradrenaline (norepinephrine) re-uptake is seen in patients who receive venlafaxine >1mg/kg/24h.[3] Only at doses of ≥350mg/day does dopamine re-uptake inhibition become apparent.

As an antidepressent, venlafaxine is more effective than SSRIs.[4] Venlafaxine also has a faster onset of action, i.e. 3 weeks compared with 4 weeks for pure SSRIs. It is a good choice for patients with psychomotor retardation. It is also of benefit in the long-term treatment of generalised anxiety disorder.[5] Venlafaxine has been shown to have an antinociceptive effect in animals.[6,7] Its antinociceptive effect is said to be mainly mediated by κ- and δ-opioid receptors and α_2-adrenergic receptors. Venlafaxine has been used successfully in chronic headache,[8] fibromyalgia[9] and neuropathic pain.[10–12] However, only one large-scale randomised controlled trial has been reported.[13] In this 6-week study in patients with painful diabetic neuropathy (n = 244), m/r venlafaxine 150–225mg o.d. was significantly better than placebo. As yet no comparative studies with **amitriptyline** have been published.

Venlafaxine is also of benefit in hot flushes associated with the menopause or hormone therapy, including androgen oblation therapy for prostate cancer.[14,15] This is not a specific effect of venlafaxine; SSRIs seem to share this property, e.g. **paroxetine** and **fluoxetine**.[16,17] Venlafaxine is metabolised to a pharmacologically active metabolite, O-desmethylvenlafaxine (ODV) which has a pharmacodynamic profile similar to that of venlafaxine.

Bio-availability 13%; 45% m/r.

Onset of action ≥2 weeks for depression.

Time to peak plasma concentration about 2.5h; 4.5–7.5h m/r and 6.5–11h ODV m/r.

Plasma halflife 5h; 11h for ODV.

Duration of effect 12–24h, situation dependent.

Cautions

Patients with epilepsy (as with all antidepressants), concurrent **cimetidine** in the elderly or if hepatic impairment. Mydriasis has been reported in association with venlafaxine; patients with raised intra-ocular pressure or at risk of narrow-angle glaucoma should be monitored closely. May increase concurrent **haloperidol** plasma concentrations (up to 70% increase in AUC and a possible doubling of the maximum plasma concentration). Concurrent use with drugs which inhibit either CYP2D6 or CYP3A4 may result in higher plasma concentrations (see Cytochrome P450, p.331). The dose of **warfarin** may need to be reduced.

With doses of ≥200mg/day, it is advisable to monitor blood pressure over the first 2–3 months; increases in diastolic pressure of 4–7mmHg have been observed in some patients. In patients with hepatic or renal impairment, a lower dose may be necessary. If taken for ≥1 week, venlafaxine should not be stopped abruptly because an antidepressant withdrawal (discontinuation) syndrome may occur (see Stopping antidepressants, p.89).

Undesirable effects

For full list, see manufacturer's SPC.

Very common: dizziness, dry mouth, insomnia, nervousness, drowsiness, constipation, nausea, abnormal ejaculation/orgasm, asthenia, headache, sweating.

Common: agitated anxiety, confusion, hypertonia, paraesthesia, tremor, dyspnoea, hypertension, palpitations, postural hypotension, vasodilation, anorexia, diarrhoea, dyspepsia, vomiting, urinary

frequency, ecchymosis, decreased libido, impotence, menstrual cycle disorders, arthralgia, myalgia, weight gain/loss, abdominal pain, abnormal dreams, chills, pyrexia, pruritus, rash, abnormal vision/ accomodation, mydriasis, tinnitus.
Uncommon: hallucinations, urinary retention, muscle spasm, hyponatraemia, increased liver enzymes, angioedema, maculopapular eruptions, urticaria.

Dose and use

It is recommended that venlafaxine is taken with or after food. If moderate to severe renal impairment or moderate to severe hepatic impairment, reduce dose by 50% and give o.d.

Depression

- starting dose 37.5mg b.d.
- increase after 2 weeks to 75mg b.d. if no benefit observed
- further dose increments may be made up to 375mg/day, with gradual dose reduction when the depression has lifted.

Neuropathic pain and hot flushes

- starting dose 37.5mg b.d.
- increase to 75mg b.d. after 1 week if necessary.

Supply

Efexor® (Wyeth 01628 604377)
Tablets 37.5mg, 50mg, 75mg, 28 days @ 75mg b.d. = £39.97.

Efexor® XL (Wyeth 01628 604377)
Capsules m/r 75mg, 150mg, 28 days @ 150mg o.d. = £39.97.

1 Horst W and Preskorn S (1998) Mechanisms of action and clinical characteristics of three atypical antidepressants: venlafaxine, nefazodone, bupropion. *Journal of Affective Disorders.* **51**: 237–254.
2 Maj J and Rogoz Z (1999) Pharmacological effects of venlafaxine, a new antidepressant, given repeatedly, on the alpha 1-adrenergic, dopamine and serotonin systems. *Journal of Neural Transmission.* **106**: 197–211.
3 Melichar J *et al.* (2001) Venlafaxine occupation at the noradrenaline reuptake site: in-vivo determination in healthy volunteers. *Journal of Psychopharmacology.* **15**: 9–12.
4 Thase M *et al.* (2001) Remission rates during treatment with venlafaxine or selective serotonin reuptake inhibitors. *British Journal of Psychiatry.* **178**: 234–241.
5 Allgulander C *et al.* (2001) Venlafaxine extended release (ER) in the treatment of generalised anxiety disorder. *British Journal of Psychiatry.* **179**: 15–22.
6 Lang E *et al.* (1996) Venlafaxine hydrochloride (Effexor) relieves thermal hyperalgesia in rats with an experimental mononeuropathy. *Pain.* **68**: 151–155.
7 Schreiber S *et al.* (1999) The antinociceptive effect of venlafaxine in mice is mediated through opioid and adrenergic mechanisms. *Neuroscience Letters.* **273**: 85–88.
8 Diamond S (1995) Efficacy and safety profile of venlafaxine on chronic headache. *Headache Quarterly.* **6**: 212–214.
9 Dwight M *et al.* (1996) Venlafaxine treatment of fibromyalgia. *Psychopharmacology Bulletin.* **32**: 435.
10 Songer D and Schulte H (1996) Venlafaxine for the treatment of chronic pain. *American Journal of Psychiatry.* **153**: 737.
11 Pernia A *et al.* (2000) Venlafaxine for the treatment of neuropathic pain. *Journal of Pain and Symptom Management.* **19**: 408–410.
12 Sumpton J and Moulin D (2001) Treatment of neuropathic pain with venlafaxine. *Annals of Pharmacotherapy.* **35**: 557–559
13 Kunz N *et al.* (2000) Diabetic neuropathic pain management with venlafaxine XR. *Poster presented at the CINP, July 2000.*
14 Barlow D (2000) Venlafaxine for hot flushes. *Lancet.* **356**: 2025–2026.
15 Loprinzi C *et al.* (2000) Venlafaxine in management of hot flashes in survivors of breast cancer: a randomised controlled trial. *Lancet.* **356**: 2059–2063.
16 Stearns V *et al.* (1997) A pilot trial assessing the efficacy of paroxetine hydrochloride (Paxil) in controlling hot flushes. *Breast Cancer Research Treatment.* **46**: 23–33.
17 Loprinzi C *et al.* (1999) Preliminary data from a randomized evaluation of fluoxetine (Prozac) for treating hot flushes in breast cancer survivors. *Breast Cancer Research Treatment.* **57**: 34.

PSYCHOSTIMULANTS — BNF 4.4

Psychostimulants increase alertness and motivation, and have antidepressant and mood-elevating properties.[1] Psychostimulants include **cocaine, dexamfetamine** (dextro-amfetamine), **methylphenidate** and **modafinil**. Of these, **methylphenidate** is the most used in palliative care. In the USA, a consensus panel concluded that a psychostimulant is the drug of choice for treating depression in patients with a prognosis of less than 3 months.[2] It is often possible to achieve a response in a few days, increasing the dose steadily until a response or toxicity occurs.[2] Psychostimulants are particularly useful in medically ill patients including patients with brain tumours, and they have been used to treat depression in HIV+ patients.[3–5] They are not as effective as conventional antidepressants in primary depressive illness,[6] and these should be used in patients with a projected lifespan of 3–6 months or more.

Psychostimulants can reduce opioid-related drowsiness, improve psychomotor performance and allow opioid dose escalation to a higher level than would otherwise be possible, thereby improving the relief of incident pain.[7–10] A comprehensive review of animal and clinical data is available.[11] Undesirable effects have been reported in up to 30% of patients. The most common are insomnia, agitation and anorexia. These generally settle in time if the drug is continued or resolve after several days if the drug is discontinued. Psychostimulants may also raise blood pressure and cause tachyarrhythmias; caution is necessary in those with cardiac disease.

1 Homsi J *et al.* (2000) Psychostimulants in supportive care. *Supportive Care in Cancer.* **8**: 385–397.
2 Block S (2000) Assessing and managing depression in the terminally ill patient. *Annals of Internal Medicine.* **132**: 209–218.
3 Fernandez F *et al.* (1995) Effects of methylphenidate in HIV-related depression: a comparative trial with desipramine. *International Journal of Psychiatry and Medicine.* **25**: 53–67.
4 Emptage R and Semla T (1996) Depression in the medically ill elderly: a focus on methylphenidate. *Annals of Pharmacotherapy.* **30**: 151–157.
5 Weitzner M and Meyers C (1997) Cognitive functioning and quality of life in malignant glioma patients: a review of the literature. *Psycho-Oncology.* **6**: 169–177.
6 Satel S and Nelson J (1989) Stimulants in the treatment of depression: A critical overview. *Journal of Clinical Psychiatry.* **50**: 241–249.
7 Bruera E *et al.* (1989) Use of methylphenidate as an adjuvant to narcotic analgesics in patients with advanced cancer. *Journal of Pain and Symptom Management.* **4**: 3–6.
8 Bruera E *et al.* (1992) Neuropsychological effects of methylphenidate in patients receiving a continuous infusion of narcotics for cancer pain. *Pain.* **48**: 163–166.
9 Bruera E *et al.* (1992) The use of methylphenidate in patients with incident cancer pain receiving regular opiates: a preliminary report. *Pain.* **50**: 75–77.
10 Wilwerding M *et al.* (1995) A randomized, crossover evaluation of methylphenidate in cancer patients receiving strong narcotics. *Supportive Care in Cancer.* **3**: 135–138.
11 Dalal S and Melzack R (1998) Potentiation of opioid analgesia by psychostimulant drugs: a review. *Journal of Pain and Symptom Management.* **16**: 245–253.

*METHYLPHENIDATE — BNF 4.4

Class: Psychostimulant.

Indications: †Depression, †opioid-related drowsiness.

Contra-indications: Anxiety, pre-existing prescription of an antipsychotic drug.

Pharmacology

Methylphenidate is a CNS stimulant structurally related to **amfetamine** but is less potent and has a shorter halflife (2h vs 10h).[1] It is used at some centres to treat depression in patients with a prognosis of less than 3 months. In HIV+ patients, methylphenidate 30mg daily was as effective

as **desipramine** 150mg.[2] In this group of patients, both drugs acted equally quickly with increasing benefit over 6 weeks. Surprisingly, anxiety, nervousness and insomnia occurred more frequently with **desipramine** than with methylphenidate. It is also used to permit higher doses of opioids without excessive drowsiness in patients with incident movement-related pain (see Psychostimulants, p.101). The mechanism of action appears to be mediated by blockade of presynpatic neurone dopamine re-uptake.[3] Multiple neurotransmitters are likely to be involved in the behavioural and cardiovascular effects.[4] Absorption from the gastro-intestinal tract is reduced by food.[5] Although methylphenidate is absorbed from the buccal mucosa, this route is not used clinically because of the higher risk of undesirable effects.[6] Methylphenidate undergoes extensive first-pass metabolism. Its major metabolite, ritalinic acid, is mainly excreted in the urine.[7] Like **dexamfetamine**, little relation exists between plasma levels and behavioural or physiological effects.[8]
Bio-availability 30%.
Onset of action 20–40min.
Time to peak plasma concentration 1–3h.
Plasma halflife 2–7h.
Duration of action 4–8h.

Cautions

Methylphenidate may antagonise the anti-epileptic effect of **phenytoin**,[9] and the action of antihypertensive drugs. It also inhibits the metabolism of **warfarin** and tricyclic antidepressants.[10] Antipsychotics and benzodiazepines antagonise the alerting action of methylphenidate.

Undesirable effects

For full list, see manufacturer's SPC.
Very common: nervousness and insomnia (at the beginning of treatment but can be controlled by reducing the dosage).
Common: headache, dizziness, dyskinesia, tachycardia, palpitations, arrythmias, increase in blood pressure and heart rate, abdominal pain, nausea, vomiting (when starting treatment and may be alleviated by concurrent food intake), decreased appetite (transient), dry mouth, rash, pruritus, urticaria, fever, arthralgia, scalp hair loss.

Dose and use

Depression
Individual dose titration is necessary to maximise benefit and minimise undesirable effects:
- starting dose 5mg b.d. (on waking/breakfast time and noon/lunchtime)
- increase after 3 days if necessary to 10mg b.d.
- increase after a further 3 days if necessary to 15mg b.d.
- occasionally higher doses are required, up to 30mg b.d. or 20mg t.d.s.[11–13]

Supply

Unless indicated otherwise, all preparations are **CD**.

Equasym® (Celltech 01753 534655)
Tablets 5mg, 10mg, 20mg, 28 days @ 10mg b.d. = £ 9.31.

Ritalin® (Cephalon 0800 783 4869)
Tablets 10mg, 28 days @ 10mg b.d. = £10.40.

M/r preparations are available (licensed for use in children with attention-deficit hyperactivity disorder), but are not appropriate as day-time stimulants in palliative care.

1 Hoffman B and Lefkowitz R (1990) Catecholamines, sympathomimetic drugs, and adrenergic receptor antagonists. In: A Gilman *et al.* (eds) *Goodman & Gilman's The Pharmacologic Basis of Therapeutics* (8e). Pergamon Press, New York, pp.187–220.

2 Fernandez F *et al.* (1995) Effects of methylphenidate in HIV-related depression: a comparative trial with desipramine. *International Journal of Psychiatry and Medicine*. **25**: 53–67.

3 Gelman CR *et al.* (eds) (2001) *Drugdex®* System Micromedex, Inc., Englewood, Colorado. Edition expires 12/2001.

4 Volkow N *et al.* (1996) Temporal relationships between the pharmacokinetics of methylphenidate in the human brain and its behavioral and cardiovascular effects. *Psychopharmacology.* **123**: 26–33.
5 Yoss R and Daly D (1968) On the treatment of narcolepsy. *Medical Clinics of North America.* **52**: 781–787.
6 Pleak R (1995) Adverse effects of chewing methylphenidate. *American Journal of Psychiatry.* **152**: 811.
7 Martindale (1996) *Martindale: The Extra Pharmacopoeia* (31e). Royal Pharmaceutical Society, London.
8 Little K (1993) d-Amphetamine versus methylphenidate effects in depressed inpatients. *Journal of Clinical Psychiatry.* **54**: 349–355.
9 Ghofrani M (1988) Possible phenytoin-methylphenidate interaction. *Developmental Medicine and Child Neurology.* **30**: 267–268.
10 American Hospital Formulary Service (1999) *Drug Information.* American Society of Health-System Pharmacists, Bethesda, pp.2028–2050.
11 Fernandez F *et al.* (1987) Methylphenidate for depressive disorders in cancer patients. An alternative to standard antidepressants. *Psychosomatics.* **28**: 455–461.
12 Macleod A (1998) Methylphenidate in terminal depression. *Journal of Pain and Symptom Management.* **16**: 193–198.
13 Homsi J *et al.* (2000) Psychostimulants in supportive care. *Supportive Care in Cancer.* **8**: 385–397.

CANNABINOIDS — BNF 4.6

Cannabinoids (and marijuana) are classified as psychodysleptics. There are two known endogenous cannabinoid receptors:

- CB_1, expressed by central and peripheral neurones[1,2]
- CB_2, expressed mainly by immune cells.[3]

Several endogenous ligands (endocannabinoids) have been identified, notably anandamide (arachidonylethanolamide),[4] an eicosanoid (i.e. a derivative of arachidonic acid) produced in the brain and peripheral tissues such as the spleen. It is also produced by macrophages and other leukocytes. Other endogenous ligands include 2-arachidonyl glycerol (2-AG) and palmitoylethanolamide (PEA). PEA is generated in inflammatory conditions and is believed to down-regulate inflammation.[4] Release of endocannabinoids is stimulated by neurotransmitters and requires the enzymatic cleavage of phospholipid precursors in the membranes of neurones and other cells. Once released, the endocannabinoids activate cannabinoid receptors on nearby cells and are rapidly inactivated by transport and subsequent enzymatic hydrolysis. These compounds might act near their site of synthesis to serve a variety of regulatory functions.[5] The modulatory role of cannabinoids appears to be parallel to the opioid system functionally, and analogous biochemically to other lipid mediators, such as the eicosanoids.[5]

A range of exogenous ligands have been identified, either naturally occurring cannabinoids, from marijuana (*Cannabis sativa*) e.g. **tetrahydrocannabinol** (**THC**), or synthetic substances, e.g. **nabilone**. Marijuana smoking and **THC** modulate the cytokine response of various immune cells.[4,6] Likewise anandamide modulates cellular responses to prolactin, IL-3 and IL-6; it also modulates the production of different cytokines such as IL-6 and IFN_γ.[7]

Cannabinoids have been shown to be of therapeutic value as analgesics and anti-emetics. Other claims relate to migraine, cachexia-anorexia in HIV+ disease, muscle spasticity in multiple sclerosis or after spinal cord injury, Parkinson's disease, epilepsy and glaucoma.[8] Studies of SL cannabinoids are in progress for some of these conditions. A systematic review of cannabinoids as analgesics for mainly postoperative and cancer pain showed that cannabinoids are no more effective than **codeine** 60mg in relieving acute and chronic pain but had more undesirable effects.[9] Undesirable effects were common and sometimes severe; the most common being sedation. However, in a rat model of neuropathic pain (constriction injury of the sciatic nerve), a CB_1 agonist has been shown to alleviate allodynia (pain from a non-noxious stimulus) and hyperalgesia (increased sensitivity to noxious stimuli).[10] Other studies have yielded similar results.[11–13] These findings suggest that cannabinoids might be useful adjuvant analgesics in neuropathic pain.

A systematic review of chemotherapy-induced nausea and vomiting found that cannabinoids had some anti-emetic efficacy in moderate emetogenic settings when compared with placebo, similar to that seen with dopamine antagonists.[14] However, in highly emetogenic settings, cannabinoids were indistinguishable from placebo. Most of these studies were performed before the introduction of specific $5HT_3$-receptor antagonists which have a high therapeutic index. Compared with $5HT_3$-receptor antagonists, the undesirable effects of cannabinoids outweigh their benefits.[15,16]

Studies of the effects of smoking marijuana cigarettes or inhaling **THC** have shown a bronchodilator effect together with either an increase in CO_2 sensitivity[17] or a slight respiratory depressant effect.[18,19] However, the potential benefits that could accrue from these actions are overshadowed by the finding that long-term cannabis smoking is associated with a form of chronic bronchitis.

1 Matsuda L *et al.* (1990) Structure of a cannabinoid receptor and functional expression of the cloned cDNA. *Nature.* **346**: 561–564.

2 Morisset V and Urban L (2001) Cannabinoid-induced presynaptic inhibition of glutamatergic EPSCs in substantia gelatinosa neurons of the rat spinal cord. *Journal of Neurophysiology.* **86**: 40–48.

3 Munro S *et al.* (1993) Molecular characterization of a peripheral receptor for cannabinoids. *Nature.* **365**: 61–65.

4 Klein T *et al.* (2000) The cannabinoid system and cytokine network (44546). *Proceedings of the Society for Experimental Biology and Medicine.* **225**: 1–8.

5 Piomelli D *et al.* (2000) The endocannabinoid system as a target for therapeutic drugs. *Trends in Pharmacological Science.* **21**: 218–224.

6 Berdyshev E *et al.* (1997) Influence of fatty acid ethanolamides and delta-9 tetrahydrocannabinol on cytokine and arachidonate release by mononuclear cells. *European Journal of Pharmacology.* **330**: 231–240.

7 Molina-Holgado F *et al.* (1998) The endogenous cannabinoid anandamide potentiates interleukin-6 production by astrocytes infected with Theiler's murine encephalomyelitis virus by a receptor-mediated pathway. *FEBS Letter.* **433**: 139–142.

8 Kalso E (2001) Cannabinoids for pain and nausea. *British Medical Journal.* **323**: 2–3.

9 Campbell F *et al.* (2001) Are cannabinoids an effective and safe treatment option in the management of pain? A qualitative systematic review. *British Medical Journal.* **323**: 13–16.

10 Herzberg U *et al.* (1997) The analgesic effects of R(+)-WIN 55,212-2 mesylate, a high affinity cannabinoid agonist, in a rat model of neuropathic pain. *Neuroscience Letters.* **221**: 157–160.

11 Richardson J *et al.* (1998) Cannabinoids reduce hyperalgesia and inflammation via interaction with CB1 receptors. *Pain.* **75**: 111–119.

12 Li J *et al.* (1999) The cannabinoid receptor agonist WIN 55, 212-2 mesylate blocks the development of hyperalgesia produced by capsaicin in rats. *Pain.* **81**: 25–33.

13 Martin W *et al.* (1999) Spinal cannabinoids are anti-allodynic in rats with persistent inflammation. *Pain.* **82**: 199–205.

14 Tramer M *et al.* (2001) Cannabinoids for control of chemotherapy induced nausea and vomiting: quantitative systemic review. *British Medical Journal.* **323**: 16–21.

15 Institute of Medicine (1999) *Marijuana and Medicine.* National Academy Press, Washington.

16 Hall W and Solowij N (1998) Adverse effects of cannabis. *Lancet.* **352**: 1611–1616.

17 Vachon L *et al.* (1973) Single-dose effect of marihuana smoke. *New England Journal of Medicine.* **288**: 985–989.

18 Bellville J *et al.* (1975) Respiratory effects of delta-9-tetrahydrocannabinol. *Clinical Pharmacology and Therapeutics.* **17**: 541–548.

19 Tashkin D *et al.* (1977) Bronchial effects of aerosolized 9-tetrahydrocannabinol in healthy and asthmatic subjects. *American Review of Respiratory Disease.* **115**: 57–65.

*NABILONE BNF 4.6

Class: Cannabinoid.

Indications: Nausea and vomiting caused by cytotoxic chemotherapy unresponsive to conventional anti-emetics, †breathlessness, †spasticity.

Pharmacology

Nabilone is the only synthetic cannabinoid licensed for use in the UK. It has significant anti-emetic activity in patients receiving moderately emetogenic cytotoxic chemotherapy.[1,2] Its mechanism of action is not fully understood but there are several points where nabilone could act to block emesis.[3] Nabilone is well absorbed orally. The main metabolite, 9-hydroxynabilone, is pharmacologically active with a plasma halflife up to 5 times longer than that of nabilone itself.[4] Like other cannabinoids, nabilone may cause sedation and, less often, hallucinations and other psychotomimetic effects. Undesirable effects on mental state can last 48–72h after the last dose. Since the advent of specific $5HT_3$-receptor antagonists, used alone or with **dexamethasone**, there has been little justification for nabilone as an anti-emetic.[1]

At a typical anti-emetic dose of 2mg b.d, nabilone has bronchodilator activity in normal subjects and increases the ventilatory response to CO_2.[5] This respiratory stimulation occurs at the time of maximal cortical sedation. Both the bronchodilation and the ventilatory enhancement may be a reflection of a widespread non-specific sympathetic arousal. Thus subjects taking nabilone can feel relaxed and sleepy, and may have demonstrable reduction in PO_2 as a result but, paradoxically, sensitivity to CO_2 is increased. This combination of effects has led to its occasional use in the relief of breathlessness in terminally ill patients.[6] Nabilone should be reserved for patients who:

- are frequently or continuously breathless
- exhibit great anxiety
- would be in danger of slipping into hypercapnic respiratory failure with other conventional respiratory sedatives.

Nabilone and other potentially sedative drugs (e.g. benzodiazepines, opioids, alcohol) have additive CNS depressant events.

Bio-availability 85% PO.

Onset of action 60–90min.

Time to peak plasma concentration 2h.

Plasma halflife 2h; active metabolite 9-hydroxynabilone 5–10h.

Duration of action 8–12h.

Cautions

Because of possible hypotension and reflex tachycardia, nabilone is unsuitable for patients with atrial fibrillation or in heart failure, and possibly the elderly. History of psychoses, severe hepatic impairment.

Undesirable effects

For full list, see manufacturer's SPC.

Most common: drowsiness, vertigo/dizziness, euphoria, dry mouth, ataxia, visual disturbances, concentration difficulties, sleep disturbance, dyspnoea, hypotension, headache, nausea.

Less common: confusion, disorientation, hallucinations, psychosis, depression, tremors, tachycardia, decreased appetite and abdominal pain.

Tolerence to CNS effects generally develops after a few days.

Dose and use

Nausea and vomiting

Should be given immediately before, during and for 48h after each pulse of chemotherapy:

- starting dose 1mg b.d.
- increase if necessary to 2–3mg b.d.
- maximum recommended dose 6mg daily.[7]

Breathlessness

The doses are much lower than for anti-emesis:

- starting dose 100microgram b.d.
- increase if necessary to 250microgram q.d.s.[8]

Above this dose, most patients with advanced cancer find the sedation unacceptable.

Spasticity
The use of nabilone for spasticity in multiple sclerosis is under investigation.[9]

Supply

Nabilone (Cambridge 0191 296 9369)
Capsules 250microgram, 20 = £39.79. (Hospital only, unlicensed, available as a named patient supply from Cambridge; see Special orders and named patient supplies, p.349.)
Capsules 1mg, 20 = £114.40 (hospital only). A lower dose capsule can be extemporaneously prepared by diluting with lactose powder.

1 Gralla R *et al.* (1999) Recommendations for the use of antiemetics: evidence-based, clinical practice guidelines. *Journal of Clinical Oncology.* **17**: 2971–2994.
2 Tramer M *et al.* (2001) Cannabinoids for control of chemotherapy induced nausea and vomiting: quantitative systemic review. *British Medical Journal.* **323**: 16–21.
3 Piomelli D *et al.* (2000) The endocannabinoid system as a target for therapeutic drugs. *Trends in Pharmacological Science.* **21**: 218–224.
4 Rubin A *et al.* (1977) Physiologic disposition of nabilone, a cannabinol derivative, in man. *Clinical Pharmacology and Therapeutics.* **22**: 85–91.
5 McAlpine L and Thomson N (1989) Lidocaine-induced bronchoconstriction in asthmatic patients. Relation to histamine airway responsiveness and effect of preservative. *Chest.* **96**: 1012–1015.
6 Ahmedzai S (1988) Respiratory distress in the terminally ill patient. *Respiratory Disease in Practice.* **5**: 21–29.
7 Mannix K (1997) Palliation of nausea and vomiting. In: D Doyle *et al.* (eds) *Oxford Textbook of Palliative Medicine.* Oxford University Press, Oxford, pp.489–499.
8 Ahmedzai S (1997) Palliation of respiratory symptoms. In: D Doyle *et al.* (eds) *Oxford Textbook of Palliative Medicine.* Oxford University Press, Oxford, pp.583–616.
9 Martyn C *et al.* (1995) Nabilone in the treatment of multiple sclerosis. *Lancet.* **345**: 579.

ANTI-EMETICS — BNF 4.6

Important factors to consider when prescribing anti-emetics include:
- mechanism of action of anti-emetic drugs (Figure 4.4; Tables 4.10 & 4.11)[1–4]
- response to anti-emetics already given
- when more than one anti-emetic drug is needed, a combination of drugs with different actions should be used (e.g. **cyclizine** and **haloperidol**)
- combinations with antagonistic actions should not be used (e.g. **cyclizine** and **metoclopramide**)[5]
- **levomepromazine** (methotrimeprazine) has multiple receptor effects and is sometimes more effective than drug combinations
- effects of anti-emetics on gastro-intestinal motility, i.e.
  prokinetic (**metoclopramide**, **domperidone**, **cisapride**)
  antikinetic (antimuscarinics)
- adjuvant use of antisecretory drugs (e.g. **hyoscine butylbromide**, **glycopyrronium**, **octreotide**)
- adjuvant use of corticosteroids (e.g. **dexamethasone**, **prednisolone**)
- undesirable effects of drugs
- cost of drugs ($5HT_3$-receptor antagonists and **octreotide** are expensive)
- role of non-drug treatments.

Generally, the initial choice of an anti-emetic in palliative care lies between three drugs, namely **metoclopramide** (see p.113), **haloperidol** (see p.76) and **cyclizine** (see p.115).[6] One of these should be prescribed both regularly and as needed (Box 4.H).

In bowel obstruction with large volume vomiting or associated intestinal colic, an antisecretory agent (which acts partly by reducing the volume of gastro-intestinal secretions) may be used either alone as a first-line manoeuvre, e.g. **hyoscine butylbromide** 60–120mg/24h CSCI, or in conjunction with **cyclizine**. If this proves inadequate, a trial of **octreotide** should be considered (see p.230).

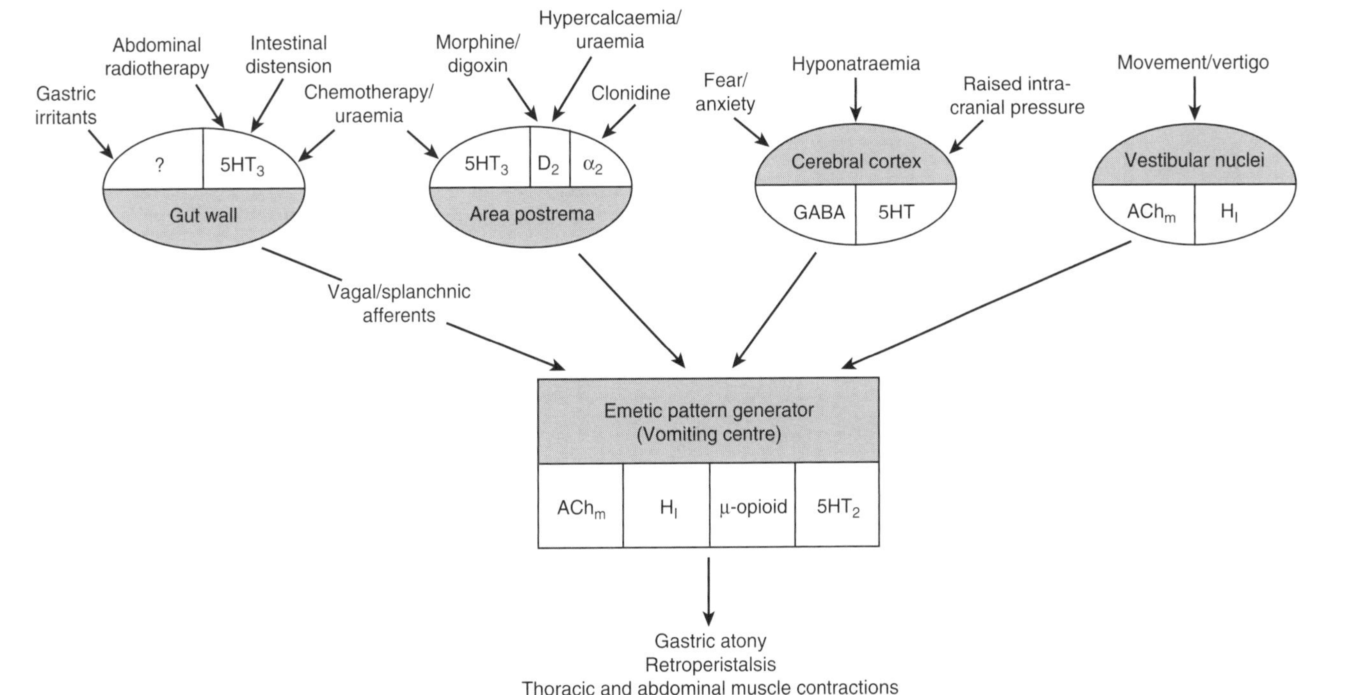

Figure 4.4 Diagram of the neural mechanisms controlling vomiting. Based on Twycross *et al.*, 1997.[1]

Abbreviations refer to receptor types: ACh_m = muscarinic cholinergic; α_2 = α_2-adrenergic; D_2 = dopamine type 2; GABA = gamma-aminobutyric acid; 5HT, $5HT_2$, $5HT_3$ = 5-hydroxytriptamine (serotonin) type undefined, type 2, type 3; H_I = histamine type I. Anti-emetics act as antagonists at these receptors, whereas the central anti-emetic effects of clonidine and opioids are agonistic.

Table 4.10 Classification of drugs used to control nausea and vomiting

Putative site of action	*Class*	*Example*
Central nervous system		
Vomiting centre	Antimuscarinic	Hyoscine hydrobromide
	Antihistaminic antimuscarinic[a]	Cyclizine, dimenhydrinate, prochlorperazine
	$5HT_2$-receptor antagonist	Levomepromazine (methotrimeprazine)
Area postrema	D_2-receptor antagonist	Haloperidol, prochlorperazine, metoclopramide, domperidone
	$5HT_3$-receptor antagonist	Granisetron, ondansetron, tropisetron
Cerebral cortex	Benzodiazepine	Lorazepam
	Cannabinoid	Nabilone
	Corticosteroid	Dexamethasone
Gastro-intestinal tract		
Prokinetic	$5HT_4$-receptor agonist	Metoclopramide, cisapride
	D_2-receptor antagonist	Metoclopramide, domperidone
Antisecretory	Antimuscarinic	Hyoscine butylbromide, glycopyrronium
	Somatostatin analogue	Octreotide, vapreotide
Vagal $5HT_3$-receptor blockade	$5HT_3$-receptor antagonist	Granisetron, ondansetron, tropisetron
Anti-inflammatory	Corticosteroid	Dexamethasone

a. antihistamines and phenothiazines both have H_1-receptor antagonistic and antimuscarinic properties (see Table 4.11, p.109).

Corticosteroids and **levomepromazine** (methotrimeprazine) are both useful options when first-line anti-emetics fail to relieve nausea and vomiting satisfactorily. **Dexamethasone** is normally *added* to an existing regimen, whereas **levomepromazine** is normally *substituted*. Sometimes it is necessary to use **dexamethasone** and **levomepromazine** concurrently. Other phenothiazines are still often used as anti-emetics, notably **promethazine**, **prochlorperazine** and **chlorpromazine**. **Promethazine** is used as an alternative to **cyclizine** and **haloperidol** in some countries, in doses similar to **cyclizine** both PO and CSCI. **Prochlorperazine** is often effective against moderate chemical emetogenic stimuli in a dose of 5–10mg t.d.s. PO; suppositories and injections are also available. **Chlorpromazine** has an even broader spectrum of receptor affinity (Table 4.11) but does not share the potent $5HT_2$ antagonism of **levomepromazine** which should be used in preference to **chlorpromazine** when a broad-spectrum drug is indicated.

$5HT_3$-receptor antagonists, developed primarily to control chemotherapeutic vomiting, have a definite but limited role in palliative care (see p.116). Drug-induced nausea and vomiting can be problematic. It may be caused by several different mechanisms (Table 4.12), each of which calls for a distinct therapeutic response.

Table 4.11 Receptor site affinities of selected anti-emetics[2–4]

	D_2-receptor antagonist	*H_1-receptor antagonist*	*Muscarinic antagonist*	*$5HT_2$-receptor antagonist*	*$5HT_3$-receptor antagonist*	*$5HT_4$-receptor agonist*
Metoclopramide	++	0	0	0	+	++
Domperidone	++[a]	0	0	0	0	0
Cisapride	0	0	0	0	0	+++
Ondansetron[b]	0	0	0	0	+++	0
Cyclizine	0	++	++	0	0	0
Hyoscine hydrobromide	0	0	+++	0	0	0
Haloperidol	+++	0	0	0	0	0
Prochlorperazine	++	+	0	0	0	0
Chlorpromazine	++	++	+	0	0	0
Levomepromazine (methotrimeprazine)	++	+++	++	+++	0	0

Pharmacological activity: 0 = none or insignificant; + = slight; ++ = moderate; +++ = marked.

a. domperidone does not cross the blood-brain barrier and therefore does not cause extrapyramidal effects

b. other $5HT_3$-receptor antagonists, e.g. granisetron and tropisetron, have comparable receptor affinity.

Box 4.H Guidelines for the management of nausea and vomiting

1 After clinical evaluation, document the most likely cause(s) of the nausea and vomiting in the patient's case notes.

2 Ask the patient to record symptoms and response to treatment, preferably using a diary.

3 Correct correctable causes/exacerbating factors, e.g. drugs, severe pain, infection, cough, hypercalcaemia. (*Correction of hypercalcaemia is not always appropriate in a dying patient.*) Anxiety exacerbates nausea and vomiting from any cause and may need specific treatment.

4 Prescribe the most appropriate anti-emetic stat, regularly and p.r.n. (see below). Give by SC injection if continuous nausea or frequent vomiting, preferably by CSCI.

Commonly used anti-emetics

Prokinetic anti-emetic (about 50% of prescriptions)
For gastritis, gastric stasis, functional bowel obstruction (peristaltic failure):
metoclopramide 10mg PO (orally) stat & q.d.s. or 10mg SC stat & 40–100mg/24h CSCI, & 10mg p.r.n. up to q.d.s.

Anti-emetic acting principally in chemoreceptor trigger zone (about 25% of prescriptions)
For most chemical causes of vomiting, e.g. morphine, hypercalcaemia, renal failure:
haloperidol 1.5–3mg PO stat & o.n. or 2.5–5mg SC stat & 2.5–10mg/24h CSCI, & 2.5–5mg p.r.n. up to q.d.s.
Metoclopramide also has a central action.

Antispasmodic and antisecretory anti-emetic
If bowel colic and/or need to reduce gut secretions:
hyoscine butylbromide 20mg SC stat, 80–200mg/24h CSCI, & 20mg SC hourly p.r.n.

Anti-emetic acting principally in the vomiting centre
For raised intracranial pressure (in conjunction with dexamethasone), motion sickness and in organic bowel obstruction:
cyclizine 50mg PO stat & b.d.–t.d.s. or 50mg SC stat & 100–150mg/24h CSCI, & 50mg p.r.n. up to q.d.s.

Broad-spectrum anti-emetic
For organic bowel obstruction and when other anti-emetics are unsatisfactory:
levomepromazine (methotrimeprazine) 6–12.5mg PO/SC stat, o.n. & p.r.n. up to q.d.s.

5 Review anti-emetic dose every 24h, taking note of p.r.n. use and the patient's diary.

6 If little benefit despite optimising the dose, have you got the cause right?
- if no, change to an alternative anti-emetic and optimise
- if yes, provided the anti-emetic has been optimised, add or substitute a second anti-emetic.

continued

Box 4.H Continued

7 Anti-emetics for inoperable bowel obstruction are best given by CSCI. Levomepromazine (methotrimeprazine) is the exception; it can be given as a single SC dose o.n.:

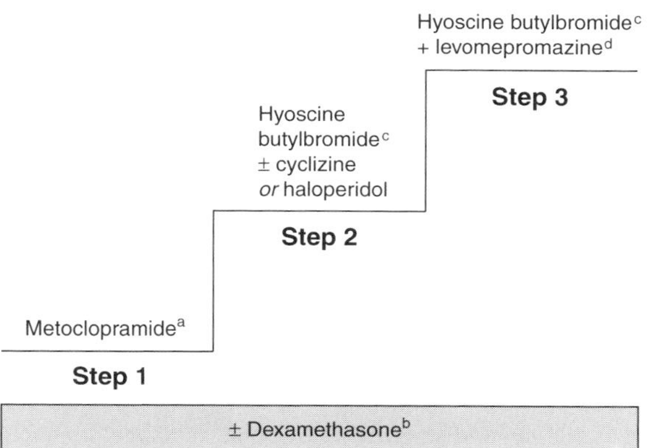

± Dexamethasone[b]

a. if colic, omit step 1
b. the place of dexamethasone in inoperable bowel obstruction is controversial; for dose see below
c. alternatively, use glycopyrronium 600–1200microgram/24h
d. if levomepromazine is too sedative, consider using olanzapine 1.25–2.5mg o.d. PO instead; or revert to step 2 but give both cyclizine and haloperidol.

8 In patients who fail to respond to the commonly used anti-emetics, consider:

Other drugs for nausea and vomiting
Corticosteroid
Adjuvant anti-emetic for bowel obstruction and when all else fails:
dexamethasone 8–16mg PO/SC stat & o.d.; consider reducing the dose after 7 days.

$5HT_3$-receptor antagonist
Use when massive release of 5HT (serotonin) from enterochromaffin cells or platelets, e.g. chemotherapy, abdominal radiation, bowel obstruction (distension), renal failure:
tropisetron 5mg PO/SC stat & o.d.

Somatostatin analogue
An anti-secretory agent without antispasmodic effects; use in obstruction if hyoscine inadequate:
octreotide 100microgram stat, 300–600microgram/24h CSCI, & 100microgram p.r.n. up to q.d.s.

9 Some patients with nausea and vomiting need more than one anti-emetic.

10 *Antimuscarinic drugs block the cholinergic pathway through which prokinetics act; concurrent use antagonises the prokinetic effect of metoclopramide and is best avoided.*

11 Continue anti-emetics unless the cause is self-limiting.

12 Except in organic bowel obstruction, consider changing to PO after 72h of good control with CSCI.

Table 4.12 Causes of drug-induced nausea and vomiting

Mechanism	*Drugs*
Gastric irritation	Antibiotics Iron supplements NSAIDs Tranexamic acid
Gastric stasis	Antimuscarinics Opioids Phenothiazines Tricyclics
Area postrema stimulation (chemoreceptor trigger zone)	Antibiotics Cytotoxics Digoxin Imidazoles Opioids
$5HT_3$-receptor stimulation	Antibiotics Cytotoxics SSRIs

1 Twycross R *et al.* (1997) The use of low dose levomepromazine (methotrimeprazine) in the management of nausea and vomiting. *Progress in Palliative Care.* **5**: 49–53.

2 Dollery C (1991) *Therapeutic Drugs.* Churchill Livingstone, Edinburgh.

3 Dollery C (1992) *Therapeutic Drugs: Supplement 1.* Churchill Livingstone, Edinburgh.

4 Peroutka SJ and Snyder SH (1982) Antiemetics: neurotransmitter receptor binding predicts therapeutic actions. *Lancet.* **1**: 658–659.

5 Schuurkes JAJ *et al.* (1986) Stimulation of gastroduodenal motor activity: dopaminergic and cholinergic modulation. *Drug Development Research.* **8**: 233–241.

6 Twycross R and Back I (1998) Nausea and vomiting in advanced cancer. *European Journal of Palliative Care.* **5**: 39–45.

METOCLOPRAMIDE BNF 4.6

Class: Prokinetic anti-emetic.

Indications: Nausea and vomiting, particularly in gastro-intestinal disorders (e.g. gastric irritation and delayed gastric emptying), and with chemotherapy and radiotherapy.

Contra-indications: Concurrent administration with antimuscarinics (block the cholinergic final common pathway of prokinetics),[1] concurrent IV administration with $5HT_3$-receptor antagonists (risk of cardiac arrhythmia).[2]

Pharmacology

Metoclopramide is a combined D_2-receptor antagonist and $5HT_4$-receptor agonist. In daily doses above 100mg SC, it manifests $5HT_3$-receptor antagonism. Metoclopramide is therefore a broad-spectrum anti-emetic but its clinical value mainly resides in its prokinetic properties (see Prokinetics, p.7). As a centrally-acting D_2-receptor antagonist, it is second to **haloperidol** (see p.76) and, as a $5HT_3$-receptor antagonist, it is second to the specific $5HT_3$-receptor antagonists (see p.116).

Prokinetics act by triggering a cholinergic system in the gut wall. Opioids impede this action but antimuscarinics block it competitively.[1] *Prokinetics and antimuscarinics should therefore not be given concurrently.* However, if given together, metoclopramide (or **domperidone**) would still exert an antagonistic effect at the dopamine receptors in the area postrema, although **haloperidol** is generally a better choice in this situation because of the advantage of o.d. administration.

D_2-receptor antagonists block the dopaminergic 'brake' on gastric emptying induced by stress, anxiety and nausea from any cause. In contrast, $5HT_4$-receptor agonists have a direct excitatory effect which in theory gives them an advantage over the D_2-receptor antagonists particularly for patients with gastric stasis or functional bowel obstruction. However, when used for dysmotility dyspepsia, metoclopramide is no more potent than **domperidone** in standard doses.

Along with other drugs which block central dopamine receptors, there is a risk of developing acute dystonic reactions with facial and skeletal muscle spasms and oculogyric crises. These are more common in the young (particularly girls and young women), generally occur within a few days of starting treatment, and subside within 24h of stopping the drug. Because of this, metoclopramide is generally not used in children. An antimuscarinic will abort an attack, e.g. **procyclidine** 5–10 mg IV.

Bio-availability 50–80% PO.
Onset of action 10–15min IM; 15–60min PO.
Time to peak plasma concentration 1–2.5h PO.
Plasma halflife 2.5–5h.
Duration of action 1–2h (data for single dose and relating to gastric emptying).

Cautions

Serious drug interactions: a combination of IV metoclopramide and IV **ondansetron** occasionally causes cardiac arrhythmias.[2] $5HT_3$-receptors influence various aspects of cardiac function, including inotropy, chronotropy and coronary arterial tone,[3] effects which are mediated by both parasympathetic and sympathetic nervous systems. Thus in any given patient, blockade of $5HT_3$-receptors will produce effects dependent on the pre-existing serotoninergic activity in both arms of the autonomic nervous system.

Metoclopramide is known to enhance the effects of catecholamines in patients with phaeochromocytomas and with essential hypertension.[4,5] Acute dystonic reactions occur in $<5\%$ of patients receiving metoclopramide in standard doses; the risk is greater if also receiving other drugs known to cause extrapyramidal effects, e.g. antipsychotics, $5HT_3$-receptor antagonists and antidepressants (see Drug-induced movement disorders, p.339).

Undesirable effects

For full list, see manufacturer's SPC.

Extrapyramidal effects, neuroleptic (antipsychotic) malignant syndrome. Occasionally drowsiness, restlessness, depression and diarrhoea.

Dose and use

Gastric irritation

- 10mg PO q.d.s. *or* 40–60mg/24h CSCI and 10mg PO/SC p.r.n.; also reduce or remove cause of gastritis and prescribe appropriate gastroprotective drugs.

Delayed gastric emptying

- as above, consider increasing to 100mg/24h CSCI or substitute **cisapride** 10–20mg b.d. PO (available on a named patient basis).

Stimulation of area postrema

- as above, but **haloperidol** generally preferable.

For nausea and vomiting associated with 5HT release, a selective $5HT_3$-receptor antagonist should be used rather than high-dose metoclopramide (see BNF 4.6).

Supply

Metoclopramide (non-proprietary)
Tablets 10mg, 28 days @ 10mg q.d.s. = £3.44.
Oral solution 5mg/5ml, 28 days @ 10mg q.d.s. = £12.32.
Injection 5mg/ml, 2ml amp = £0.34.

Maxolon® (Shire 01256 894000)
Tablets 10mg, 28 days @ 10mg q.d.s. = £12.51.
Oral syrup 5mg/5ml, 28 days @ 10mg q.d.s. = £21.45.
Injection 5mg/ml, 2ml amp = £0.27.

1 Schuurkes JAJ *et al.* (1986) Stimulation of gastroduodenal motor activity: dopaminergic and cholinergic modulation. *Drug Development Research.* **8**: 233–241.
2 Baguley W *et al.* (1997) Cardiac dysrhythmias associated with the intravenous administration of ondansetron and metoclopramide. *Anesthesia and Analgesia.* **84**: 1380–1381.
3 Saxena P and Villalon C (1991) 5-Hydroxytryptamine: a chameleon in the heart. *Trends in Pharmacological Sciences.* **12**: 223–227.
4 Kuchel O *et al.* (1985) Effect of metoclopramide on plasma catecholamine release in essential hypertension. *Clinical Pharmacology and Therapeutics.* **37**: 372–375.
5 Agabiti-Rosei E (1995) Hypertensive crises in patients with phaeochromocytoma given metoclopramide. *Annals of Pharmacology.* **29**: 381–383.

DOMPERIDONE — BNF 4.6

Class: Prokinetic anti-emetic.

Indications: Nausea and vomiting, particularly when there is need for a prokinetic anti-emetic with D_2 antagonism but without risk of extrapyramidal effects.

Pharmacology

Domperidone is a D_2-receptor antagonist which does not cross the blood-brain barrier. Its prokinetic effect is limited to the oesophagus, stomach and duodenum; it also acts in the area prostrema. Domperidone can only correct the gastric dopamine brake; it has no positive prokinetic effect in its own right. It is therefore not as useful a prokinetic drug as **metoclopramide**. Its use is further limited by the absence of a parenteral formulation; it is available, however, as a suppository. Its prokinetic effect is blocked by antimuscarinics (see p.4).[1]
Bio-availability 13–17% PO; 12% PR.
Onset of action 30min.
Time to peak plasma concentration 0.5–2h PO; 1h PR.
Plasma halflife 14h.
Duration of action 8–16h.

Undesirable effects

For full list, see manufacturer's SPC.
Acute dystonia (rare), rashes, reduced libido, gynaecomastia (raised prolactin concentration).

Dose and use

Given its long plasma halflife, domperidone can be prescribed b.d. even though the SPC recommends more frequent administration:

- starting dose 20mg PO b.d.
- increase if necessary to 30mg PO q8h *or* 20mg PO q6h (these doses differ from BNF recommendations)
- 30mg PR = 10mg PO.

Supply

Domperidone (non-proprietary)
Tablets 10mg, 28 days @ 20mg b.d. = £9.31.

Motilium® (Sanofi-Synthelabo 01483 505515)
Tablets 10mg, 28 days @ 20mg b.d. = £8.77.
Oral suspension 5mg/5ml, 28 days @ 20mg b.d. = £10.08.
Suppositories 30mg, 28 days @ 60mg b.d. = £29.68.

1 Schuurkes JAJ *et al.* (1986) Stimulation of gastroduodenal motor activity: dopaminergic and cholinergic modulation. *Drug Development Research.* **8**: 233–241.

CYCLIZINE — BNF 4.6

Class: Antihistaminic antimuscarinic anti-emetic.

Indications: Nausea and vomiting, particularly if associated with motion sickness, †mechanical bowel obstruction and †raised intracranial pressure.

Pharmacology

Antihistaminic anti-emetics were originally introduced to control motion sickness following the observation that a patient with urticaria no longer became car sick during treatment with **dimenhydrinate**.[1] Studies were conducted in American servicemen crossing the Atlantic in the *General Ballou*, a modified freight ship without stabilisers which allowed the agents tested to be classified according to relative efficacy. There is no correlation between efficacy in motion sickness and antihistamine potency. Antihistaminic anti-emetics exert their effect by acting upon the vomiting centre. Cyclizine is effective for many causes of vomiting, including opioid-induced.[2–4] However, in practice **haloperidol** and **metoclopramide** are often used in preference, either because of convenience (**haloperidol**) or to avoid antimuscarinic effects.
Bio-availability no data.
Onset of action 30min; maximal effects 1–2h.
Time to peak plasma concentration 2h PO.
Plasma halflife 20h.
Duration of action 4–6h, probably longer in some patients.

Undesirable effects

For full list, see manufacturer's SPC.
Drowsiness and antimuscarinic effects (see p.4).

Dose and use
Depending on circumstances, cyclizine can be given either PO or SC:
- 50–100mg PO b.d.–t.d.s. & p.r.n.
- 100–300mg/24h CSCI (typically 100mg) & 50mg SC p.r.n.
- usual maximum daily dose 200mg PO and CSCI.

Supply
Valoid® (CeNeS 0870 241 3674)
Tablets 50mg, 28 days @ 50mg t.d.s. = £3.99.
Injection 50mg/ml, 1ml amp = £0.54.

1 Gay L and Carliner P (1949) The prevention and treatment of motion sickness. *Bulletin of John Hopkins Hospital.* **49**: 470–491.
2 Gutner B *et al.* (1952) The effects of potent analgesics upon vestibular function. *Journal of Clinical Investigations.* **31**: 259–266.
3 Dundee J and Jones P (1968) The prevention of analgesic-induced nausea and vomiting by cyclizine. *British Journal of Clinical Practice.* **22**: 379–382.
4 Walder A and Aitkenhead A (1995) A comparison of droperidol and cyclizine in the prevention of postoperative nausea and vomiting associated with patient-controlled analgesia. *Anaesthesia.* **50**: 654–656.

$5HT_3$-RECEPTOR ANTAGONISTS — BNF 4.6

Indications: Nausea and vomiting after surgery, chemotherapy and radiotherapy, †intractable vomiting due to chemical, abdominal and cerebral causes when usual approaches have failed, †pruritus associated with opioids.[1,2]

Contra-indications: Concurrent IV administration with IV **metoclopramide** (see p.113).

Pharmacology
$5HT_3$-receptor antagonists were developed specifically to control emesis associated with highly emetogenic chemotherapy, e.g. **cisplatin**. They block the amplifying effect of excess 5HT on vagal nerve fibres and are therefore of specific value in situations where excessive amounts of 5HT are released from the body's stores (enterochromaffin cells and platelets) following chemotherapy or radiation-induced damage of the gut mucosa, bowel distension and renal failure (leaky platelets).

$5HT_3$-receptor antagonists also relieve nausea and vomiting after head injury, brain stem radiotherapy,[3,4] and in multiple sclerosis with brain stem disease;[5] leakage of 5HT from the raphe nucleus probably accounts for the benefit seen in these circumstances. $5HT_3$-receptor antagonists are also effective in nausea and vomiting associated with acute gastro-enteritis.[6] In one patient who experienced persistent nausea after the insertion of an endo-oesophageal tube, a $5HT_3$-receptor antagonist brought about relief after failure with **metoclopramide** and **cyclizine**, and only temporary relief with **domperidone**.[7]

Ondansetron relieves itch associated with spinal opioids.[1] Intravenous **ondansetron** 4–8mg relieves itch induced by spinal opioids in 3–30min.[8,9] In chronic cholestasis, two double-blind, placebo-controlled trials of **ondansetron** showed either no benefit (IV 8mg stat + tablets 8mg b.d. for 5 days)[10] or minimal benefit (tablets 8mg t.d.s. for 1 week).[11] Ondansetron is also ineffective in uraemic itch.[12] Although trials have not been conducted with other $5HT_3$-receptor antagonists, it is reasonable to conclude that the benefit shown with **ondansetron** is a class effect.[13]

Ondansetron, the first $5HT_3$-receptor antagonist to be marketed, has been superseded as an anti-emetic by **granisetron** and **tropisetron**; these need only be given o.d., are as effective

PO as by injection and are cheaper than recommended IV **ondansetron** regimens.[14,15] However, all $5HT_3$-receptor antagonists are expensive, and it is important not to price palliative care 'out of the market' by using them unnecessarily. Thus, if a $5HT_3$-receptor antagonist is not clearly effective within 3 days, it should be discontinued.[16,17] **Levomepromazine** (methotrimeprazine) is a much cheaper drug and can often substitute effectively for $5HT_3$-receptor antagonists (see p.116). For pharmacokinetic details see Table 4.13.

Table 4.13 Pharmacokinetic characteristics of $5HT_3$-receptor antagonists

		Ondansetron	*Granisetron*	*Tropisetron*
Bio-availability	PO	56–71% (60% PR)	60%	>95%
Onset of action	PO IV	<30min <5min	<30min <15min	<30min <15min
Plasma halflife		3–5h (6h PR)	10–11h	24h[a]
Time to peak plasma concentration	PO IM PR	1.5h 10min 6h	No data	3h
Duration of action		12h	24h	24h

a. 32–45h in poor metabolisers; 8h in extensive metabolisers.

Undesirable effects

For full list, see manufacturer's SPC.
Common: constipation, headache.
Rare: dystonic reactions (**ondansetron**), sensation of warmth or flushing, hiccup.

Dose and use

For chemotherapeutic vomiting, see BNF section 4.6. In palliative care, **granisetron** 1–2 mg PO/SC o.d. *or* **tropisetron** 5mg PO/SC o.d. for 3 days initially; if of benefit, continue indefinitely unless cause self-limiting. For intractable vomiting, a $5HT_3$ antagonist may need to be co-administered with **haloperidol**.[16,18] Doses in pruritus are comparable.[19]

Supply

Granisetron

Kytril® (Roche 01707 366000)
Tablets 1mg, 2mg, 28 days @ 1mg o.d. = £244.50.
Oral solution (paediatric, sugar-free) 1mg/5ml, 28 days @ 1mg o.d. = £244.49.
Injection 1mg/ml, for dilution and use as injection or infusion, 1ml vial = £11.46; 3ml amp = £34.38.

Tropisetron

Navoban® (Novartis 01276 698370)
Capsules 5mg, 28 days @ 5mg o.d. = £301.62.
Injection 1mg/ml, 2ml and 5ml amp = £4.86 and £12.16 respectively.

Ondansetron

Zofran® (GSK 0800 221441)
Tablets 4mg, 8mg, 28 days @ 8mg b.d. = £433.22.
Dispersible tablets (Zofran Melt®) 4mg, 8mg, 28 days @ 8mg b.d. = £433.22.
Oral syrup 4mg/5ml, 28 days @ 8mg b.d. = £433.22.
Suppositories 16mg, 28 days @ 16mg o.d. = £433.16.
Injection 2mg/ml, 2ml and 4ml amp = £6.45 and £12.89 respectively.

1 Borgeat A and Stimemann H-R (1999) Ondansetron is effective to treat spinal or epidural morphine-induced pruritus. *Anesthesiology.* **90**: 432–436.
2 Kyriakides K *et al.* (1999) Management of opioid-induced pruritus: a role for 5HT antagonists? *British Journal of Anaesthesia.* **82**: 439–441.
3 Kleinerman K *et al.* (1993) Use of ondansetron for control of projectile vomiting in patients with neurosurgical trauma: two case reports. *Annals of Pharmacotherapy.* **27**: 566–568.
4 Bodis S *et al.* (1994) The prevention of radiosurgery-induced nausea and vomiting by ondansetron: evidence of a direct effect on the central nervous system chemoreceptor trigger zone. *Surgery and Neurology.* **42**: 249–252.
5 Rice G and Ebers G (1995) Ondansetron for intractable vertigo complicating acute brainstem disorders. *Lancet.* **345**: 1182–1183.
6 Cubeddu L *et al.* (1997) Antiemetic activity of ondansetron in acute gastroenteritis. *Alimentary Pharmacology and Therapeutics.* **11**: 185–191.
7 Fair R (1990) Ondansetron in nausea. *Pharmaceutical Journal.* **245**: 514.
8 Arai L *et al.* (1996) The use of ondansetron to treat pruritus associated with intrathecal morphine in two paediatric patients. *Paediatric Anaesthesia.* **6**: 337–339.
9 Larijani G *et al.* (1996) Treatment of opioid-induced pruritus with ondansetron: report of four patients. *Pharmacotherapy.* **16**: 958–960.
10 O'Donohue J *et al.* (1997) Ondansetron in the treatment of pruritus of cholestasis: a randomised controlled trial. *Gastroenterology.* **112**: A1349.
11 Muller C *et al.* (1998) Treatment of pruritus in chronic liver disease with the 5-hydroxytryptamine receptor type 3 antagonist ondansetron: a randomized, placebo-controlled, double-blind cross-over trial. *European Journal of Gastroenterology.* **10**: 865–870.
12 Murphy M *et al.* (2001) A randomised double blind trial of ondansetron in renal itch. *British Journal of Dermatology.* **145 (suppl 59)**: 20–21.
13 Quigley C and Plowman PN (1996) 5HT3 receptor antagonists and pruritus due to cholestasis. *Palliative Medicine.* **10**: 54.
14 Gralla R *et al.* (1997) Can an oral antiemetic regimen be as effective as intravenous treatment against cisplatin: results of a 1054 patient randomized study of oral granisetron versus IV ondansetron. *Proceedings of the American Society of Clinical Oncology.* **16**: 178.
15 Perez E *et al.* (1997) Efficacy and safety of oral granisetron versus IV ondansetron in prevention of moderately emetogenic chemotherapy-induced nausea and vomiting. *Proceedings of the American Society of Clinical Oncology.* **16**: 149.
16 Cole R *et al.* (1994) Successful control of intractable nausea and vomiting requiring combined ondansetron and haloperidol in a patient with advanced cancer. *Journal of Pain and Symptom Management.* **9**: 48–50.
17 Currow D *et al.* (1997) Use of ondansetron in palliative medicine. *Journal of Pain and Symptom Management.* **13**: 302–307.
18 Pereira J and Bruera E (1996) Successful management of intractable nausea with ondansetron: a case study. *Journal of Palliative Care.* **12**: 47–50.
19 Sanger GJ and Twycross R (1996) Making sense of emesis, pruritus, 5HT and 5HT3 receptor antagonists. *Progress in Palliative Care.* **4**: 7–8.

HYOSCINE HYDROBROMIDE — BNF 4.6

Class: Antimuscarinic.

Indications: Motion sickness, †drying secretions (e.g. sialorrhoea, drooling, death rattle), †intestinal colic, †inoperable bowel obstruction.

Contra-indications: Narrow-angle glaucoma (unless moribund).

Pharmacology

Hyoscine (scopolamine) is a naturally occurring belladonna alkaloid with smooth muscle relaxant (antispasmodic) and antisecretory properties. It is available as *hydrobromide* and *butylbromide* (Buscopan) salts. Unlike hyoscine *hydrobromide*, **hyoscine *butylbromide*** does not cross the blood-brain barrier and so does not cause drowsiness or have a central anti-emetic action. Repeated administration of hyoscine *hydrobromide* leads to cumulation and sedation; occasionally this results paradoxically in an agitated delirium. Despite a plasma halflife of several hours, the duration of the antisecretory effect in volunteers after a single dose is only about 1h (*butylbromide*) and 2h (*hydrobromide*).[1] However, particularly after repeat injections and in moribund patients, a duration of effect of up to 9h has been observed.[2] Both **hyoscine *butylbromide*** and hyoscine *hydrobromide* relieve death rattle in 50–60% of patients.[3] However, provided time is taken to explain the cause of the rattle to the relatives and there is ongoing support, relatives' distress is relieved in >90% of cases.[2] Hyoscine *hydrobromide* can also be used in other situations where an antimuscarinic effect is needed.

For pharmacokinetic details see Table 4.14.

Table 4.14 Pharmacokinetic characteristics of hyoscine salts

		Hyoscine hydrobromide	*Hyoscine butylbromide*
Bio-availability	PO	(?) 60–80% SL	8–10%
Onset of action	PO	–	1–2h
	SL	10–15min	–
	IM	3–5min	3–5min
Plasma halflife		5–6h	5–6h
Duration of action IM			
(spasmolytic)		15min	15min
(antisecretory)		1–9h	1–9h

Cautions

As for all antimuscarinics (see p.4). Blocks the final common (cholinergic) pathway through which prokinetics act,[4] avoid concurrent use.

Undesirable effects

For full list, see manufacturer's SPC.

Antimuscarinic effects (see p.4). Central anticholinergic syndrome (excitement, ataxia, hallucinations, behavioural abnormalities and drowsiness).

Dose and use

Drooling

An alternative oral antimuscarinic may be better and more convenient, e.g. **amitriptyline** (see p.94), **propantheline** (see p.6), **thioridazine** (see p.79).

- **hyoscine *hydrobromide*** transdermal patch 1mg/72h.

Death rattle

With death rattle, an antisecretory drug is best started sooner rather than later because it does not affect existing pharyngeal secretions. There is less impact when the rattle is secondary to pneumonia[5] and little effect in pulmonary oedema.

- 400microgram SC stat
- 1200microgram CSCI
- repeat 400microgram p.r.n.

Some centres use **hyoscine *butylbromide*** (see p.5) or **glycopyrronium** (see p.287) instead;[6] both are cheaper than hyoscine *hydrobromide*.[7]

Hyoscyamine: an alternative SL preparation in some countries where hyoscine *hydrobromide* is not available. **Hyoscyamine** is the laevo-isomer of **atropine**; because the dextro-isomer is virtually inactive, **hyoscyamine** is approximately twice as potent as **atropine.**

Supply

Kwells® (Roche 01707 366000)
Tablets SL 300microgram, available OTC.

Scopoderm TTS® (Novartis Consumer Health 01276 692255)
Transdermal patch 1mg/72h, 28 days = £19.35.

Hyoscine hydrobromide (non-proprietary)
Injection 400microgram and 600microgram/ml, 1ml amp = £2.70 and £2.81 respectively.

1 Herxheimer A and Haefeli L (1966) Human pharmacology of hyoscine butylbromide. *Lancet.* **ii:** 418–421.
2 Hughes A *et al.* (1997) Management of 'death rattle'. *Palliative Medicine.* **11**: 80–81.
3 Hughes A *et al.* (2000) Audit of three antimuscarinic drugs for managing retained secretions. *Palliative Medicine.* **14**: 221–222.
4 Schuurkes JAJ *et al.* (1986) Stimulation of gastroduodenal motor activity: dopaminergic and cholinergic modulation. *Drug Development Research.* **8**: 233–241.
5 Bennett M (1996) Death rattle: an audit of hyoscine (scopolamine) use and review of management. *Journal of Pain and Symptom Management.* **12**: 229–233.
6 Bennett M *et al.* (2002) Using anti-muscarinic drugs in the management of death rattle: evidence based guidelines for palliative care. *Palliative Medicine.* **16**: 120.
7 Bausewein C and Twycross R (1995) Comparative cost of hyoscine injections. *Palliative Medicine.* **9**: 256.

ANTI-EPILEPTICS — BNF 4.8

Indications: Epilepsy, neuropathic pain (**gabapentin**), terminal agitation (**phenobarbital**).

Pharmacology

Anti-epileptic drugs act mainly by two mechanisms:

- reducing electrical excitability of cell membranes, possibly through use-dependent block of sodium channels ('membrane stabilisers')
- enhancing GABA-mediated synaptic inhibition. This may be achieved by an enhanced post-synaptic action of GABA (Figure 4.5),[1] by inhibiting GABA-transaminase, or by drugs with direct GABA-agonist properties (Box 4.I).[2–4]

A few drugs appear to act by inhibition of calcium channels, e.g. **ethosuximide** and **gabapentin. Ethosuximide** is effective in petit mal absences and myoclonic seizures but is ineffective against grand mal (tonic-clonic) seizures. However, if given alone to patients experiencing seizures of mixed type, it may precipitate grand mal seizures. There is no evidence that the newer anti-epileptic drugs are more effective in seizure control than traditional drugs.[5]

Anti-epileptics are used extensively as adjuvant analgesics in the treatment of analgesic-resistant neuropathic pain, particularly **carbamazepine** and **sodium valproate.**[6–8] **Phenytoin** was the first anti-epileptic to be used for neuropathic pain but is no longer used much.[9] Although generally not used for *nociceptive* pain, **phenytoin**, **lamotrigine** and **gabapentin** have a demonstrable antinociceptive/analgesic effect.[10,11]

The pharmacokinetic details of anti-epileptics are summarised in Table 4.15.

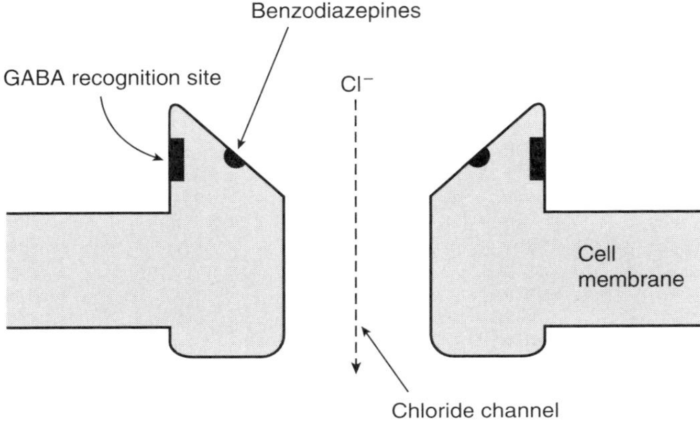

Figure 4.5 Diagram of GABA (inhibitory) receptor-channel complex.[1]

Box 4.1 Mechanisms of action of some anti-epileptics

Non-synaptic action
Sodium-channel blockers ('membrane stabilisers'):

- carbamazepine
- lamotrigine
- phenytoin

Presynaptic action

- carbamazepine
- gabapentin
- lamotrigine
- phenytoin
- sodium valproate

Increased release of GABA:

- sodium valproate

Postsynaptic action
Activation of inhibitory receptor-channel complex (Figure 4.5):

- benzodiazepines (via receptor)
- phenobarbital (activates chloride channel)
- sodium valproate (? GABA agonist)

Perisynaptic action
Inhibition of GABA transaminase:

- vigabatrin

Interactions

Interactions between anti-epileptics are complex and may enhance toxicity without a corresponding increase in anti-epileptic effect. Interactions are generally caused by hepatic enzyme induction or inhibition (Box 4.J). These interactions are highly variable and unpredictable. Plasma monitoring is therefore often advisable with combination therapy.

Table 4.15 Pharmacokinetics of anti-epileptics

Drug	*Bio-availability PO (%)*	T_{max} *(h)*	*Plasma binding (%)*	*Plasma halflife (h)*
Carbamazepine	80	4–8	75	8–24
Clobazam	100	0.5–2	85	10–30
Clonazepam	80–100	1–4	80–90	30–40
Diazepam	80–100	1–3	95–98	24–48
Gabapentin	60[a]	2–3	0	6
Lamotrigine	95–100	1–3	56	23–36
Phenobarbital	95–100	4–12	50	72–144
Phenytoin	90–95	4–8	90	9–40[a]
Sodium valproate	100	1–2[b]	90	7–17
Vigabatrin	80–90	1	0	6

a. dose or plasma concentration dependent
b. 3–8h for e/c tablets.

Box 4.J Drug interactions between anti-epileptics[a]

Carbamazepine, often lowers plasma concentration of clonazepam, lamotrigine, phenytoin (but may also raise), topiramate and sodium valproate. Sometimes lowers plasma concentration of ethosuximide, and primidone (± corresponding increase in phenobarbital concentration).

Ethosuximide, sometimes raises plasma concentration of phenytoin.

Lamotrigine, sometimes raises plasma concentration of an active metabolite of carbamazepine.

Phenobarbital or primidone, often lowers plasma concentration of carbamazepine, clonazepam, lamotrigine, phenytoin (but may also raise), and sodium valproate. Sometimes lowers plasma concentration of ethosuximide.

Phenytoin, often lowers plasma concentration of carbamazepine, clonazepam, lamotrigine, topiramate and sodium valproate. Often raises plasma concentration of phenobarbital. Sometimes lowers plasma concentration of ethosuximide, and primidone (± corresponding increase in phenobarbital concentration).

Sodium valproate, often raises plasma concentration of an active metabolite of carbamazepine and of lamotrigine, phenobarbital and phenytoin (but may also lower). Sometimes raises plasma concentration of ethosuximide, and primidone (± corresponding increase in phenobarbital concentration).

Topiramate, sometimes raises plasma concentration of phenytoin.

Vigabatrin, often lowers plasma concentration of phenytoin. Sometimes lowers plasma concentration of phenobarbital and primidone.

a. Also see Cytochrome P450, p.331.

Other important interactions include:
- effect of **carbamazepine** enhanced by **dextropropoxyphene** (in co-proxamol)
- some SSRIs increase plasma **carbamazepine** concentration; ***paroxetine*** *and* ***sertraline*** *do not*[12]
- some SSRIs increase valproic acid concentration; ***paroxetine*** *does not*[13] but no specific interaction studies have been done with **sertraline** and **sodium valproate**
- **carbamazepine** accelerates the metabolism of tricyclic antidepressants
- **sodium valproate** inhibits the metabolism of tricyclic antidepressants[14]
- effect of **tramadol** decreased by **carbamazepine**.

Cautions

Driving: patients suffering from epilepsy may drive a motor vehicle (but not a heavy goods or public service vehicle) provided that they have had a seizure-free period of one year or, if subject to seizures only while asleep, have sustained a 3-year period without seizures while awake. Patients affected by drowsiness should not drive or operate machinery.

Undesirable effects

For full list, see manufacturer's SPC.

Drug-induced psychosis has been reported with several anti-epileptics.

Carbamazepine: generally fewer adverse effects than **phenytoin** or **phenobarbital**: dose-related reversible diplopia, blurring of vision, nystagmus, dizziness, ataxia, drowsiness, headache.[15] Undesirable effects may be reduced by giving a smaller dose more often (see below).

Phenobarbital: drowsiness, mental depression, ataxia, allergic skin reactions; paradoxical excitement, restlessness and delirium in the elderly.

Phenytoin: nausea and vomiting, nystagmus, delirium, dizziness, slurred speech, ataxia, coarse facies, acne, hirsutism, gingivial hypertrophy and tenderness.

Sodium valproate: gastric irritation, nausea, tremor, ataxia, drowsiness, impaired liver function leading rarely to fatal hepatic failure.

Dose and use

Combination therapy should be avoided because:
- no evidence of additive therapeutic effect
- drug interactions
- toxicity may be enhanced.

Epilepsy

Carbamazepine is a drug of choice for simple and complex partial seizures and for tonic-clonic seizures secondary to a focal discharge. It has a wider therapeutic index than **phenytoin** and the relationship between dose and plasma concentration is linear, but monitoring of plasma concentrations may be helpful in determining optimum dose. With regular administration, the plasma halflife reduces from about 36h to 16–24h as a result of auto-induction by hepatic enzymes. Plasma concentrations increase after each dose even when a steady-state has been attained, sufficent to cause or exacerbate adverse effects.[16] It is therefore better to give **carbamazepine** in a lower dose more frequently than a higher dose less often, e.g. 50–100mg q.d.s. initially, rather than 100–200mg b.d.:
- starting dose 100–200mg o.d.–b.d.
- increments of 100–200mg every 2 weeks
- usual maximum daily dose 800–1200mg in divided doses, occasionally 1.6–2g
- m/r preparations are best taken b.d.

Neuropathic pain
- **gabapentin** is the only anti-epileptic licensed in the UK for the treatment of neuropathic pain
- **carbamazepine** is used in the same way as for epilepsy
- **sodium valproate** 200–500mg o.n. initially, increasing if necessary to 1g daily[17,18]
- **phenytoin** is now rarely prescribed for pain relief.

Terminal agitation

Phenobarbital is needed on rare occasions for terminal anguish not responding to CSCI of **midazolam** 60mg and *either* **haloperidol** 30mg/24h *or* **levomepromazine** (methotrimeprazine) 200mg/24h:
- dilute 200mg/1ml (in propylene glycol) injection to 10ml with WFI
- give a stat dose of 100–200mg IV
- then 600–1200mg/24h CSCI.

Also used as an anti-epileptic in patients who cannot swallow but in whom sedation with **midazolam** is inappropriate:
- if a stat dose is indicated, give 100mg SC/IM
- then 200–400mg/24h CSCI.

Stopping anti-epileptics

Abrupt cessation of long-term anti-epileptic therapy, particularly barbiturates and benzodiazepines, should be avoided because rebound seizures may be precipitated. If it is decided to discontinue anti-epileptic therapy, it should be done *slowly over six months or more* (Table 4.16). In adults the risk of relapse on stopping treatment is 40–50%.[19] Substituting one anti-epileptic drug regimen for another should also be done cautiously, withdrawing the first drug only when the new regimen has been introduced.

Table 4.16 Recommended monthly reductions of anti-epileptics[20]

Drug	*Reduction*
Carbamazepine	100mg
Clobazam	10mg
Clonazepam	0.5mg
Ethosuximide	250mg
Gabapentin	400mg
Lamotrigine	25mg
Phenobarbital	15mg
Phenytoin	50mg
Sodium valproate	200mg
Topiramate	25mg
Vigabatrin	500mg

Supply

Carbamazepine (non-proprietary)
Tablets 100mg, 200mg, 400mg, 28 days @ 200mg b.d. = £3.00.

Tegretol® (Cephalon 0800 783 4869)
Tablets 100mg, 200mg, 400mg, 28 days @ 200mg b.d. = £3.00.
Tablets (chewable) 100mg, 200mg, 28 days @ 200mg b.d. = £6.59.
Oral solution (sugar-free) 100mg/5ml, 28 days @ 200mg b.d. = £12.81.
Suppositories 125mg (equivalent to 100mg PO), 250mg (equivalent to 200mg PO), 28 days @ 250mg b.d. = £141.12.

Modified-release
Tegretol® Retard (Cephalon 0800 783 4869)
Tablets m/r 200mg, 400mg, 28 days @ 200mg b.d. = £5.26.

Teril® CR (Taro 01279 859100)
Tablets m/r 200mg, 400mg, 28 days @ 200mg b.d. = £3.85.

Timonil® Retard (CP 01978 661261)
Tablets m/r 200mg, 400mg, 28 days @ 200mg b.d. = £4.76.

Phenobarbital (non-proprietary)
Injection 200mg/ml, 1ml amp = £1.57.

Phenytoin (non-proprietary)
Capsules **phenytoin sodium** 50mg, 100mg, 28 days @ 100mg b.d. = £1.57.
Tablets **phenytoin sodium** 100mg, 28 days @ 100mg b.d. = £3.39.
Injection **phenytoin sodium** 50mg/ml, 5ml amp = £3.63.

Epanutin® (Pfizer 01304 616161)
Capsules **phenytoin sodium** 50mg, 100mg, 300mg, 28 days @ 100mg b.d. = £1.57.
Tablets (chewable) phenytoin 50mg, 28 days @ 100mg b.d. = £6.16.
Oral suspension phenytoin 30mg/5ml, 28 days @ 90mg b.d. = £5.96 (*phenytoin 90mg/15ml =* ***phenytoin sodium*** *100mg capsules or tablets*).
Injection **phenytoin sodium** 50mg/ml, 5ml amp = £4.07.

Sodium valproate (non-proprietary)
Tablets e/c 200mg, 500mg, 28 days @ 500mg o.n. = £4.14.
Oral solution 200mg/5ml, 28 days @ 500mg o.n. = £6.37.

Epilim® (Sanofi-Synthelabo 01483 505515)
Tablets (crushable) 100mg, 28 days @ 500mg o.n. = £5.46.
Tablets e/c 200mg, 500mg, 28 days @ 500mg o.n. = £4.49.
Oral solution 200mg/5ml, 28 days @ 500mg o.n. = £6.87.
Oral syrup 200mg/5ml, 28 days @ 500mg o.n. = £6.87.

Modified-release
Epilim® Chrono (Sanofi-Synthelabo 01483 505515)
Tablets m/r 200mg, 300mg, 500mg, 28 days @ 500mg o.n. = £5.66.

1 Richens A (1991) The basis of the treatment of epilepsy: neuropharmacology. In: M Dam (ed) *A Practical Approach to Epilepsy*. Pergamon Press, Oxford, pp.75–85.
2 Meldrum B (1996) Update on the mechanism of action of antiepileptic drugs. *Epilepsia*. **37 (suppl 6)**: S6–S11.
3 Macdonald R and Greenfield L (1997) Mechanisms of action of new antiepileptic drugs. *Current Opinion in Neurology*. **10**: 121–128.
4 Moshe S (2000) Mechanisms of action of anticonvulsant agents. *Neurology*. **55 (suppl 1)**: S32–S40.
5 Chadwick D (1999) The use of new antiepileptic drugs. *Journal of the Royal College of Physicians London*. **33**: 328–332.
6 Hansen H (1999) Treatment of chronic pain with antiepileptic drugs. *Southern Medical Journal*. **92**: 642–649.
7 Backonja M-M (2000) Anticonvulsants (antineuropathics) for neuropathic pain syndromes. *Clinical Journal of Pain*. **16**: S67–S72.
8 Collins S *et al.* (2000) Antidepressants and anticonvulsants for diabetic neuropathy and post-herpetic neuralgia: a quantitative systematic review. *Journal of Pain and Symptom Management*. **20**: 449–458.
9 McCleane G (1999) Intravenous infusion of phenytoin relieves neuropathic pain: a randomized, double-blinded, placebo-controlled, crossover study. *Anesthesia and Analgesia*. **89**: 985–988.
10 Webb J and Kamali F (1998) Analgesic effects of lamotrigine and phenytoin on cold-induced pain: a crossover placebo-controlled study in healthy volunteers. *Pain*. **76**: 357–363.
11 Lu Y and Westlund K (1999) Gabapentin attenuates nociceptive behaviors in an acute arthritis model in rats. *Pharmacology*. **290**: 214–219.
12 *Invicta Pharmaceuticals Study 226, data on file.*
13 Andersen B *et al.* (1991) No influence of the antidepressant paroxetine on carbamazepine, valproate and phenytoin. *Epilepsy Research*. **10**: 201–204.
14 Fu C *et al.* (1994) Valproate/nortriptyline interaction. *Journal of Clinical Psychopharmacology*. **14**: 205–206.
15 Hoppener R *et al.* (1980) Correlation between daily fluctuations of carbamazepine serum levels and intermittent side effects. *Epilepsia*. **21**: 341–350.
16 Tomson T (1984) Interdosage fluctuations in plasma carbamazepine concentration determine intermittent side effects. *Archives of Neurology*. **41**: 830–834.
17 Budd K (1989) Sodium valproate in the treatment of pain. In: D Chadwick (ed) *Fourth International Symposium on Sodium Valproate and Epilepsy*. Royal Society of Medicine, London, pp.213–216.
18 Twycross R and Wilcock A (2001) *Symptom Management in Advanced Cancer* (3e). Radcliffe Medical Press, Oxford.
19 Hopkins A and Shorvon S (1995) Definitions and epidemiology of epilepsy. In: A Hopkins *et al.* (eds) *Epilepsy*. Chapman & Hall, London, pp.1–24.
20 Chadwick D (1995) The withdrawal of antiepileptic drugs. In: A Hopkins *et al.* (eds) *Epilepsy*. Chapman & Hall, London, pp.215–220.

GABAPENTIN — BNF 4.8.1

Class: Anti-epileptic.

Indications: Adjunctive treatment for partial seizures with or without secondary generalisation;[1,2] neuropathic pain of any cause.[3–6]

Contra-indications: Absence seizures (may worsen).

Pharmacology

Gabapentin is a chemical analogue of GABA but does not act as a GABA-receptor agonist. It binds to a specific site in the CNS, gabapentin-binding protein, and interacts with $\alpha 2\delta$ calcium channels in the CNS.[7] It increases GABA synthesis and release but its exact mechanism of action is not fully understood. Absorption is by a saturable mechanism and bio-availability is halved as the dose increases. Antacids containing **aluminium** or **magnesium** reduce gabapentin bio-availability by 10–25%. It is not protein-bound and freely crosses the blood-brain barrier. It is excreted unchanged by the kidneys and cumulates in renal impairment. The halflife increases to 50h when creatinine clearance is <30ml/min and to over 5 days in anuria. In contrast to many other anti-epileptics, gabapentin is well tolerated and has few drug interactions. **Cimetidine** impairs the renal excretion of gabapentin but not to a clinically important extent. It does not interact with anti-retroviral antibiotics. Gabapentin is increasingly used for neuropathic pain.[3–6,8,9] However, there is no evidence that it is more effective than older anti-epileptics.[10] Although in an open study in diabetic neuropathy, gabapentin provided better relief than **amitriptyline,**[11] in a randomised controlled trial no difference was detected.[12] In motor neurone disease (amyotrophic lateral sclerosis), gabapentin 800mg t.d.s slowed decrease in arm strength marginally ($p > 0.5$) over a 6-month period.[13] It reduces spasticity and muscle spasm in multiple sclerosis.[14] There is a report of gabapentin abolishing opioid-related myoclonus.[15]
Bio-availability PO 100mg, 74%; 300mg, 60%; 1600mg, 35%.
Onset of action 1–3h.
Time to peak plasma concentration 2–3h PO.
Plasma halflife 5–7h, increasing to 2–5 days in severe renal failure.
Duration of action probably 8–12h.

Cautions

Renal impairment; false positive readings for urinary protein with Ames N-Multistix SG®; aluminium- and magnesium-containing compounds reduce bio-availability.

Undesirable effects

For full list, see manufacturer's SPC.
Common: Drowsiness, dizziness, ataxia, fatigue.
Uncommon: Headache, nystagmus, tremor, anxiety, diplopia, amblyopia, dysarthria, amnesia, weight gain, dyspepsia, rhinitis, pharyngitis, myalgia, arthralgia, gynaecomastia.[16]

Dose and use

Gabapentin should be given at least 2h after antacids containing **aluminium** or **magnesium**. For both epilepsy and neuropathic pain, a rapid upward titration is suggested in the SPC (Table 4.17). However, a slower titration of the dose of gabapentin is advisable in elderly patients, those with renal impairment (see below) or if receiving other CNS depressant drugs. If required the capsules can be opened and the contents mixed with water, fruit juice, apple sauce, etc.[17] The maintenance dose of gabapentin should be adjusted in adults with renal impairment (Table 4.18).

Table 4.17 Dose escalation for gabapentin

Rapid		*Slow*	
Day 1	300mg o.n	Day 1	100mg t.d.s
Day 2	300mg b.d	Day 7	300mg t.d.s
Day 3	300mg t.d.s	Day 14	600mg t.d.s
Day 4	400mg t.d.s	Day 21	900mg t.d.s
Then add 300mg/day as needed up to 600–1200mg t.d.s		Day 28	1200mg t.d.s

Table 4.18 Dose adjustment of initial maintenance dose in renal impairment

Creatinine clearance (ml/min)	*Dose (mg)*
>60	400mg t.d.s.
31–60	300mg b.d.
15–30	300mg o.d.
<15	300mg o.d. alternate days
Haemodialysis	loading dose of 300–400mg followed by 200–300mg after every 4h of dialysis

Stopping gabapentin

To avoid precipitating seizures or pain, gabapentin should be withdrawn gradually over at least 1 week. Also see Stopping anti-epileptics, p.123.

Supply

Neurontin (Pfizer 01304 616161)
Capsules 100mg, 300mg, 400mg, 28 days @ 300mg t.d.s. = £44.52.
Tablets 600mg, 800mg, 28 days @ 600mg t.d.s. = £89.04.

1 Anonymous (1994) Gabapentin – a new antiepileptic drug. *Drug and Therapeutics Bulletin.* **32**: 29–30.
2 Chadwick D (1994) Gabapentin. *Lancet.* **343**: 89–91.
3 Caraceni A *et al.* (1999) Gabapentin as an adjuvant to opioid analgesia for neuropathic cancer pain. *Journal of Pain and Symptom Management.* **17**: 441–445.
4 Rosner H *et al.* (1996) Gabapentin adjunctive therapy in neuropathic pain states. *Clinical Journal of Pain.* **12**: 56–68.
5 Schachter S and Sauter M (1996) Treatment of central pain with gabapentin: case reports. *Journal of Epilepsy.* **9**: 223–225.
6 Segal A and Rodorf G (1996) Gabapentin for the novel treatment of post-herpetic neuralgia. *Neurology.* **46**: 1175–1176.
7 Taylor C *et al.* (1998) A summary of mechanistic hypotheses of gabapentin pharmacology. *Epilepsy and Research.* **29**: 233–249.
8 Backonja M *et al.* (1998) Gabapentin for the symptomatic treatment of painful neuropathy in patients with diabetes mellitus: a randomized controlled trial. *Journal of the American Medical Association.* **280**: 1831–1836.
9 Rowbotham M *et al.* (1998) Gabapentin for the treatment of postherpetic neuralgia. *Journal of the American Medical Association.* **280**: 1837–1842.
10 Collins S *et al.* (2000) Antidepressants and anticonvulsants for diabetic neuropathy and post-herpetic neuralgia: a quantitative systematic review. *Journal of Pain and Symptom Management.* **20**: 449–458.
11 Dallocchio C *et al.* (2000) Gabapentin vs. amitriptyline in painful diabetic neuropathy: an open-label pilot study. *Journal of Pain and Symptom Management.* **20**: 280–285.
12 Morello CM *et al.* (1999) Randomized double-blind study comparing the efficacy of gabapentin with amitriptyline on diabetic peripheral neuropathic pain. *Archives of Internal Medicine.* **159**: 1931–1937.
13 Miller R *et al.* (1996) Placebo-controlled trial of gabapentin in patients with amyotrophic lateral sclerosis. Western Amyotrophic Lateral Sclerosis Study Group. *Neurology.* **47**: 1383–1388.
14 Bryans J and Wustrow D (1999) 3-substituted GABA analogs with central nervous system activity: a review. *Medicinal Research Reviews.* **19**: 149–177.
15 Mercadante S *et al.* (2001) Gabapentin for opioid-related myoclonus in cancer patients. *Support Care Cancer.* **9**: 205–206.
16 Zylicz Z (2000) Painful gynecomastia: an unusual toxicity of gabapentin? *Journal of Pain and Symptom Management.* **20**: 2–3.
17 Gidal B *et al.* (1998) Gabapentin absorption: effect of mixing with foods of varying macronutrient composition. *Annals of Pharmacotherapy.* **32**: 405–409.

ORPHENADRINE BNF 4.9.2

Class: Antimuscarinic antiparkinsonian.

Indications: Parkinson's disease, parkinsonism, †sialorrhoea (drooling), †extrapyramidal dystonic reactions.

Contra-indications: Glaucoma, prostatic hypertrophy, tardive dyskinesia (see Drug-induced movement disorders, p.339).

Pharmacology

Orphenadrine and other antimuscarinic antiparkinsonian drugs are used primarily in Parkinson's disease. They are less effective than **levodopa** in established Parkinson's disease although they often usefully supplement its action. Patients with mild symptoms, particularly where tremor predominates, may be treated initially with antimuscarinics (alone or with **selegiline**), **levodopa** being added or substituted as symptoms progress. Antimuscarinics exert their antiparkinsonian effect by correcting the relative central cholinergic excess which occurs in parkinsonism as a result of dopamine deficiency. In most patients their effects are only moderate, reducing tremor and rigidity to some extent but without significant action on bradykinesia. They exert a synergistic effect when used with **levodopa** and are also useful in reducing sialorrhoea.

Antimuscarinics reduce the symptoms of drug-induced parkinsonism (seen mainly with antipsychotics) but there is no justification for giving them prophylactically. *Tardive dyskinesia is not improved by the antimuscarinic drugs and may be made worse.* No major differences exist between antimuscarinics but orphenadrine sometimes has a mood-elevating effect. Some people tolerate one antimuscarinic better than another. **Procyclidine** and **benzatropine** may be given parenterally and are effective emergency treatment for severe acute drug-induced dystonic reactions (see Drug-induced movement disorders, p.339).

Bio-availability no data.

Onset of action 30–60min.

Time to peak plasma concentration 2–4h PO.

Plasma halflife 18h.

Duration of action 12–24h.

Cautions

Hepatic or renal impairment, cardiovascular disease. Avoid abrupt discontinuation.

Undesirable effects

For full list, see manufacturer's SPC.

Antimuscarinic effects (see p.4). Nervousness, euphoria, insomnia occasionally. In a psychotic patient receiving a phenothiazine, the addition of orphenadrine to reverse a drug-induced movement disorder may precipitate a toxic confusional psychosis as a result of the summation of antimuscarinic effects.

Dose and use

- starting dose 50mg b.d.–t.d.s.
- increase by 50mg every 3 days if necessary
- maximum recommended daily dose 400mg.

Supply

Disipal® (Yamanouchi 01932 342291)
Tablets 50mg, 28 days @ 50mg t.d.s. = £2.90.

Orphenadrine (non-proprietary)
Oral solution 50mg/5ml, 28 days @ 50mg t.d.s. = £19.89.

Biorphen® (Alliance 01249 466966)
Oral solution 25mg/5ml, 28 days @ 50mg t.d.s. = £30.45.

5: ANALGESICS

PRINCIPLES OF USE OF ANALGESICS

Analgesics comprise three classes, namely non-opioid, opioid and adjuvant (Figure 5.1). The principles governing the use of analgesics are encapsulated in the WHO Method for Relief of Cancer Pain:[1,2]

'By the mouth'
'By the clock'
'By the ladder' (Figure 5.2)
'Individual dose titration'
'Use adjuvant drugs'
'Attention to detail'.

As a general rule, the combined effect of a non-opioid (particularly an NSAID) and a strong opioid should be exploited before introducing adjuvant analgesics.

Some patients require additional p.r.n. doses for episodic pain.[3] It is important to differentiate between:

- *predictable (incident) pain*, an exacerbation of pain caused by weight-bearing and activity which may or may not be associated with a background of constant (through controlled) pain at the same location[4]
- *unpredictable (unexpected) pain*, spontaneous pain unrelated to weight-bearing or activity, e.g. colic, stabbing pain associated with nerve injury

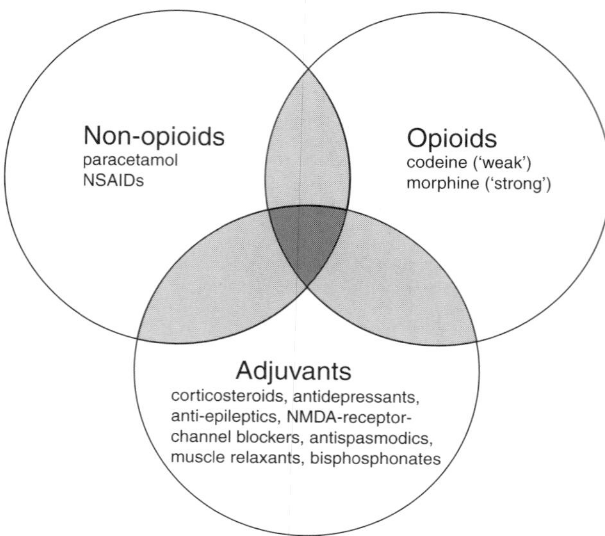

Figure 5.1 Broad-spectrum analgesia; drugs from different categories are used singly or in combination according to the type of pain and response to treatment.

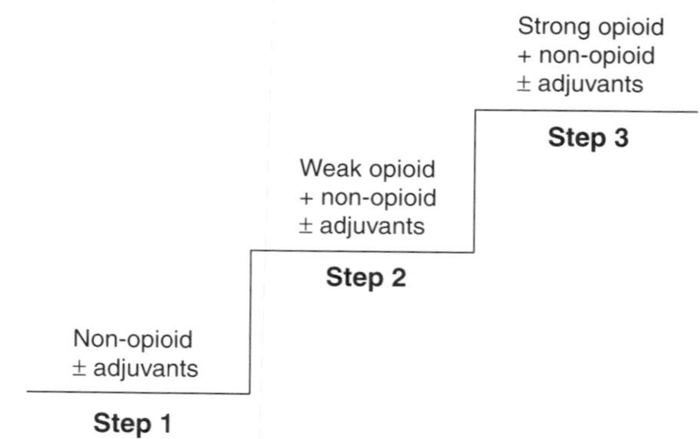

Figure 5.2 The World Health Organization 3-step analgesic ladder.[1]

- *end-of-dose failure*, occurs shortly before the next dose of regular analgesics is due; it generally responds to an increase in the analgesic dose.

If these pains occur in patients taking a regular strong opioid (see p.168), they are often called breakthrough pain.

Various strategies are used to reduce the impact of episodic pain, including the use of **morphine** and **transmucosal fentanyl** p.r.n. With **morphine** PO, in the UK and elsewhere, 1/6 of the total daily dose has been traditionally recommended. However, in some countries, smaller doses are used, e.g. 1/10 of the total daily dose. Clearly, if a patient experiences undesirable effects with 1/6 of the total daily dose, a lower dose should be considered. With **transmucosal fentanyl,** the dose is individually titrated; there is no correlation between the regular dose of **morphine** or TD **fentanyl** and p.r.n requirements.

1 World Health Organization (1986) *Cancer Pain Relief.* WHO, Geneva.
2 World Health Organization (1996) *Cancer Pain Relief: with a guide to opioid availability* (2e). WHO, Geneva.
3 Swanwick M *et al.* (2001) The prevalence of episodic pain in cancer: a survey of hospice patients on admission. *Palliative Medicine.* **15**: 9–18.
4 Douglas I *et al.* (2000) Central issues in the management of temporal variation in cancer pain. In: R Hillier *et al.* (eds) *The Effective Management of Cancer Pain.* Aesculapius Medical Press, London, pp.93–106.

ADJUVANT ANALGESICS

Adjuvant analgesics are a miscellaneous group of drugs which relieve pain in specific circumstances. They include:
- corticosteroids
- antidepressants
- anti-epileptics
- NMDA-receptor-channel blockers
- antispasmodics
- muscle relaxants
- bisphosphonates.

Corticosteroids

Corticosteroids (see p.219) are helpful for pain and weakness associated with:
- nerve root/nerve trunk compression, e.g. dexamethasone 4–8mg o.d.
- spinal cord compression, e.g. dexamethasone 12–16mg o.d.[1,2]

Corticosteroids are not helpful in pure non-cancer nerve injury pain, e.g. chronic postoperative scar pain, postherpetic neuralgia. However, with cancer-related nerve injury pain, if there is associated limb weakness a 5–7 day trial of **dexamethasone** may be beneficial.

Antidepressants and anti-epileptics

Nerve injury pains do not always respond to the combined use of an NSAID and a strong opioid.[3] Antidepressants (see p.85) and anti-epileptics (see p.120) are often of benefit.[4–7] The number needed to treat (NNT) to have one patient achieve 50% relief with tricyclics collectively is 2.4, for 'balanced' tricyclics (e.g. **amitriptyline** and **imipramine**) it is 2, whereas for SSRIs it is 7.[5,8–10] Remarkably, in one trial in which the dose of **imipramine** was titrated to achieve a combined plasma concentration of >400nM for **imipramine** and **desipramine** (the active metabolite), the NNT was 1.4.[5]

In comparison, for anti-epileptics, the NNT for **carbamazepine** in painful polyneuropathy is 3.3 and for **gabapentin** (which is specifically licensed for neuropathic pain) it is about 3.5.[7] Surprisingly, although **sodium valproate** is widely used to treat neuropathic pain, no controlled trials have been published. **Carbamazepine** has been evaluated mostly in trigeminal neuralgia but is often disappointing in other situations.[7] (For details about the use of antidepressants and anti-epileptics in the management of neuropathic pain, see their respective sections and/or individual drug monographs.)

The analgesic effect of tricyclic antidepressants may depend on several pharmacological mechanisms:
- pre-synaptic re-uptake inhibition of serotonin and noradrenaline (norepinephrine; Figure 5.3)
- postsynaptic receptor antagonism
  - α-adrenergic
  - histamine type I (H_1)
  - μ-opioid (low affinity)
- channel blockade
  - NMDA-receptor
  - sodium
  - calcium.[5]

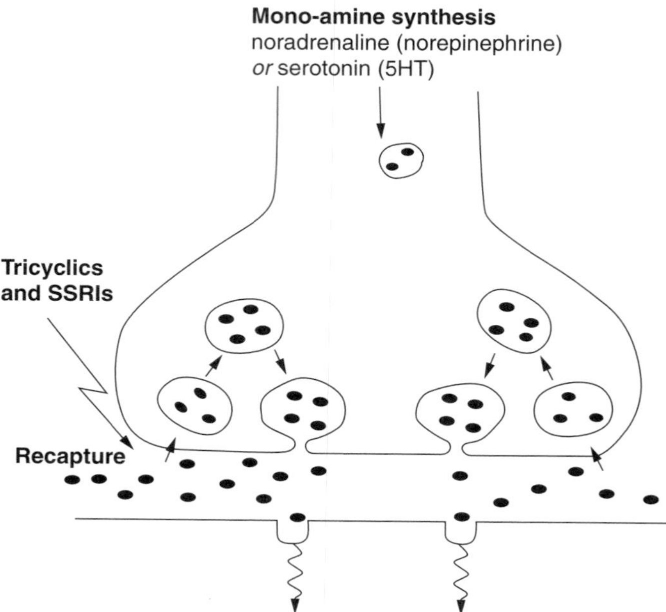

Figure 5.3 Tricyclic antidepressants and SSRIs potentiate one or other or both of the two descending spinal inhibitory pathways by blocking presynaptic re-uptake (one noradrenergic, the other serotoninergic). They also potentiate opioid analgesia by a serotoninergic mechanism in the brain stem.

Venlafaxine, a non-tricyclic antidepressant, is a relatively 'balanced' mono-amine re-uptake inhibitor in doses above 1mg/kg/24h. However, it does not possess the other properties possessed by tricyclics. It may therefore turn out to be less efficacious (bigger NNT) than **amitriptyline** and **imipramine**, despite several impressive case reports.

In contrast, some anti-epileptics act as peripheral sodium-channel blockers (Figure 5.4). Others impact mainly on the dorsal horn by inhibiting the glutamate (excitatory) system or activating the GABA (inhibitory) system, or both, in one of several ways. It is now generally agreed that gabapentin, although a structural analogue of GABA, acts principally as an $\alpha 2\delta$-type calcium channel blocker.[7] It makes sense, therefore, to combine an antidepressant with an anti-epileptic in those patients who fail to achieve satisfactory relief with either class of drug individually.

Response may also vary with the duration of the pain. For example, in postherpetic neuralgia, if **amitriptyline** is commenced within 6 months of onset, there is a response rate of about 75%, but if delayed more than 2 years the response rate drops to 25%.[11,12]

It is important to establish a practical protocol for neuropathic pain management, selecting only one or two drugs from each category of drugs (Figure 5.5).[13,14] For example, in Steps 2 and 3, **amitriptyline** 25–75mg o.n (an antidepressant) and **sodium valproate** 400–1000mg o.n. (an anti-epileptic) are often used.[15,16] Adjuvant analgesics may be effective alone in 'pure' non-cancer nerve injury pain, e.g. chronic surgical incision pain, postherpetic neuralgia. However, if the nerve injury pain is associated with an infiltrating cancer, **morphine** and an NSAID should be tried first before *adding* an antidepressant, or an anti-epileptic or both.[17–19] About 90% of patients with nerve injury pain respond to the systematic use of non-opioids, opioids and adjuvant analgesics.[3] The remainder require spinal analgesia (e.g. **morphine** + **bupivacaine** ± **clonidine**) or a neurolytic procedure to obtain adequate relief. Some patients derive benefit from other non-drug measures, e.g. TENS.

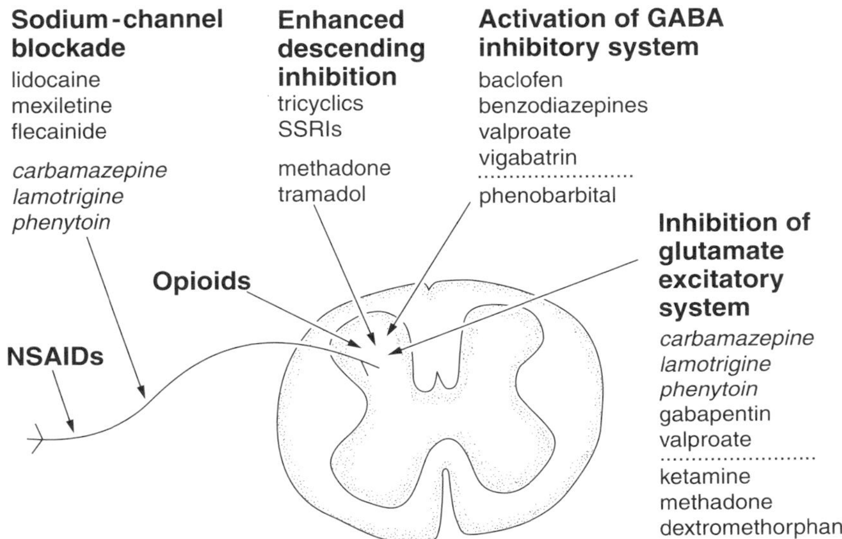

Figure 5.4 Primary sites of action of analgesics and adjuvant analgesics on peripheral nerves and the dorsal horn of the spinal cord. Drugs in italics act both peripherally and centrally. Drugs below the dotted lines are channel blockers at their respective receptor-channel complex.

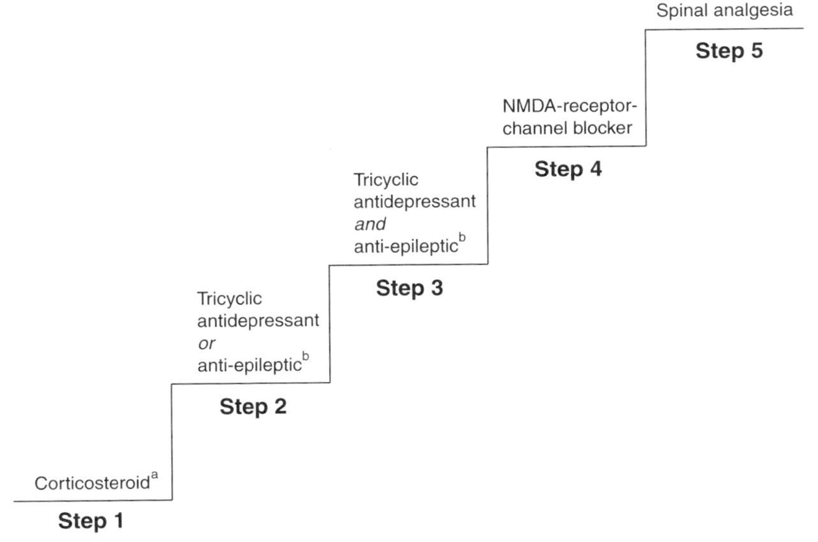

Figure 5.5 Adjuvant analgesics for neuropathic pain. If caused by cancer, use only if the pain does not respond to the combined use of a NSAID and a strong opioid.

a. important when neuropathic pain is associated with limb weakness
b. some centres use mexiletine, a local anaesthetic congener and cardiac anti-arrhythmic drug which blocks sodium channels, as an alternative to an anti-epileptic.[13,14]

Relief is not an 'all or none' phenomenon. The crucial first step in many cases is to help the patient obtain a good night's sleep. The second is to reduce pain intensity and allodynia associated with nerve injury pain to a bearable level during the day. Initially there may be marked diurnal variation in relief, with more prolonged periods with less or no pain rather than a decrease in worst pain intensity round-the-clock. The patient should be warned that major benefit often takes a week or more to manifest, although improvement in sleep should occur immediately. Undesirable drug effects are often a limiting therapeutic factor.

NMDA-receptor-channel blockers

NMDA-receptor-channel blockers are most commonly used when neuropathic pain does not respond well to standard analgesics together with an antidepressant and an anti-epileptic. They have also been used in inflammatory pain, e.g. severe mucositis.[20] NMDA-receptor-channel blockers include:

- **ketamine** (see p.289)[21–23]
- **methadone** (see p.194)[24,25]
- **amantadine**.[26,27]

As with other classes of drugs, NMDA-receptor-channel blockers are not always beneficial. Controlled data show significant but modest benefit with **amantidine** 200mg IV over 3h, whereas earlier case reports indicated dramatic benefit.[27,28]

Antispasmodics

Antispasmodics is the term given to antimuscarinics used to relieve visceral distension pain and colic. In advanced cancer, there is little place for 'weak' antispasmodics such as **dicycloverine** (dicyclomine) and **mebeverine**. In the UK, **hyoscine butylbromide** (see p.5) is widely regarded as the antispasmodic of choice. In countries where **hyoscine butylbromide** is not available, **glycopyrronium** (see p.287) can be substituted.

Muscle relaxants

For painful muscle spasm (cramp) and myofascial pain, the correct approach is:

- explanation and physical therapy (local heat, massage)
- **diazepam** (see p.69) and relaxation therapy
- injection of trigger points with local anaesthetic and a corticosteroid, e.g. **bupivacaine** 0.5% and depot **methylprednisolone** 80mg).[29,30]

*However severe, **morphine** is ineffective for the relief of cramp and trigger point pains.*

Bisphosphonates

Bisphosphonates (see p.215) are osteoclast inhibitors and are used to relieve metastatic bone pain which persists despite analgesics and radiotherapy ± orthopaedic surgery. Published data relate mainly to breast cancer and myeloma; benefit is also seen with other cancers.[31–37] About 50% of patients benefit, typically in 7–14 days, and this may last for 2–3 months. Benefit may be seen only after a second treatment but, if there is no response after two treatments, nothing is gained by further use.[37] In those who respond, continue to treat p.r.n. for as long as there is benefit.

---

1 Vecht C *et al.* (1989) Initial bolus of conventional versus high-dose dexamethasone in metastatic spinal cord compression. *Neurology.* **39**: 1255–1257.

2 Loblaw D and Laperriere N (1998) Emergency treatment of malignant extradural spinal cord compression: an evidence-based guideline. *Journal of Clinical Oncology.* **16**: 1613–1624.

3 Grond S *et al.* (1999) Assessment and treatment of neuropathic cancer pain following WHO guidelines. *Pain.* **79**: 15–20.

4 Anonymous (2000) Drug treatment of neuropathic pain. *Drug and Therapeutics Bulletin.* **38**: 89–93.

5 Sindrup S and Jensen T (2001) Antidepressants in the treatment of neuropathic pain. In: PT Hansson *et al.* (eds) *Neuropathic Pain: pathophysiology and treatment.* IASP, Seattle, pp. 169–183.

6 Collins S *et al.* (2000) Antidepressants and anticonvulsants for diabetic neuropathy and post-herpetic neuralgia: a quantitative systematic review. *Journal of Pain and Symptom Management.* **20**: 449–458.

7 Backonja M (2001) Anticonvulsants and antiarrhythmics in the treatment of neuropathic pain syndromes. In: PT Hansson *et al.* (eds) *Neuropathic Pain: pathophysiology and treatment.* IASP, Seattle, pp. 185–201.
8 Onghena P and Houdenhove BV (1992) Antidepressant-induced analgesia in chronic nonmalignant pain: a meta-analysis of 39 placebo-controlled trials. *Pain.* **49**: 205–219.
9 Sindrup S and Jensen T (1999) Efficacy of pharmacological treatments of neuropathic pain: an update and effect related to mechanism of drug action. *Pain.* **83**: 389–400.
10 Ansari A (2000) The efficacy of newer antidepressants in the treatment of chronic pain: a review of current literature. *Harvard Review Psychiatry.* **7**: 257–277.
11 Bowsher D (1997) The effects of pre-emptive treatment of postherpetic neuralgia with amitriptyline: a randomized, double-blind, placebo-controlled trial. *Journal of Pain and Symptom Management.* **13**: 327–331.
12 Bowsher D (2000) The important time parameter is missing. Comment on Sindrup and Jensen 1999. *Pain.* **88**: 313.
13 Chabal C *et al.* (1992) The use of oral mexiletine for the treatment of pain after peripheral nerve injury. *Anaesthesiology.* **76**: 513–517.
14 Chong S *et al.* (1997) Pilot study evaluating local anesthetics administered systemically for treatment of pain in patients with advanced cancer. *Journal of Pain and Symptom Management.* **13**: 112–117.
15 McQuay H *et al.* (1995) Anticonvulsant drugs for management of pain: a systematic review. *British Medical Journal.* **311**: 1047–1052.
16 McQuay H *et al.* (1996) A systematic review of antidepressants in neuropathic pain. *Pain.* **68**: 217–227.
17 Dellemijn P *et al.* (1994) Medical therapy of malignant nerve pain. A randomised double-blind explanatory trial with naproxen versus slow-release morphine. *European Journal of Cancer.* **30A**: 1244–1250.
18 Ripamonti C *et al.* (1996) Continuous subcutaneous infusion of ketorolac in cancer neuropathic pain unresponsive to opioid and adjuvant drugs. A case report. *Tumori.* **82**: 413–415.
19 Dellemijn P (1999) Are opioids effective in relieving neuropathic pain? *Pain.* **80**: 453–462.
20 Jackson K *et al.* (2001) 'Burst' ketamine for refractory cancer pain: an open-label audit of 39 patients. *Journal of Pain and Symptom Management.* **22**: 834–842.
21 Enarson M *et al.* (1999) Clinical experience with oral ketamine. *Journal of Pain and Symptom Management.* **17**: 384–386.
22 Fine P (1999) Low-dose ketamine in the management of opioid nonresponsive terminal cancer. *Journal of Pain and Symptom Management.* **17**: 296–300.
23 Finlay I (1999) Ketamine and its role in cancer pain. *Pain Reviews.* **6**: 303–313.
24 Gannon C (1997) The use of methadone in the care of the dying. *European Journal of Palliative Care.* **4**: 152–158.
25 Morley J and Makin M (1998) The use of methadone in cancer pain poorly responsive to other opioids. *Pain Reviews.* **5**: 51–58.
26 Kornhuber J *et al.* (1995) Therapeutic brain concentration of the NMDA receptor antagonist amantadine. *Neuropharmacology.* **34**: 713–721.
27 Pud D *et al.* (1998) The NMDA receptor antagonist amantadine reduces surgical neuropathic pain in cancer patients: a double blind, randomized, placebo controlled trial. *Pain.* **75**: 349–354.
28 Eisenberg E and Pud D (1998) Can patients with chronic neuropathic pain be cured by acute administration of the NMDA receptor antagonist amantadine? *Pain.* **74**: 337–339.
29 Rowell NP (1988) Intralesional methylprednisolone for rib metastases: an alternative to radiotherapy? *Palliative Medicine.* **2**: 153–155.
30 Twycross R (1994) *Pain Relief in Advanced Cancer.* Churchill Livingstone, Edinburgh, pp.442–443.
31 Ernst OS *et al.* (1992) A double-blind, crossover trial of intravenous clodronate in metastatic bone pain. *Journal of Pain and Symptom Management.* **7**: 4–11.
32 Vorreuther R (1993) Biphosphonates as an adjunct to palliative therapy of bone metastases from prostatic carcinoma. A pilot study on clodronate. *British Journal of Urology.* **72**: 792–795.
33 Robertson AG *et al.* (1995) Effect of oral clodronate on metastatic bone pain: a double-blind, placebo-controlled study. *Journal of Clinical Oncology.* **13**: 2427–2430.

34 Ernst D *et al.* (1997) A randomized, controlled trial of intravenous clodronate in patients with metastatic bone disease and pain. *Journal of Pain and Symptom Management.* **13**: 319–326.
35 Hillner B *et al.* (2000) American Society of Clinical Oncology guideline on the role of bisphosphonates in breast cancer. American Society of Clinical Oncology Bisphosphonates Expert Panel. *Journal of Clinical Oncology.* **18**: 1378–1391.
36 Lipton A *et al.* (2000) Pamidronate prevents skeletal complications and is effective palliative treatment in women with breast carcinoma and osteolytic bone metastases. *Cancer.* **88**: 1082–1090.
37 Mannix K *et al.* (2000) Using bisphosphonates to control the pain of bone metastases: evidence-based guidelines for palliative care. *Palliative Medicine.* **14**: 455–461.

PARACETAMOL — BNF 4.7.1

Class: Non-opioid analgesic.

Indications: Mild-to-moderate pain, migraine, headache, pyrexia.

Pharmacology

Paracetamol (acetaminophen USA) is a synthetic centrally-acting non-opioid analgesic. Although some studies have suggested a peripheral action,[1,2] most evidence points to a purely central effect.[3] Because it is centrally acting, it has been suggested that paracetamol should not be used with opioids.[4] However, the central mechanisms of paracetamol and that of opioids are distinct, and the likelihood of an additive effect should not be discounted. Paracetamol inhibits the production of CNS PGs,[5,6] and thereby helps to counter the central sensitisation which occurs as a consequence of inflammation.[7,8] It also interacts with the L-arginine-nitric oxide, serotonin and opioid systems.[9,10] Like NSAIDs, paracetamol is antipyretic; unlike NSAIDs, it has no peripheral anti-inflammatory effect. Paracetamol can be taken by 2/3 of patients who are hypersensitive to aspirin.[11] Paracetamol metabolism is age and dose-dependent. Only 2–5% of a therapeutic dose of paracetamol is excreted unchanged in the urine; the remainder is metabolised mainly by the liver. At therapeutic dosages, >80% of paracetamol is metabolised to glucuronide and sulphate conjugates. About 10% is converted by cytochrome P450-dependent hepatic mixed-function oxidase to a highly reactive metabolite. In turn, this metabolite is rapidly inactivated by conjugation with glutathione and excreted in the urine after further metabolism. The recommended dose limit for paracetamol of 4 g/day is more traditional than scientific. However, although a single therapeutic dose of 1.5–2g is not harmful, the effects of taking paracetamol at >4g/day over a long period could be dangerous in debilitated patients. Little is known about the relationship between paracetamol dose and body weight; 1g equates to 25mg/kg in a 40kg person, but only 12.5mg/kg in someone weighing 80kg. The clinical significance of this is not clear. Hepatotoxicity and acute liver failure have been reported in patients treating themselves for dental pain, notably in a 21-year old man who took >9g/day for 4 days.[12] Animal data suggest that a high dose may be more toxic when divided than when given as a single dose.

Single overdoses of paracetamol below 125mg/kg (7.5g or 15 tablets in a 60kg person) are unlikely to result in hepatic damage. At twice this dose, the probability of hepatic damage is around 50%, but the individual may remain well. A dose of 500mg/kg (30g or 60 tablets in a 60kg person) is almost certain to produce life-threatening liver damage. Hepatotoxicity results from the production of a toxic metabolite, N-acetyl-p-benzoquinoneimine (NAPQI; Figure 5.6). Normally this is detoxified by conjugation with glutathione but, in paracetamol overdose, the body's glutathione store becomes exhausted and the resulting large quantity of NAPQI reacts with liver parenchymal cells, leading to cell death. Overdose can be treated using a glutathione precursor, either IV **N-acetylcysteine** or oral **methionine**. **Acetylcysteine** should ideally be given within 15h of the overdose, when it prevents NAPQI from reacting with liver cell proteins, but may well be beneficial up to 72h because it has a protective effect against apoptosis (programmed cell death).[13]

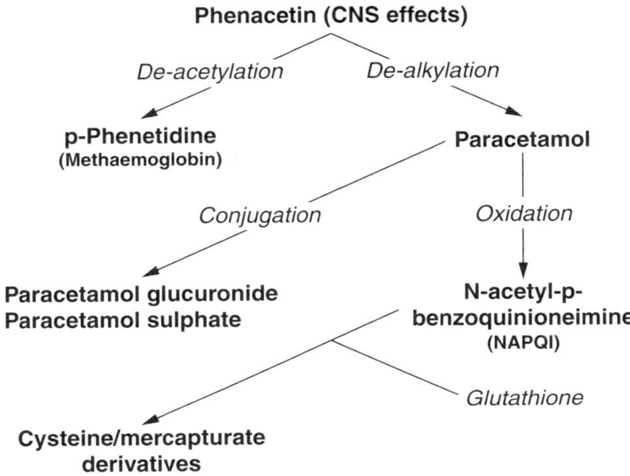

Figure 5.6 Metabolism of phenacetin and paracetamol.

Factors which may place a patient at increased risk of hepatotoxicity from an overdose include:

- old age
- poor nutritional status
- fasting/anorexia

} lower glutathione stores[14]

- concurrent use of enzyme-inducing drugs, e.g. **phenobarbital**
- chronic alcohol abuse.[15]

Acute alcohol intake does not increase the risk of hepatotoxicity. In fact, because alcohol and paracetamol compete for the same oxidative enzymes, acute alcohol consumption at the time of a paracetamol overdose may be protective. In patients on **warfarin**, a regular intake of paracetamol ≥1300mg/day for a week may result in an increase in the INR to >6, and necessitate a reduction in the dose of concurrently administered coumarin anticoagulants.[16,17] However, a total weekly dose of paracetamol of ≤2g does not affect the INR. The underlying mechanism is not clear, but may relate to interference with the hepatic synthesis of factors II, VII, IX and X.

Although there are conflicting views, there is no hard evidence that paracetamol precipitates asthma in asthmatics.[18,19] However, in patients with a history of aspirin/NSAID-induced asthma, about 5% will develop bronchospasm after taking paracetamol.[20]

Bio-availability 60% after 500mg PO, 90% after 1g PO; PR is about 2/3 of PO, but is higher with two 500mg suppositories than with one 1g suppository.

Onset of action 15–30min.

Time to peak plasma concentration 40–60min.

Plasma halflife 2–4h.

Duration of action 4–6h.

Cautions

In people with a history of aspirin/NSAID-induced asthma, give a test dose of 250mg (half a tablet) and observe for 2–3h. If no undesirable effects, paracetamol can safely be used in standard doses. Severe hepatic impairment, particularly if associated with alcohol dependence and malnutrition.

Undesirable effects

For full list, see manufacturer's SPC.

Overdose causes hepatic damage and, less frequently, renal damage.[21]

Rare: rash, cholestatic jaundice,[22,23] acute pancreatitis after prolonged use, thrombocytopenia, agranulocytosis, anaphylaxis.[24–26]

Dose and use

Typical oral dose regimens range from 500–1000mg q6h–q4h: *the latter dose exceeds the 4g maximum daily dose recommended in the BNF but is sometimes given q4h with normal-release morphine.* Paracetamol is available in several combination preparations with weak opioids.

Supply

Paracetamol (non-proprietary)
Tablets 500mg, 28 days @ 1g q.d.s. = £1.68.
Tablets dispersible 500mg, 28 days @ 1g q.d.s. = £10.53.
Capsules and ***caplets*** 500mg are available OTC; many patients find these easier to swallow.
Oral suspension 120mg/5ml, 250mg/5ml, 28 days @ 1g q.d.s. = £16.35.
Suppositories 500mg, 28 days @ 1g q.d.s. = £213.47.
Injection 150mg/2ml ampoules for IM/IV use, 10 ampoules = £20. (Unlicensed, available as a named patient supply from IDIS 020 8410 0800, see Special orders and named patient supplies, p.349)

Permission from the MCA to import this product can take up to 28 days.

1 Lim R *et al.* (1964) Site of action of narcotic and non-narcotic analgesics determined by blocking bradykinin-evoked visceral pain. *Archives Internationales de Pharmacodynamie et de Therapie.* **152**: 25–58.
2 Moore U *et al.* (1992) The efficacy of locally applied aspirin and acetaminophen in post-operative pain after third molar surgery. *Clinical Pharmacology and Therapeutics.* **52**: 292–296.
3 Twycross R *et al.* (2000) Paracetamol. *Progress in Palliative Care.* **8**: 198–202.
4 Axelsson B and Christensen B (2001) Is there an additive analgesic effect of paracetamol in morphine therapy of pain in cancer patients? A double-blind randomized study. In: B Axelsson (ed) *The Incurable Cancer Patient at the End of Life.* Acta Universitatis Upsaliensis, Uppsala.
5 Flower RJ and Vane JR (1972) Inhibition of prostaglandin synthetase in brain explains the anti-pyretic activity of paracetamol. *Nature.* **240**: 410–411.
6 Simmons D *et al.* (1999) Induction of an acetaminophen-sensitive cyclooxygenase with reduced sensitivity to nonsteroidal antiinflammatory drugs. *Proceedings of the National Academy of Science USA.* **96**: 3275–3280.
7 Baba H *et al.* (2001) Direct activation of rat spinal dorsal horn neurons by prostaglandin E2. *Journal of Neuroscience.* **21**: 1750–1756.
8 Samad T *et al.* (2001) Interleukin-1B-mediated induction of COX-2 in the CNS contributes to inflammatory pain hypersensitivity. *Nature.* **410**: 471–475.
9 Bjorkman R *et al.* (1994) Acetaminophen (paracetamol) blocks spinal hyperalgesia induced by NMDA and substance P. *Pain.* **57**: 259–264.
10 Pini L *et al.* (1997) Naloxone-reversible antinociception by paracetamol in the rat. *Journal of Pharmacology and Experimental Therapeutics.* **280**: 934–940.
11 Settipane R *et al.* (1995) Prevalence of cross-sensitivity with acetaminophen in aspirin-sensitive asthmatic subjects. *Journal of Allergy and Clinical Immunology.* **96**: 480–485.
12 Sivaloganathan K *et al.* (1993) Pericoronitis and accidental paracetamol overdose: a cautionary tale. *British Dental Journal.* **174**: 69–71.
13 British National Formulary (2001) Emergency treatment of poisoning. In: *British National Formulary* (No. 41). British Medical Association and Royal Pharmaceutical Society of Great Britain, London, pp.22–23.
14 Horsmans Y *et al.* (1998) Paracetamol-induced liver toxicity after intravenous administration. *Liver.* **18**: 294–295.
15 Zimmerman H and Maddrey W (1995) Acetaminophen (paracetamol) hepatotoxicity with regular intake of alcohol: analysis of instances of therapeutic misadventure. *Hepatology.* **22**: 767–773.
16 Bell W (1998) Acetaminophen and warfarin: undesirable synergy. *Journal of the American Medical Association.* **279**: 702–703.
17 Hylek E *et al.* (1998) Acetaminophen and other risk factors for excessive warfarin in anti-coagulation. *Journal of the American Medical Association.* **279**: 657–662.
18 Shaheen S *et al.* (2000) Frequent paracetamol use and asthma in adults. *Thorax.* **55**: 266–270.
19 Shin G *et al.* (2000) Paracetamol and asthma. *Thorax.* **55**: 882–884.

20 Szczeklik A (1986) Analgesics, allergy and asthma. *Drugs.* **32**: 148–163.
21 D'Arcy P (1997) Paracetamol. *Adverse Drug Reaction Toxicology Review.* **16**: 9–14.
22 Waldum H *et al.* (1992) Can NSAIDs cause acute biliary pain and cholestasis? *Journal of Clinical Gastroenterology.* **14**: 328–330.
23 Wong V *et al.* (1993) Paracetamol and acute biliary pain with cholestasis. *Lancet.* **342**: 869.
24 Stricker B *et al.* (1985) Acute hypersensitivity reactions to paracetamol. *British Medical Journal.* **291**: 938–939.
25 Leung R *et al.* (1992) Paracetamol anaphylaxis. *Clinical and Experimental Allergy.* **22**: 831–833.
26 Mendizabal S and Gomez MD (1998) Paracetamol sensitivity without aspirin intolerance. *Allergy.* **53**: 457–458.

NON-STEROIDAL ANTI-INFLAMMATORY DRUGS (NSAIDs) BNF 4.7.1, 10.1.1

NSAIDs are essential analgesics for most forms of cancer pain, including neuropathic pain.[1] They are of particular benefit for pains associated with inflammation. Inflammation is associated with increased prostaglandin (PG) production locally and also in the CNS. Increased PGs in the CNS results in central sensitisation, and increased pain.[2,3] NSAIDs inhibit cyclo-oxygenase (COX), the main enzyme in the synthesis of PGs from arachidonic acid. NSAIDs inhibit PG production both at the site of injury and in the CNS, i.e. they have both a peripheral and central action.

COX exists in two forms; COX-1 is present in all tissues and is often referred to as 'constitutive' (i.e. part of the body's constitution), whereas COX-2 is generally detectable only in discrete locations in various tissues but is massively induced by inflammation (Figure 5.7).

The classification of NSAIDs is now generally based on their relative ability to inhibit COX-1 and COX-2.[4] However, classifications differ, mainly according to whether COX-1 inhibition is measured at IC_{50} or IC_{80}.[5] Because IC_{80} better reflects clinical reality, this parameter is used in *PCF2* (Box 5.A). The incentive for developing selective COX-2 inhibitors was to obtain an NSAID devoid of gastroduodenal toxicity. The coxib class of NSAID has partly fulfilled this hope but how much this relates to COX-2 selectivity is uncertain. Gastroduodenal toxicity depends on multiple factors, and dual COX inhibitors such as **ibuprofen** and **nabumetone** have a low propensity for causing serious gastro-intestinal events, i.e. perforation, ulceration, bleeding (PUB; Box 5.B).

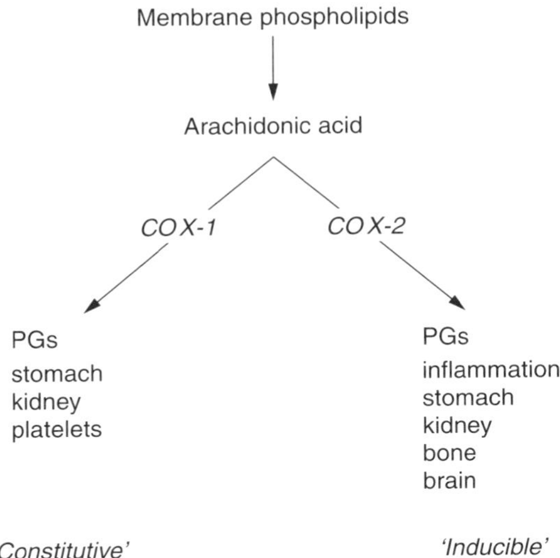

Figure 5.7 Cyclo-oxygenase (COX) and the production of prostaglandins (PGs).

Box 5.A NSAID classification

Dual COX inhibitors (Inhibition COX-1 = COX-2)
e.g. diclofenac, flurbiprofen, ibuprofen, naproxen

COX-1 sparing (COX-2 selective)
e.g. nimesulide, celecoxib, meloxicam, etodolac

Specific COX-2 inhibitors (Inhibition of COX-2 only)
e.g. rofecoxib

Box 5.B Factors intrinsic to NSAIDs which result in low gastroduodenal toxicity[6]

Competitive masking of gastric COX-1 by inactive forms, e.g. R-ibuprofen, R-etodolac.

Weak/no uncoupling of oxidative phosphorylation; Low disruption of phospholipids in protective mucus and mucus membranes } non-acidic compounds, e.g. nabumetone, coxibs.

High protein-binding (less available).

Weak/no inhibition of platelet aggregation, e.g. non-acetylated salicylates, diclofenac, meloxicam, coxibs.

Inhibition of PG synthesis does not account for the total analgesic effect of NSAIDs. In dental extraction pain, most weak COX inhibitors are significantly superior to aspirin and most strong inhibitors inferior (Table 5.1). NSAIDs differ in their effect on platelet function. In patients undergoing chemotherapy or with thrombocytopenia from other causes, it is best to use an NSAID which has no effect on platelet function and which has low intrinsic gastrotoxity (Table 5.2).

Table 5.1 Analgesic efficacy of oral NSAIDs in dental pain compared to aspirin 650mg[11]

Significantly superior[a]	*Not significantly different*	*Significantly inferior*
Azapropazone (3)	Diclofenac (1)	Fenbufen (1)
Diflunisal (3)	Etodolac (1)	Nabumetone (1)
Flurbiprofen (1)	Sulindac (1)	
Ketoprofen (2)		
Ketorolac (3)		
Naproxen (3)		
Tolmetin (3)		

a. numbers in parentheses indicate capacity to inhibit PG synthesis: 1 = strong; 2 = moderate; 3 = weak.

Activated platelets synthesise thromboxane A_2 (TXA_2) which is COX-1 mediated (potent platelet aggregant and vasoconstrictor, i.e. is pro-thrombotic). In contrast, endothelial cells synthesise PGI_2 which is COX-2 mediated (inhibits platelet activation and induces vasodilation, i.e. is anti-thrombotic). **Aspirin**, via COX-1 and COX-2 inhibition, reduces both TXA_2 production and PGI_2 production, i.e. produces a balanced reduction of prostanoids with opposing actions. In contrast, specific COX-2 inhibitors will block PGI_2 production but have no impact on TXA_2 production, i.e. will lead to an imbalance between anti-thrombotic and pro-thrombotic states. In a study comparing long-term **rofecoxib** with **naproxen**, the rate of serious thrombotic events

Table 5.2 NSAIDs and impairment of platelet function

Drug	*Effect*	*Comment*
Dual COX inhibitors		
Aspirin	+	*Irreversible* platelet dysfunction as a result of acetylation of platelet COX-1
Non-acetylated salicylates e.g. choline magnesium trisalicylate, diflunisal, salsalate	–	No effect at recommended doses
Classical NSAIDs *except diclofenac* e.g. ibuprofen, flurbiprofen, ketorolac, naproxen	+	Reversible platelet dysfunction
Diclofenac	–	Although diclofenac *in vitro* is a potent reversible inhibitor of platelet aggregation, typical oral doses of diclofenac *in vivo* do not affect platelet function[12]
COX-1 sparing NSAIDs		
Nimesulide,[13] celecoxib,[14] meloxicam[15]	–	
Specific COX-2 inhibitors		
Rofecoxib[16]	–	

was significantly higher in the patients who received **rofecoxib**.[7] Further, several case reports suggest that specific COX-2 inhibitors may be dangerously pro-thrombotic in patients with a predisposition to thrombosis, e.g. in connective tissue disorders.[8] Because cancer is often associated with a pro-thrombotic tendency,[9,10] pending further postmarketing surveillance, *caution should be exercised when prescribing specific COX-2 inhibitors to cancer patients.*

Cautions

Recent peptic ulceration (e.g. within 3–6 months), hypovolaemia, cardiac failure, renal impairment and hepatic impairment. Most NSAIDs can cause gastroduodenal injury and many interfere with platelet aggregation (Table 5.2); concurrent administration of a classical NSAID with coumarin anticoagulants increases the risk of bleeding >10 times. Some NSAIDs also inhibit **warfarin** metabolism and may cause an increase in INR (Table 5.3). Drug interactions are summarised in Tables 5.3 and 5.4. Also see Cytochrome P450, p.331. Of particular importance is the interaction with **methotrexate**, a weak organic acid which is 60–80% excreted unchanged by the kidney.[17] *Concurrent administration of* ***methotrexate*** *and an NSAID decreases the excretion of* ***methotrexate*** *and increases its toxicity.* In most patients concurrent treatment is safe in the absence of renal impairment. However, two deaths have occurred with **aspirin**, and life-threatening neutropenia has been reported with several other NSAIDs.[18] Toxicity is dose-related; it is much less likely with chronic low-dose **methotrexate** in rheumatoid arthritis than with high-dose pulses of cancer chemotherapy.

Undesirable effects

For full list, see manufacturer's SPC.
The undesirable effects have been categorised as type A ('augmented') and type B ('bizarre'). Type A effects are predictable and dose-dependent, whereas type B are unpredictable and dose-independent (Tables 5.5 and 5.6).

Gastro-intestinal toxicity is by far the most serious undesirable class effect of NSAIDs (Box 5.C).[22] Various risk factors have been identified (Table 5.7). Being over 60 years old may not be a true risk factor; it may relate to the fact that many elderly people take **aspirin** as prophylaxis against thrombosis. This might also explain why heart disease was found to be a risk factor (odds ratio ≈ 2) in another study.[23] Antidepressants which inhibit presynaptic serotonin re-uptake,

Table 5.3 Pharmacokinetic interactions: NSAIDs affecting other drugs[19]

Drug affected	*NSAIDs implicated*	*Effect*	*Clinical implications*
Aminoglycosides	All NSAIDs	Reduce renal function in susceptible individuals, reducing aminoglycoside clearance and increasing plasma concentration	Monitor plasma concentration and adjust dose
Baclofen	Ibuprofen ? other NSAIDs	Reduced excretion of baclofen with increased risk of toxicity	Reduce dose of baclofen
Digoxin	All NSAIDs	In cardiac failure, NSAIDS may precipitate renal failure, reducing digoxin excretion with increased risk of toxicity	In cardiac failure, avoid NSAIDs if possible; if not, check digoxin and creatinine plasma concentrations
Hypoglycaemics	Azapropazone	Inhibits metabolism of sulphonylureas and prolongs halflife with increased risk of hypoglycaemia	Use an alternative NSAID
Lithium	All NSAIDs (?except sulindac, aspirin)	Inhibit renal excretion of lithium and increase plasma concentration with increased risk of severe toxicity	Halve dose of lithium and monitor lithium concentration
Methotrexate	Salicylates Other NSAIDs less so	Competitively inhibit the tubular excretion of methotrexate increasing its plasma concentration with risk of severe toxicity	Avoid aspirin and other salicylates during chemotherapy; probably safe between pulses Use other NSAIDs with caution *Generally not a problem with low-dose chronic methotrexate therapy used in rheumatoid arthritis*
Phenytoin	All NSAIDs	Displace phenytoin from plasma proteins	Phenytoin toxicity can develop even when the plasma concentration is still within the therapeutic range

continued

Table 5.3 Continued

Drug affected	*NSAIDs implicated*	*Effect*	*Clinical implications*
Sodium valproate	Aspirin ? other NSAIDS	Displaces valproate from plasma proteins, inhibits valproate metabolism and increases plasma concentration	Avoid aspirin; with other NSAIDs reduce the dose of sodium valproate if toxicity suspected
Warfarin	Azapropazone Flurbiprofen Celecoxib Rofecoxib	Inhibits metabolism of warfarin and increases INR	Isolated cases also reported with several other NSAIDs, including diclofenac and ibuprofen; reduce dose of warfarin and check INR; do not use azapropazone concurrently
Zidovudine	All NSAIDs	Increased haematological toxicity	Monitor blood count

Table 5.4 Pharmacokinetic interactions: other drugs affecting NSAIDs[19]

Drug implicated	*NSAIDs affected*	*Effect*	*Clinical implications*
Antacids	All e/c NSAIDs	Destruction of enteric-coating	Administer at different times
Antacids	Aspirin	Decreased absorption and reduced plasma concentration	Use an alternative NSAID
Antacids	Indometacin	Variable effects aluminium-containing antacids reduce rate and extent of absorption of indometacin sodium bicarbonate increases rate and extent of absorption of indometacin	Use an alternative NSAID[20]
Barbiturates	Possibly all NSAIDs	Increased metabolic clearance of NSAIDs	May need higher dose of NSAID
Ciclosporin	Diclofenac	Increased plasma concentration of diclofenac	Halve the dose of diclofenac
Colestyramine	Naproxen ? other NSAIDs	Anion exchange resin binds NSAIDs in gut reducing absorption	Separate administration by 4h; may need higher dose of NSAID
Fluconazole	Celecoxib	Reduced celecoxib metabolism	Halve the dose of celecoxib
Metoclopramide	Aspirin	Increased rate and extent of absorption of aspirin in patients with migraine	Can be used therapeutically to speed onset of action of aspirin
Probenecid	Probably all NSAIDs	Reduced metabolism and renal clearance of NSAIDs and glucuronide metabolites which are hydrolysed back to parent drug; *NSAIDs also reduce the uricosuric effect of probenecid*	Consider a reduction in the dose of NSAID but could be used therapeutically to increase the response
Rifampicin	Rofecoxib	600mg/day reduces plasma concentration by 50%	Increase dose of rofecoxib if pain returns
Ritonavir	Piroxicam ? other NSAIDs	Increased plasma concentration with increased risk of toxicity	Avoid concurrent use

Table 5.5 Type A reactions to NSAIDs[21]

Organ/system	*Clinical reaction*
Blood	Decreased platelet aggregation (see Table 5.2)
Gastro-intestinal tract	Dyspepsia Peptic ulceration Haemorrhage Perforation
Kidney	Salt and water retention Interstitial nephritis
Lung	Bronchospasm (asthma)

Table 5.6 Type B reactions to NSAIDs[21]

Organ/system	*Clinical reaction*	*NSAIDs*
Immunological	Anaphylaxis	Most NSAIDs
Skin	Morbilliform rash Angioedema	Fenbufen Ibuprofen Azapropazone Piroxicam
Blood	Thrombocytopenia	Diclofenac Ibuprofen Piroxicam
	Haemolytic anaemia	Mefenamic acid Diclofenac
Gastro-intestinal	Diarrhoea	Mefenamic acid Flufenamic acid
Liver	Reye's syndrome Hepatitis	Aspirin Diclofenac Piroxicam
CNS	Aseptic meningitis	Ibuprofen

Box 5.C Risk of NSAID-related gastroduodenal toxicity

Minimal	**Low**	**Intermediate**	**Highest**
Celecoxib Rofecoxib	Diclofenac Ibuprofen Meloxicam Nimesulide	Diflunisal Flurbiprofen Indometacin Ketoprofen Naproxen Piroxicam	Aspirin Azapropazone Ketorolac

notably SSRIs, **clomipramine**, **amitriptyline**, **venlafaxine**, decrease serotonin uptake from the blood by platelets.[24] Because platelets do not synthesise serotonin, re-uptake inhibitors which decrease platelet serotonin concentration may adversely affect platelet aggregation. In elderly patients, particularly those over 80 years, serotonin re-uptake inhibitors are an independent risk factor for gastro-intestinal bleeding; concurrent use with an NSAID increases the risk.[25]

Table 5.7 Risks of complicated peptic ulcer in patients taking NSAIDs compared with non-users of NSAIDs[22,26,27]

	Relative risk
Use of NSAID (overall risk)	4
Past history peptic ulcer disease	17
Age >60 years	3–13[28]
Azapropazone	23–31[29]
Low dose NSAID:high dose	2:8[29,30]
Multiple NSAID use	9
Co-prescription of	
corticosteroids	10[31]
anticoagulants	13[32]
aspirin (75–300mg daily)	8 (odds ratio)[33]
antidepressants[a] (in elderly)	2.8

a. if high inhibition of serotonin re-uptake, particularly SSRIs, clomipramine, amitriptyline and venlafaxine.[25]

Aspirin-induced asthma is related to COX inhibition. Aspirin-sensitive subjects possibly differ from other people with asthma by depending more on the bronchodilating activity of PGE_2 than on the β-adrenergic system. **Aspirin** inhibits the production of PGE_2 with the result that more arachidonic acid is available as a substrate for leukotriene production. Leukotrienes C_4 and D_4 are potent bronchoconstrictors and mucus secretagogues. Other unidentified bronchoconstrictors could also be involved.[34] Although a class effect, bronchospasm has not been observed with **choline salicylate**, **sodium salicylate**, **azapropazone** and **benzydamine**. It also does not occur with **rofecoxib**, a specific COX-2 inhibitor[35] and probably not with **celecoxib**.[36]

All NSAIDs cause salt and water retention which may result in ankle oedema; they therefore antagonise the action of diuretics. NSAIDs may also cause acute or acute-on-chronic renal failure particularly in patients with hypovolaemia from any cause, e.g. diuretics, fever, dehydration, vomiting, diarrhoea, haemorrhage, surgery. The risk of NSAID-induced renal failure increases in situations where the plasma concentrations of vasoconstrictor substances such as angiotensin II, noradrenaline (norepinephrine) and vasopressin are increased, e.g. in heart failure, cirrhosis and nephrotic syndrome. The inhibition of renal PG production by NSAIDs prevents the protective vasodilatory mechanism for safeguarding renal blood flow from functioning effectively.[37] Early studies which suggested that **sulindac** has little or no effect on renal PG synthesis have not been substantiated by subsequent reports.[38] Sporadic cases of interstitial nephritis (± nephrotic syndrome or ± papillary necrosis) have been reported with most NSAIDs.

Choice of NSAID

Choice of NSAID depends on:

- availability
- efficacy
- safety
- special requirements
- cost
- fashion.

Ibuprofen (see p.152), **diclofenac** (see p.149) and **naproxen** (see p.156) are probably the most widely used NSAIDs in palliative care. **Flurbiprofen** (see p.151) is the NSAID of choice at Sir Michael Sobell House, and **diclofenac** at Hayward House. The central analgesic effects of NSAIDs have not been fully elucidated and it is possible that clinically important differences may emerge when more data are available. Further, it is still unclear whether some cancer patients obtain more benefit from one particular NSAID as is anecdotally reported in rheumatoid arthritis, or whether apparent differences relate simply to a relative increase in the dose of NSAID (Box 5.D).

Box 5.D Typical NSAID regimens

Celecoxib 200mg o.d.–b.d.

Diclofenac sodium 50mg t.d.s.

Diclofenac sodium m/r 150–200mg o.d.[a] *or* 75–100mg b.d.[a]

Diflunisal 250–500mg b.d.

Flurbiprofen 50–100mg b.d.

Flurbiprofen m/r 200mg o.d.

Ibuprofen 400–600mg q.d.s.

Meloxicam 15mg o.d.

Naproxen 250–500mg b.d.

Nimesulide 100mg b.d.

Rofecoxib 25–50mg o.d.[b]

a. the UK licence is for ≤150mg/24h
b. the UK licence for 50mg o.d. is for short-term use only.

Generally, apart from biliary and renal colic,[39] NSAIDS should be given PO in patients who can swallow because, except in the case of **ketorolac**,[40,41] there is no evidence of greater efficacy by other routes.[42] Topical NSAIDs are of value for the relief of pain associated with soft tissue trauma, e.g. strains and sprains.[43]

Diclofenac 150mg or **ketorolac** 30–90mg/24h by CSCI is used at some centres when parenteral administration is necessary.[40,41] **Tenoxicam** 20mg SC/IM o.d. is a useful alternative and may obviate the need for a second syringe driver in a patient requiring multiple parenteral drugs.

Piroxicam 20mg, given as a Feldene Melt® tablet, is another option; this dissolves rapidly and completely if placed on the tongue or in the mouth. However, absorption is gastro-intestinal, which means that Feldene Melt® tablets can be used only in patients who can swallow their saliva.

1 Shah S and Hardy J (2001) Non-steroidal anti-inflammatory drugs in cancer pain: a review of the literature as relevant to palliative care. *Progress in Palliative Care*. **9**: 3–7.
2 Baba H *et al.* (2001) Direct activation of rat spinal dorsal horn neurons by prostaglandin E2. *Journal of Neuroscience*. **21**: 1750–1756.
3 Samad T *et al.* (2001) Interleukin-1B-mediated induction of COX-2 in the CNS contributes to inflammatory pain hypersensitivity. *Nature*. **410**: 471–475.
4 Shah S and Hardy J (2001) A review of the COX-2 inhibitors. *Progress in Palliative Care*. **9**: 47–52.
5 Warner T *et al.* (1999) Nonsteroidal drug selectivities for cyclo-oxygenase-1 rather than cyclo-oxygenase-2 are associated with human gastrointestinal toxicity: a full in vitro analysis. *Proceedings of the National Academy of Science USA*. **96**: 7563–7568.
6 Rainsford K (1999) Profile and mechanisms of gastrointestinal and other side effects of non-steroidal anti-inflammatory drugs (NSAIDs). *American Journal of Medicine*. **107 (6A)**: 27s–36s.
7 Bombardier C *et al.* (2000) Comparison of upper gastrointestinal toxicity of rofecoxib and naproxen in patients with rheumatoid arthritis. *New England Journal of Medicine*. **343**: 1520–1528.
8 Crofford L *et al.* (2000) Thrombosis in patients with connective tissue diseases treated with specific cyclooxygenase 2 inhibitors. A report of four cases. *Arthritis and Rheumatism*. **43**: 1891–1896.
9 Levine M and Hirsh J (1990) The diagnosis and treatment of thrombosis in the cancer patient. *Seminars in Oncology*. **17**: 160–171.
10 Piccioli A *et al.* (1996) Cancer and venous thromboembolism. *American Heart Journal*. **132**: 850–855.
11 McCormack K and Brune K (1991) Dissociation between the antinociceptive and anti-inflammatory effects of the nonsteroidal anti-inflammatory drugs: a survey of their analgesic efficacy. *Drugs*. **41**: 533–547.
12 Todd P and Sorkin E (1988) Diclofenac sodium: a reappraisal of its pharmacodynamic and pharmacokinetic properties, and therapeutic efficacy. *Drugs*. **35**: 244–285.
13 Cullen L *et al.* (1997) Selective suppression of cyclooxygenase-2 during chronic administration of nimesulide in man. *Presented at the Fourth International Congress on essential fatty acids and eicosanoids. Edinburgh.*

14 Clemett D and Goa K (2000) Celecoxib: a review of its use in osteoarthritis, rheumatoid arthritis and acute pain. *Drugs*. **59**: 957–980.
15 Guth B *et al.* (1996) Therapeutic doses of meloxicam do not inhibit platelet aggregation in man. *Rheumatology in Europe*. **25**: Abstract 443.
16 vanHecken A *et al.* (2000) Comparative inhibitory activity of rofecoxib, meloxicam, diclofenac, ibuprofen and naproxen on COX-2 versus COX-1 in healthy volunteers. *Journal of Clinical Pharmacology*. **40**: 1109–1120.
17 Stockley I (1996) *Drug Interactions* (4e). Pharmaceutical Press, London, pp.505–506.
18 Patrignani P *et al.* (1997) Differential inhibition of human prostaglandin endoperoxide synthase-1 and -2 by nonsteroidal anti-inflammatory drugs. *Journal of Physiology and Pharmacology*. **48**: 623–31.
19 Tonkin A and Wing L (1988) Interactions of nonsteroidal anti-inflammatory drugs. In: P Brooks (ed) *Bailliere's Clinical Rheumatology. Anti-rheumatic drugs*. Bailliere Tindall, London, pp.455-483.
20 Stockley I (1996) *Drug Interactions* (4e). Pharmaceutical Press, London, p.278.
21 Rawlins M (1997) Non-opioid analgesics. In: D Doyle *et al.* (eds) *Oxford Textbook of Palliative Medicine*. Oxford University Press, Oxford, pp.355–361.
22 Hawkins C and Hanks G (2000) The gastroduodenal toxicity of nonsteroidal anti-inflammatory drugs. A review of the literature. *Journal of Pain and Symptom Management*. **20**: 140–151.
23 Silverstein FE *et al.* (1995) Misoprostol reduces serious gastrointestinal complications in patients with rheumatoid arthritis receiving nonsteroidal anti-inflammatory drugs. *Annals of Internal Medicine*. **123**: 241–249.
24 Ross S *et al.* (1980) Inhibition of 5-hydroxytryptamine uptake in human platelets by anti-depressant agents in vivo. *Psychopharmacology*. **67**: 1–7.
25 vanWalraven C *et al.* (2001) Inhibition of serotonin reuptake by antidepressants and upper gastrointestinal bleeding in elderly patients: retrospective cohort study. *British Medical Journal*. **323**: 655–657.
26 Garcia-Rodriguez L and Jick H (1994) Risk of upper gastrointestinal bleeding and perforation associated with individual non-steroidal anti-inflammatory drugs. *Lancet*. **343**: 769–772.
27 Hawkey C (1996) Nonsteroidal anti-inflammatory drug gastropathy: causes and treatment. *Scandinavian Journal of Gastroenterology*. **31 (suppl 220)**: 124–127.
28 Henry D *et al.* (1993) Variability in the risk of major gastrointestinal complications from non-aspirin nonsteroidal anti-inflammatory drugs. *Gastroenterology*. **105**: 1078–1088.
29 Langman MJS *et al.* (1994) Risks of bleeding peptic ulcer associated with individual non-steroidal anti-inflammatory drugs. *Lancet*. **343**: 1075–1078.
30 Garcia-Rodriguez L (1997) Nonsteroidal anti-inflammatory drugs, ulcers and risk: a collaborative metanalysis. *Seminars in Arthritis and Rheumatism*. **26 (suppl 1)**: 16–20.
31 Piper JM *et al.* (1991) Corticosteroid use and peptic ulcer disease: role of nonsteroidal anti-inflammatory drugs. *Annals of Internal Medicine*. **114**: 735–740.
32 Shorr R *et al.* (1993) Concurrent use of nonsteroidal anti-inflammatory drugs and oral anti-coagulants places elderly persons at high risk for hemorrhagic peptic ulcer disease. *Archives of Internal Medicine*. **153**: 1665–1670.
33 Weil J *et al.* (1995) Prophylactic aspirin and risk of peptic ulcer bleeding. *British Medical Journal*. **310**: 827–830.
34 Capron A *et al.* (1985) New functions for platelets and their pathological implications. *International Archives of Allergy and Applied Immunology*. **77**: 107–114.
35 Anonymous (2001) The 'coxibs' don't cross-react in aspirin sensitive asthmatics. *Journal of Allergy and Clinical Immunology*. **108**: 47–51.
36 Dicpinigaitis P (2001) Effect of the cyclooxygenase-2 inhibitor celecoxib on bronchial responsiveness and cough reflex sensitivity in asthmatics. *Pulmonary Pharmacology and Therapeutics*. **14**: 93–97.
37 MacDonald T (1994) Selected side-effects: 14. Non-steroidal anti-inflammatory drugs and renal damage. *Prescribers' Journal*. **34**: 77–80.
38 Eriksson L-O *et al.* (1990) Effects of sulindac and naproxen on prostaglandin excretion in patients with impaired renal function and rheumatoid arthritis. *American Journal of Medicine*. **89**: 313–321.
39 Lundstam SOA *et al.* (1982) Prostaglandin-synthetase inhibition with diclofenac sodium in treatment of renal colic: comparison with use of a narcotic analgesic. *Lancet*. **1**: 1096–1097.

40 Middleton RK *et al.* (1996) Ketorolac continuous infusion: a case report and review of the literature. *Journal of Pain and Symptom Management.* **12**: 190–194.
41 Hughes A *et al.* (1997) Ketorolac: continuous subcutaneous infusion for cancer pain. *Journal of Pain and Symptom Management.* **13**: 315–317.
42 Tramer M *et al.* (1998) Comparing analgesic efficacy of non-steroidal anti-inflammatory drugs given by different routes in acute and chronic pain: a qualitative systematic review. *Acta Anaesthesiologica Scandinavica.* **42**: 71–79.
43 Moore R *et al.* (1998) Quantitative systematic review of topically applied non-steroidal anti-inflammatory drugs. *British Medical Journal.* **316**: 333–338.

DICLOFENAC BNF 10.1.1

Class: Non-opioid analgesic, NSAID.

Indications: Pain and inflammation in rheumatoid arthritis and other musculoskeletal disorders, dysmenorrhoea, acute gout, postoperative pain, †cancer pain, †neoplastic fever.

Contra-indications: Active peptic ulceration, hypersensitivity to **aspirin** or other NSAID (urticaria, rhinitis, asthma, angioedema).

Pharmacology

Diclofenac is an acetate NSAID.[1] It is traditionally classed as a dual COX inhibitor although in some assays it appears to be COX-1 sparing.[2] Although diclofenac is a potent reversible inhibitor of platelet aggregation *in vitro*, typical oral doses have no effect on platelet adhesiveness or bleeding time.[3] Further, although IV diclofenac has a measurable effect on bleeding time, most subjects remain within the normal range. About 10% of patients experience undesirable effects (mainly gastric intolerance) which are generally mild and transient; diclofenac needs to be withdrawn in only 2%.[3] Age and renal or hepatic impairment do not have any significant effect on plasma concentrations of diclofenac, although metabolite concentrations increase in severe renal impairment. The principal metabolite, hydroxydiclofenac, possesses little anti-inflammatory effect. Diclofenac does not normally interact with coumarin anticoagulants or oral hypoglycaemic agents. Diclofenac is never, or hardly ever, associated with certain sporadic undesirable effects seen with many other NSAIDs, e.g. acute pancreatitis, aseptic meningitis, cutaneous reactions and photosensitivity. Diclofenac sodium is the NSAID of choice at Hayward House. Diclofenac *potassium* is also available; it is absorbed more quickly and peak plasma concentration is reached sooner.
Bio-availability Voltarol® e/c and suppositories 50%; dispersible and m/r 82% of Voltarol® e/c; reduced 16% by food.
Onset of action 20–30min.
Time to peak plasma concentration 20min Voltarol® IM; 1h Voltarol® dispersible and suppository PR; 2h Voltarol® e/c; 2.5h Diclomax® m/r caps 75mg and 100mg; 4h Voltarol® m/r tabs 75mg and 100mg; 20–60min Voltarol® Rapid (diclofenac potassium).
Plasma halflife 1–2h.
Duration of action 8h.

Cautions and undesirable effects

For full list, see manufacturer's SPC.
Also see NSAIDs, p.139.

Dose and use

- 50mg b.d.–t.d.s.
- m/r 100mg o.d.
- m/r 75mg b.d. *or* 150mg o.d.

Although the manufacturer's UK licence is for ≤150mg/24h, some patients obtain greater benefit with no increase in undesirable effects from 200mg/24h, e.g. m/r 100mg b.d. Diclofenac is also given by injection:

- 75mg SC/IM stat and 150mg/24h by CSCI in patients unable to take oral medication
- 75mg IM p.r.n. for biliary and renal colic.[4,5]

In some centres diclofenac is given by CSCI if a non-oral route is necessary. It is immiscible with other drugs and must be given in a separate syringe driver. **Tenoxicam** may be a more convenient option for some patients who need a parenteral NSAID; this has a plasma halflife of 72h and can be given 20mg o.d. as a bolus injection.

Supply

Diclofenac sodium (non-proprietary)
Tablets e/c 50mg, 28 days @ 50mg t.d.s. = £3.67.
Suppositories 100mg, 10 = £3.70.
Injection 25mg/ml, 3ml amp = £0.80.

Voltarol® (Novartis 01276 698370)
Tablets e/c 50mg, 28 days @ 50mg t.d.s. = £6.13.
Tablets dispersible 50mg, 28 days @ 50mg t.d.s. = £22.52.

Voltarol Rapid® (Novartis 01276 698370)
***Tablets* diclofenac potassium** 25mg, 50mg, 28 days @ 50mg t.d.s. = £19.32.

Modified-release
Diclomax SR® (Pfizer 01304 616161)
Capsules m/r, 75mg, 28 days @ 75mg b.d. = £13.01.

Diclomax Retard® (Pfizer 01304 616161)
Capsules m/r 100mg, 28 days @ 100mg o.d. = £9.36.

Motifene® 75mg (Sankyo 01494 766866)
Capsules m/r, e/c 75mg, 28 days @ 75mg b.d. = £14.99.

Voltarol® 75mg SR (Novartis 01276 698370)
Tablets m/r 75mg, 28 days @ 75mg b.d. = £17.35.

Voltarol® Retard (Novartis 01276 698370)
Tablets m/r 100mg, 28 days @ 100mg o.d. = £12.72.

With **misoprostol**
Arthrotec® 50 (Pharmacia 01908 661101)
Tablets e/c diclofenac sodium 50mg + **misoprostol** 200microgram, 28 days @ 1 t.d.s. = £18.63.

Arthrotec® 75 (Pharmacia 01908 661101)
Tablets e/c diclofenac sodium 75mg + **misoprostol** 200microgram, 28 days @ 1 b.d. = £16.42.

1 John V (1979) The pharmacokinetics and metabolism of diclofenac sodium (Voltarol) in animals and man. *Rheumatology and Rehabilitation.* **Suppl 2**: 22–37.
2 Patrignani P *et al.* (1997) Differential inhibition of human prostaglandin endoperoxide synthase-1 and -2 by nonsteroidal anti-inflammatory drugs. *Journal of Physiology and Pharmacology.* **48**: 623–631.
3 Todd P and Sorkin E (1988) Diclofenac sodium: a reappraisal of its pharmacodynamic and pharmacokinetic properties, and therapeutic efficacy. *Drugs.* **35**: 244–285.
4 Lundstam SOA *et al.* (1982) Prostaglandin-synthetase inhibition with diclofenac sodium in treatment of renal colic: comparison with use of a narcotic analgesic. *Lancet.* **1**: 1096–1097.
5 Thompson JF *et al.* (1989) Rectal diclofenac compared with pethidine injection in acute renal colic. *British Medical Journal.* **299**: 1140–1141.

DIFLUNISAL BNF 10.1.1

Class: Non-opioid analgesic, NSAID.

Indications: Pain and inflammation in rheumatoid arthritis and other musculoskeletal disorders, dysmenorrhoea, †cancer pain, †neoplastic fever.

Contra-indications: Active peptic ulceration, hypersensitivity to **aspirin** or other NSAID (urticaria, rhinitis, asthma, angioedema).

Pharmacology
Diflunisal is a salicylic acid derivative which causes less gastrotoxicity than equivalent doses of **aspirin**. Steady-state concentration is reached after 3–4 days with a dose of 125mg b.d., after 7–9 days with 500mg b.d. With each doubling of dose, the plasma concentration increases about 3 times.[1] Bio-availability is reduced by the regular use of aluminium-containing antacids, although this effect is less marked if taken with or after food. Diflunisal is metabolised by conjugation to glucuronide and excreted in the urine. Diflunisal decreases plasma uric acid concentration. It affects platelet function only in doses >500mg b.d.
Bio-availability 100% PO.
Onset of action 1h.
Time to peak plasma concentration 2–3h.
Plasma halflife 8–12h; up to 115h in severe renal impairment.
Duration of action 8–12h.

Cautions and undesirable effects
For full list, see manufacturer's SPC.
Also see NSAIDs, p.139.

Dose and use
- a loading dose of 500mg–1g can be given
- continue with 250–500mg b.d. *or* 500mg–1g o.d.
- increase daily dose to 1.5g if necessary.

Supply
Dolobid® (MSD 01992 467272)
Tablets 250mg, 500mg, 28 days @ 500mg b.d. = £10.10.

1 Cooper S (1983) New peripherally-acting oral analgesic agent. *Annual Review of Pharmacology and Toxicology.* **23**: 617–647.

FLURBIPROFEN — BNF 10.1.1

Class: Non-opioid analgesic, NSAID.

Indications: Pain and inflammation in rheumatoid arthritis and other musculoskeletal disorders, dysmenorrhoea, postoperative analgesia, relief of sore throat, †cancer pain, †neoplastic fever, †detrusor instability.[1]

Contra-indications: Active peptic ulceration, hypersensitivity to **aspirin** or other NSAID (urticaria, rhinitis, asthma, angioedema).

Pharmacology
Flurbiprofen is a propionic acid derivative and a highly potent COX inhibitor. In animal studies, it is 8–20 times more potent than **aspirin**. It is excreted in the urine both as unchanged drug and a number of hydroxylated metabolites. In addition to its analgesic use, flurbiprofen has been used to relieve frequency caused by instability of the detrusor muscle of the bladder.[1] Flurbiprofen is the NSAID of choice at Sir Michael Sobell House.
Bio-availability >85% PO.
Onset of action 30–60min.
Time to peak plasma concentration 1.5–2h.
Plasma halflife 3–4h.
Duration of action 8–16h.[2]

Cautions and undesirable effects
For full list, see manufacturer's SPC.
Also see NSAIDs, p.139.

Dose and use

Pain

- 50–100mg b.d.–t.d.s.
- m/r 200mg o.d.

Suppositories can be used in patients who are unable to swallow tablets.

Sore throat

Flurbiprofen lozenges 8.75mg:

- dissolve 1 lozenge slowly in the mouth every 3–6h
- not more than 5/24h for a maximum of 3 days.

Supply

Froben® (Abbott 01628 773355)
Tablets 50mg, 100mg, 28 days @ 100mg b.d. = £10.61.
Suppositories 100mg, 28 days @ 100mg b.d. = £13.53.
Froben® SR (Abbott 01628 773355)
Capsules m/r 200mg, 28 days @ 200mg o.d. = £10.15.
Strefen® (Crookes 0115 968 8922)
Lozenges 8.75mg, 16 = £2.00.

1 Cardozo L *et al.* (1980) Evaluation of flurbiprofen in detrusor instability. *British Medical Journal.* **280**: 281–282.
2 Kowanko I *et al.* (1981) Circadian variations in the signs and symptoms of rheumatoid arthritis and in the therapeutic effectiveness of flurbiprofen at different times of day. *British Journal of Clinical Pharmacology.* **11**: 477–484.

IBUPROFEN — BNF 10.1.1

Class: Non-opioid analgesic, NSAID.

Indications: Pain and inflammation in rheumatoid arthritis and other musculoskeletal disorders, dysmenorrhoea, migraine, postoperative pain, fever, †cancer pain, †neoplastic fever.

Contra-indications: Active peptic ulceration, hypersensitivity to **aspirin** or other NSAID (urticaria, rhinitis, asthma, angioedema).

Pharmacology

Ibuprofen acts predominantly as an analgesic in doses up to 1200mg/24h; its anti-inflammatory properties are more evident at higher doses. Doses of 2400mg/24h are well tolerated by most patients. Because of its good safety record, ibuprofen can be purchased OTC.[1] Ibuprofen is safe in overdose; no deaths have been reported with ibuprofen alone, even with a single dose of 40g.[2] Ibuprofen is 3 times more potent than **aspirin**, i.e. 200mg is equivalent to 600mg of **aspirin**. Higher doses of ibuprofen have a greater analgesic effect than standard doses of **aspirin**. Ibuprofen is also used topically, particularly for sprains, strains and arthritis.[3] In the UK, ibuprofen cream is available without prescription. Although application to the skin produces plasma concentrations which are only 5% of those obtained with oral administration, the underlying muscle and fascial concentrations are 25 times greater.[4,5] A randomised placebo-controlled double-blind trial showed that patients with sprains and bruises treated with transdermal ibuprofen fared better in terms of speed of resolution, relief of pain, reduction in swelling and return of function.[6]
Bio-availability 90% PO; >95% Fenbid® m/r capsules.
Onset of action 20–30min; 1h for Fenbid® m/r.
Time to peak plasma concentration 30–120min; 2–5h for Fenbid® m/r.
Plasma halflife 2h.[7]
Duration of action 4–6h; 8–12h for Fenbid® m/r; 24h for Brufen® m/r.

Cautions and undesirable effects

For full list, see manufacturer's SPC.
Also see NSAIDs, p.139.

Dose and use

Pain

- starting dose 400mg t.d.s.
- increase to 800mg t.d.s. if necessary.

Supply

Ibuprofen (non-proprietary)
Tablets 200mg, 400mg, 600mg, 28 days @ 400mg t.d.s. = £2.46.
Oral suspension 100mg/5ml, 28 days @ 400mg t.d.s. = £30.58.

Brufen® (Abbott 01628 773355)
Tablets 400mg, 600mg, 28 days @ 400mg t.d.s. = £6.47.
Oral syrup 100mg/5ml, 28 days @ 400mg t.d.s. = £27.12.
Oral granules effervescent 600mg/sachet, 28 days @ 600mg t.d.s. = £28.56; *contains* Na^+ *9mmol/sachet.*

Modified-release
Fenbid® (Goldshield 020 8649 8500)
Capsules m/r 300mg, 28 days @ 600mg b.d. = £9.00.

Brufen Retard® (Abbott 01628 773355)
Tablets m/r 800mg, 28 days @ 1600mg o.d. = £7.24.

Topical preparations
Fenbid® Forte Gel (Goldshield 020 8649 8500)
Gel 10%, 100g = £6.50.

Ibugel® (Dermal 01462 458866)
Gel 5%, 100g, available OTC.
Forte gel 10%, 100g = £6.50.

Ibumousse® (Dermal 01462 458866)
Foam 5%, 125g, available OTC.

Ibuspray® (Dermal 01462 458866)
Spray application 5%, 100ml = £6.95.

Proflex® (Novartis Consumer Health 01403 210211)
Cream 5%, 100g, available OTC.

1 Rainsford K (1999) *Ibuprofen: a critical bibliographic review.* Taylor and Francis, London.
2 Busson M (1984) Update on ibuprofen: review article. *Journal of International Medical Research.* **14**: 53–62.
3 Chlud K and Wagener H (1987) Percutaneous nonsteroidal anti-inflammatory drug (NSAID) therapy with particular reference to pharmacokinetic factors. *EULAR Bulletin.* **2**: 40–43.
4 Mondino A *et al.* (1983) Kinetic studies of ibuprofen on humans. Comparative study for the determination of blood concentrations and metabolites following local and oral administration. *Med Welt.* **34**: 1052–1054.
5 Kageyama T (1987) A double blind placebo controlled multicenter study of piroxicam 0.5% gel in osteoarthritis of the knee. *European Journal of Rheumatology and Inflammation.* **8**: 114–115.
6 Peters H *et al.* (1987) Percutaneous kinetics of ibuprofen (German). *Aktuelle Rheumatologie.* **12**: 208–211.
7 Brocks D and Jamali F (1999) The pharmacokinetics of ibuprofen. In: K Rainsford (ed) *Ibuprofen: a critical bilbiographic review.* Taylor and Francis, London.

*KETOROLAC **BNF 10.1.1**

Class: Non-opioid analgesic, NSAID.

Indications: Postoperative pain relief; †post-traumatic pain relief, †severe cancer pain poorly responsive to maximum doses of other NSAIDs combined with a strong opioid.

Contra-indications: Active peptic ulceration or history of peptic ulceration, gastro-intestinal bleeding, suspected or confirmed cerebrovascular bleeding, haemorrhagic diatheses; asthma, hypersensitivity to **aspirin** or other NSAID; syndrome of nasal polyps, angioedema and bronchospasm (partial or complete); creatinine >160micromol/L, hypovolaemia. Concurrent prescription with **warfarin**, other NSAID, **oxypentifyline**, **probenecid** and **lithium**.

Pharmacology

Ketorolac is a cyclic propionate structurally related to the acetate NSAIDs, **tolmetin** and **indometacin**.[1,2] It is available as ketorolac trometamol which is more water-soluble. Over 99% of the oral dose is absorbed and about 75% of a dose is excreted in the urine within 7h, and over 90% within 2 days, nearly 2/3 as unmodified ketorolac.[3] The rest is excreted in the faeces. Because of early reports of fatal gastro-intestinal bleeding, the licence for ketorolac is restricted to short-term postoperative use (7 days UK).[4,5] In some countries, the licence has been with-drawn: France (1998), Germany (1999). However, recent postoperative studies indicate that the short-term use of ketorolac is associated with only a small increased risk of gastro-intestinal and operative site bleeding compared with opioids.[6,7] The risk is largely related to old age but increases significantly if treatment is continued for >7 days.[6,8] Ketorolac is also used in emergency depart-ments for post-traumatic pain.[7] In palliative care, ketorolac has been used for extended periods but always with a gastroprotective drug.[9–12]

The analgesic and anti-inflammatory activity of ketorolac resides mainly in the laevorotatory isomer. The analgesic effect is far greater than the antipyretic and anti-inflammatory properties. In animal studies, ketorolac is about 350 times more potent than **aspirin** as an analgesic but only 20 times more potent as an antipyretic.[9] As an anti-inflammatory ketorolac is about 1/2 as potent as **indometacin** and twice as potent as **naproxen**. Like most NSAIDs, ketorolac inhibits platelet aggregation. Clinical experience suggests that parenteral ketorolac is effective in some patients who fail to obtain relief with classical NSAIDs PO.[9–12]

Bio-availability 100% PO.
Onset of action 30min PO.
Time to peak plasma concentration 35min.[13]
Plasma halflife 5h; 7h in the elderly;[14] 6–19h with renal impairment.[8]
Duration of action 6h PO, 4–6h IM.

Cautions

Hepatic impairment. Interacts with **furosemide** (frusemide; decreased diuretic response), ACE inhibitors (increased risk of renal impairment), **methotrexate** and **lithium** (decreased clearance), **probenecid** (increased ketorolac levels and halflife), **oxypentifyline** (increased bleeding tendency).

Undesirable effects

For full list, see manufacturer's SPC.
Also see NSAIDs, p.139. Bleeding and pain at injection site (less with CSCI).

Dose and use

Postoperative pain

In the UK, oral ketorolac is licensed for use ≤7 days:

- usual dose 10mg q.d.s. PO (maximum recommended daily dose 40mg)
- elderly patients 10mg t.d.s.

Maximum recommended duration of IM/IV therapy is 2 days:

- starting dose 10mg
- follow with 10–30mg q4h p.r.n. (maximum recommended daily dose 90mg)
- elderly patients and those weighing <50kg, limit to 60mg/day.

In some countries, e.g. USA, ketorolac is licensed for 5 days of parenteral use with a maximum dose of 120mg.

Cancer pain

Ketorolac is used at some centres when a parenteral NSAID is indicated. Alternative injectable NSAIDs include **diclofenac** and **tenoxicam**. Ketorolac can be given by intermittent injections 20–30mg SC t.d.s. but these are uncomfortable; it is better given by CSCI. It is generally given for a short period (<3 weeks) while arranging and awaiting benefit from more definitive therapy, e.g. radiotherapy. However, when all other options have been exhausted, ketorolac has been used for 6 months without undesirable effects:[12]

- start with 60mg/24h by CSCI; also the recommended maximum dose in people over 65 and those ≤50kg
- increase by 15mg/24h to 90mg/24h if necessary
- co-prescribe a gastroprotective drug, e.g. **misoprostol** 200microgram t.d.s–q.d.s,[10] **lansoprazole** 30mg o.d. or **omeprazole** 20mg o.d.

If 0.9% saline is used, ketorolac 60–120mg/10ml is miscible with **diamorphine**.[10] *Ketorolac is immiscible with **cyclizine, midazolam, haloperidol, morphine, pethidine, hydroxyzine** and **promethazine*** (see Syringe drivers, p.297).[3]

Supply

Toradol® (Roche 01707 366000)

Tablets 10mg, 28 days @ 10mg t.d.s. = £26.17.

Injection 10mg/ml and 30mg/ml, 1ml amp = £1.02 and £1.22 respectively.

1 Buckley MM-T and Brogden R (1990) Ketorolac: a review of its pharmacodynamic and pharmacokinetic properties, and therapeutic potential. *Drugs*. **39**: 86–109.

2 Gillis J and Brogden R (1997) Ketorolac: A reappraisal of its pharmacodynamic and pharmacokinetic properties and therapeutic use in pain management. *Drugs*. **53**: 139–188.

3 Litvak K and McEvoy G (1990) Ketorolac: an injectable nonnarcotic analgesic. *Clinical Pharmacy*. **9**: 921–935.

4 Choo V and Lewis S (1993) Ketorolac doses reduced. *Lancet*. **342**: 109.

5 Lewis S (1994) Ketorolac in Europe. *Lancet*. **343**: 784.

6 Strom B *et al.* (1996) Parenteral ketorolac and risk of gastrointestinal and operative site bleeding. A postmarketing surveillance study. *Journal of the American Medical Assocation*. **275**: 376–382.

7 Rainer T *et al.* (2000) Cost effectiveness analysis of intravenous ketorolac and morphine for treating pain after limb injury: double blind randomised controlled trial. *British Medical Journal*. **321**: 1247–1251.

8 Reinhart D (2000) Minimising the adverse effects of ketorolac. *Drug Safety*. **22**: 487–497.

9 Blackwell N *et al.* (1993) Subcutaneous ketorolac – a new development in pain control. *Palliative Medicine*. **7**: 63–65.

10 Myers K and Trotman I (1994) Use of ketorolac by continuous subcutaneous infusion for the control of cancer-related pain. *Postgraduate Medical Journal*. **70**: 359–362.

11 Middleton RK *et al.* (1996) Ketorolac continuous infusion: a case report and review of the literature. *Journal of Pain and Symptom Management*. **12**: 190–194.

12 Hughes A *et al.* (1997) Ketorolac: continuous subcutaneous infusion for cancer pain. *Journal of Pain and Symptom Management*. **13**: 315–317.

13 Gordon M *et al.* (1995) Ketorolac tromethamine bioavailability via tablet, capsule, and oral solution dosage forms. *Drug Development and Industry Pharmacy*. **21**: 1143–1155.

14 Greenwald R (1992) Ketorolac: an innovative nonsteroidal analgesic. *Drugs of Today*. **28**: 41–61.

NAPROXEN **BNF 10.1.1**

Class: Non-opioid analgesic, NSAID.

Indications: Pain and inflammation in rheumatoid arthritis and other musculoskeletal disorders, dysmenorrhoea, acute gout, †cancer pain, †neoplastic fever.

Contra-indications: Active peptic ulceration, hypersensitivity to **aspirin** or other NSAID (urticaria, rhinitis, asthma, angioedema).

Pharmacology

Naproxen is a propionic acid derivative. Absorption is not affected by food or antacids. A steady-state is achieved after 3 days of b.d. administration. Excretion is almost entirely urinary, mainly as conjugated naproxen, with some unchanged drug. Plasma concentrations do not increase with doses >500mg b.d. because of rapid urinary excretion.[1] Naproxen sodium 550mg is equivalent to 500mg naproxen. Naproxen sodium is more rapidly absorbed, resulting in higher plasma concentrations and an earlier onset of action.[2] Although generally given b.d., a single dose of 500mg o.n. was equal in efficacy to 250mg b.d. in patients with osteo-arthritis[3,4] and with rheumatoid arthritis.[5]

Bio-availability 99–100% PO.
Onset of action 20–30min.
Time to peak plasma concentration 1.5–5h depending on dose and formulation.[6,7]
Plasma halflife 12–15h.
Duration of action 6–8h with single dose; >12h with multiple doses.

Cautions and undesirable effects

For full list, see manufacturer's SPC.
Also see NSAIDs, p.139.

Dose and use

- typically 250–500mg b.d.
- can be taken as a single daily dose, either o.m. or o.n.
- increase to 500mg t.d.s. if necessary; this is higher than the maximum dose of 1g daily recommended in the *SPC* and the *BNF* but is comparable to doses used for severe rheumatoid arthritis.

Supply

Naproxen (non-proprietary)
Tablets 250mg, 500mg, 28 days @ 500mg b.d. = £6.16.
Tablets e/c 250mg, 375mg, 500mg, 28 days @ 500mg b.d. = £8.14.

Naprosyn® (Roche 01707 366000)
Tablets 250mg, 500mg, 28 days @ 500mg b.d. = £9.77.
Tablets e/c (Naprosyn EC®) 250mg, 375mg, 500mg, 28 days @ 500mg b.d. = £9.77.
Oral suspension 125mg/5ml, 28 days @ 500mg b.d. = £17.03; *contains Na^+ 1.7mmol/5ml.*

Synflex® (Roche 01707 366000)
***Tablets* naproxen sodium** 275mg, 28 days @ 550mg b.d. = £15.14.
(Note 275mg naproxen sodium is equivalent to 250mg naproxen.)

Modified-release
Naprosyn® S/R (Roche 01707 366000)
Tablets m/r 500mg (as **naproxen sodium** 548mg), 28 days @ 1g o.d. = £14.60.

With **misoprostol**
Napratec® (Pharmacia 01908 661101)
Tablets combination pack, naproxen 500mg + **misoprostol** 200microgram, 28 days @ 1 of each b.d. = £19.80.

1 Simon L and Mills J (1980) Nonsteroidal anti-inflammatory drugs. Part 2. *New England Journal of Medicine*. **302**: 1237–1243.
2 Sevelius H *et al.* (1980) Bioavailability of naproxen sodium and its relationship to clinical analgesic effects. *British Journal of Clinical Pharmacology*. **10**: 259–263.
3 Brooks P *et al.* (1982) Evaluation of a single daily dose of naproxen in osteoarthritis. *Rheumatology and Rehabilitation*. **21**: 242–246.
4 Mendelsohn S (1991) Clinical efficacy and tolerability of naproxen in osteoarthritis patients using twice-daily and once-daily regimens. *Clinical Therapy*. **13 (suppl A)**: 8–15.
5 Graziano F (1991) Once-daily or twice-daily administration of naproxen in patients with rheumatoid arthritis. *Clinical Therapy*. **13 (suppl A)**: 20–25.
6 Kelly J *et al.* (1989) Pharmacokinetic properties and clinical efficacy of once-daily sustained-release naproxen. *European Journal of Clinical Pharmacology*. **36**: 383–388.
7 Davies N and Anderson K (1997) Clinical pharmacokinetics of naproxen. *Clinical Pharmacokinetics*. **32**: 268–293.

ROFECOXIB — BNF 10.1.1

Class: Non-opioid analgesic, NSAID (specific COX-2 inhibitor).

Indications: Acute pain, osteo-arthritis, rheumatoid arthritis, dysmenorrhoea (USA), †alternative to classical NSAIDs in patients with gastric intolerance despite the concurrent prescription of a PPI.[1]

Contra-indications: Active peptic ulceration, hypersensitvity to **aspirin** or other NSAID (urticaria, rhinitis, asthma, angioedema), severe congestive cardiac failure.

Pharmacology

Rofecoxib is a specific COX-2 inhibitor.[2,3] When COX-2 is inhibited by 80%, inhibition of COX-1 is <20%[4,5] A steady-state is reached after 4 days of o.d. administration. Rofecoxib is 87% protein-bound. Elimination is almost entirely by metabolism by cytosolic (non-cytochrome) enzymes in the liver to inactive metabolites which are excreted in the urine. In healthy volunteers, repeated daily doses of rofecoxib 25–375mg are well tolerated.[5] Platelet aggregation and bleeding time are unaffected by such doses.[6] Faecal blood loss is equivalent to placebo.[7] Rofecoxib causes significantly fewer major gastro-intestinal adverse effects (perforations, ulcers, bleeds; PUB) than classical NSAIDs, including **diclofenac** and **ibuprofen**, and in this respect is indistinguishable from placebo.[8–10] However, 'comparable to placebo' does not mean zero incidence. In a study over 6 months in patients with osteo-arthritis, the cumulative incidence of PUB was about half that of a combined group of classical NSAIDs, namely 1.3% compared with 2.6%.[11] Patients at high-risk of NSAID-induced gastroduodenal toxicity, if prescribed rofecoxib, should therefore also be prescribed a gastroprotective drug.[12] Given relative costs, the use of rofecoxib should probably be restricted to high-risk patients who cannot tolerate a classical NSAID with concurrent gastroprotection.[1] A study of the long-term safety of rofecoxib 50mg o.d. compared with **naproxen** 500mg b.d. in rheumatoid patients showed that the rate of serious thrombotic events, e.g. myocardial infarction, was significantly higher in patients receiving rofecoxib: 1.67 events per 100 patient-years compared with 0.70 for **naproxen**.[13] So if antithrombotic precautions are required, e.g. after a myocardial infarct or cerebrovascular thrombosis, **aspirin** 75–150mg o.d. should be prescribed concurrently.

Single-dose studies in postdental extraction pain show a dose-response curve up to 50mg but, over 6–8h, no greater efficacy than **ibuprofen** 400mg or **naproxen** 500mg.[14–18] In a study

extending over 24h, pain relief from rofecoxib was maintained throughout this period, whereas with **codeine** 60mg plus **paracetamol** 600mg relief after 7–8h was indistinguishable from placebo.[18] In chronic dosing in osteo-arthritis, rofecoxib 12.5 or 25mg is as effective as **ibuprofen** 800mg t.d.s. in terms of symptomatic relief.[19] Rofecoxib does not cause bronchospasm and can be used safely in patients sensitive to **aspirin**.[20] The same appears to hold true for **celecoxib**.[21] Rofecoxib and dual COX inhibitors have a comparable effect on renal function.[22]
Bio-availability 93% PO; reduced 20% by antacids.
Onset of action 20–30 min.
Peak plasma concentration 2–4h.
Plasma halflife 17h.
Duration of action >24h.[4]

Cautions

The elderly; renal impairment; cardiac failure; hypertension; hypovolaemia. Administration with **warfarin** results in a small increase in INR. Plasma lithium concentration should be checked in patients receiving **lithium** concurrently. **Rifampicin** 600mg/day (an inducer of liver metabolism) reduces the plasma concentration of rofecoxib by 50%.[2] Rofecoxib 75mg o.d. (a supratherapeutic dose) increases the plasma concentration of **methotrexate** by about 25%.[2]

Undesirable effects

For full list, see manufacturer's SPC.
UK doctors and pharmacists should report any suspected adverse reactions to rofecoxib to the CSM.

About 25% of patients experience non-erosive dyspepsia (comparable to **ibuprofen**). Diarrhoea, headache, nausea. Indistinguishable from placebo in relation to gastric erosions and ulceration. Like other NSAIDs (see p.139), rofecoxib may cause fluid retention[19] and renal failure.[23]

Dose and use

Acute pain
- 50mg stat
- 25–50mg o.d. until pain resolves.

Osteo-arthritis
- start with 12.5mg o.d.
- increase if necessary to 25mg o.d.

Cancer pain
- start with 25mg o.d.
- consider a trial of 50mg o.d. after 1 week if pain not adequately relieved.

Supply

Vioxx® (MSD 01992 467272)
Tablets 12.5mg, 28 days @ 25mg o.d. = £43.16; 25mg, 28 days @ 25mg o.d. = £21.58 (i.e. use 25mg tablets unless prescribing only 12.5mg o.d.).
Oral suspension 12.5mg/5ml, 28 days @ 25mg o.d. = £43.16; 25mg/5ml, 28 days @ 25mg o.d. = £21.58 (i.e. use 25mg/5ml suspension).

Vioxx® Acute (MSD 01992 467272)
Tablets 25mg, 28 days @ 50mg o.d. = £43.16; 50mg, 28 days @ 50mg o.d. = £21.56; *licensed for acute pain only* (i.e. use 50mg tablets unless prescribing only 25mg o.d.).

1 Shah S and Hardy J (2001) A review of the COX-2 inhibitors. *Progress in Palliative Care*. **9**: 47–52.
2 Scott L and Lamb H (1999) Rofecoxib. *Drugs*. **58**: 499–505.
3 Matheson A and Figgitt D (2001) Rofecoxib. A review of its use in the management of osteoarthritis, acute pain and rheumatoid arthritis. *Drugs*. **61**: 833–865.
4 Warner T *et al.* (1999) Nonsteroidal drug selectivities for cyclo-oxygenase-1 rather than cyclo-oxygenase-2 are associated with human gastrointestinal toxicity: a full in vitro analysis. *Proceedings of the National Academy of Science USA*. **96**: 7563–7568.
5 Depre M *et al.* (2000) Pharmacokinetics, COX-2 specificity, and tolerability of supratherapeutic doses of rofecoxib in humans. *European Journal of Clinical Pharmacology*. **56**: 167–174.

6 vanHecken A *et al.* (2000) Comparative inhibitory activity of rofecoxib, meloxicam, diclofenac, ibuprofen and naproxen on COX-2 versus COX-1 in healthy volunteers. *Journal of Clinical Pharmacology.* **40**: 1109–1120.
7 Hunt R *et al.* (2000) A randomized trial measuring fecal blood loss after treatment with rofecoxib, ibuprofen or placebo in healthy subjects. *American Journal of Medicine.* **109**: 201–206.
8 Laine L *et al.* (1999) A randomized trial comparing the effect of rofecoxib, a cyclooxygenase 2-specific inhibitor, with that of ibuprofen on the gastroduodenal mucosa of patients with osteoarthritis. *Gastroenterology.* **117**: 776–783.
9 Lanza F *et al.* (1999) Specific inhibition of cyclooxygenase-2 with MK-0966 is associated with less gastroduodenal damage than either aspirin or ibuprofen. *Alimentary Pharmacology and Therapeutics.* **13**: 761–767.
10 Hawkey C *et al.* (2000) Comparison of the effect of rofecoxib (a cyclooxygenase 2 inhibitor), ibuprofen, and placebo on the gastroduodenal mucosa of patients with osteoarthritis. *Arthritis and Rheumatism.* **43**: 370–377.
11 Langman M *et al.* (1999) Adverse upper gastrointestinal effects of rofecoxib compared with NSAIDs. *Journal of the American Medical Association.* **282**: 1929–1933.
12 Anonymous (2000) Are rofecoxib and celecoxib safer NSAIDs? *Drug and Therapeutics Bulletin.* **38 (11)**: 81–86.
13 Bombardier C *et al.* (2000) Comparison of upper gastrointestinal toxicity of rofecoxib and naproxen in patients with rheumatoid arthritis. *New England Journal of Medicine.* **343**: 1520–1528.
14 Mehlisch D *et al.* (1998) Ex vivo assay of COX-2 inhibition predicts analgesic efficacy in postsurgical dental pain with MK-966. *Clinical Pharmacology and Therapeutics.* **63**: 139.
15 Ehrich E *et al.* (1999) Characterization of rofecoxib as a cyclooxygenase-2 isoform inhibitor and demonstration of analgesia in the dental pain model. *Clinical Pharmacology and Therapeutics.* **65**: 336–347.
16 Fricke J *et al.* (1999) MK-966 versus naproxen sodium 550mg in postsurgical dental pain. *Clinical Pharmacology and Therapeutics.* **65**: 119.
17 Morrison B *et al.* (1999) Analgesic efficacy of the cyclooxygenase-2-specific inhibitor rofecoxib in post-dental surgery pain: a randomised, controlled trial. *Clinical Therapeutics.* **21**: 943–953.
18 Chang J *et al.* (2000) Post-operative analgesia in dental surgery. *Oral presentation at the American Pain Society, Atlanta, Georgia.*
19 Saag K *et al.* (1998) MK-0966, a specific COX-2 inhibitor has clinical efficacy comparable to ibuprofen in the treatment of knee and hip osteoarthritis (OA) in a 6-week controlled trial. *Arthritis and Rheumatism.* **41 (suppl)**: S196.
20 Stevenson D and Simon R (2001) Lack of cross-reactivity between rofecoxib and aspirin in aspirin-sensitive patients with asthma. *Journal of Allergy and Clinical Immunology.* **108**: 47–51.
21 Dicpinigaitis P (2001) Effect of the cyclooxygenase-2 inhibitor celecoxib on bronchial responsiveness and cough reflex sensitivity in asthmatics. *Pulmonary Pharmacology and Therapeutics.* **14**: 93–97.
22 Swan S *et al.* (2000) Effect of cyclooxygenase-2 inhibition on renal function in elderly persons receiving a low-salt diet. *Annals of Internal Medicine.* **133**: 1–9.
23 Rocha J and Fernandez-Alonso J (2001) Acute tubulointerstitial nephritis associated with the selective COX-2 enzyme inhibitor, rofecoxib. *Lancet.* **357**: 1946–1947.

WEAK OPIOIDS — BNF 4.7.2

The division of opioids into 'weak' and 'strong' is to a certain extent arbitrary. By IM injection, all the weak opioids can provide analgesia equivalent, or nearly equivalent, to morphine 10mg. However, **codeine**, **dextropropoxyphene** and **dihydrocodeine** are not generally used parenterally. Pharmacologically, there is no absolute need to use weak opioids; small doses of **morphine** or alternative strong opioid can be used instead. Thus, there is no pharmacological need for Step 2 of the WHO Analgesic Ladder. However, because of non-availability or highly restricted supplies of oral **morphine** in many countries, Step 2 is a practical necessity when viewed from an international perspective. **Tramadol** straddles the divide between weak opioids and strong opioids; it is considered in this section for convenience.

Table 5.8 Weak opioids

Drug	*Bio-availability (%)*	*Time to peak plasma concentration (h)*	*Plasma halflife (h)*	*Duration of analgesia (h)*[a]	*Potency ratio with codeine*
Codeine	40 (12–84)	1–2	2.5–3.5	4–6	1
Dextropropoxyphene	40	2–2.5	6–12[b]	6–8	7/8[c]
Dihydrocodeine	20	1.6–1.8	3.5–4.5	3–4	4/3
Meptazinol	<10	0.5–2	2[d]	3–4	2/5[e]
Pentazocine	20	1	3	2–3	1[e]
Tramadol	75[f]	2	6[g]	4–6	2[e]

a. when used in usual doses for mild-to-moderate pain
b. increased >50% in elderly
c. multiple doses; single dose = 1/2–2/3
d. multiple doses in elderly = 3.5–5h
e. estimated on basis of potency ratio with morphine
f. multiple doses >90%
g. active metabolite (M1) 7.4h; both figures double in cirrhosis and severe renal failure.

Weak opioids are said to have a 'ceiling' effect for analgesia. This is an oversimplication; whereas mixed agonist-antagonists such as **pentazocine** have a true ceiling effect, the maximum effective dose of weak opioid agonists is arbitrary. At higher doses there are progressively more undesirable effects, notably nausea and vomiting, which outweigh any additional analgesic effect. For example, the amount of **dextropropoxyphene** in compound tablets was chosen so that only a small minority of patients would experience nausea and vomiting with two tablets. This adds a further constraint; the upper dose limit is set in practice by the number of tablets which a patient will accept, possibly only 2–3 of any preparation. There is little to choose between the weak opioids in terms of efficacy (Table 5.8). **Codeine** and **dihydrocodeine** are more constipating and, for this reason, **co-proxamol** or **tramadol** is preferred at most palliative care units in the UK. **Meptazinol** is not widely used in the UK. The following general rules should be observed:

- a weak opioid should be *added to*, not substituted for, a non-opioid
- if a weak opioid is inadequate when given regularly, change to a strong opioid (**morphine**)
- do not 'kangaroo' from weak opioid to weak opioid.

CODEINE PHOSPHATE BNF 3.9.1 & 4.7.2

Class: Opioid analgesic.

Indications: Mild-to-moderate pain, cough, diarrhoea.

Pharmacology

Codeine (methylmorphine) is an opium alkaloid, about 1/10 as potent as **morphine**. An increasing analgesic response has been reported with IM doses up to 360mg.[1] In practice, codeine is used PO in doses of 20–60mg, generally in combination with a non-opioid. Its oral to parenteral potency ratio is 2:3, about double that of **morphine**.[2] The main metabolite is codeine-6-glucuronide which binds weakly to the μ-opioid receptor, together with small amounts of norcodeine, **morphine**, morphine-3-glucuronide and morphine-6-glucuronide. Codeine is mainly a pro-drug of **morphine** and lacks significant analgesic activity if demethylation is blocked by CYP2D6 inhibitors such as **fluoxetine**, **paroxetine** and **quinidine** or the subject is a CYP2D6 poor metaboliser (7% of Caucasians).[3] Also see Cytochrome P450, p.331. The amount of codeine biotransformed to **morphine** varies from 2–10%.[4] However, in humans, at least part of the analgesic effect of codeine is a direct one.[5] Like **morphine**, codeine is antitussive and also slows gastro-intestinal motility.[6]

Bio-availability 40% (12–84%) PO.[7]

Onset of action 30–60min for analgesia; 1–2h for antitussive effect.

Time to peak plasma concentration 1–2h.

Plasma halflife 2.5–3.5h.[7]

Duration of action 4–6h.

Cautions and undesirable effects

For full list, see manufacturer's SPC.

Also see Strong opioids, p.168.

Dose and use

Pain relief

Codeine is commonly given in a compound preparation with a non-opioid, typically 2 tablets q6h–q4h. The codeine content of these preparations is either low (8mg) or high (30mg); patients with inadequate relief will therefore benefit by changing to a higher strength preparation. When given alone, the dose is generally 30–60mg q4h. Higher doses can be given but equivalent doses of **morphine** are probably less constipating.

Cough

Codeine is effective as an antitussive by any route. Administration as a linctus is not essential. The dose is tailored to need, e.g. 15–30mg p.r.n.–q4h.

Diarrhoea

To control diarrhoea, a dose of 30–60mg is used both p.r.n. and regularly, up to q4h. However, in palliative care, **morphine** tablets or solution are generally more convenient. Also see **loperamide**, p.15.

It is bad practice to prescribe codeine to patients already taking morphine; if a greater antitussive or antidiarrhoeal effect is needed, the dose of ***morphine*** *should be increased.*

Supply

Codeine (non-proprietary)
Tablets 15mg, 30mg, 60mg, 28 days @ 30mg q.d.s. = £5.82.
Oral syrup 25mg/5ml, 28 days @ 25mg q.d.s. = £4.98.
Injections **CD** are available but are not recommended.

Codeine Linctus BP
Oral solution 15mg/5ml, 28 days @ 30mg q.d.s. = £4.48.
Diabetic oral solution 15mg/5ml, 28 days @ 30mg q.d.s. = £8.18.

Compound tablets containing codeine
Co-codaprin (non-proprietary)
Tablets codeine 8mg + **aspirin** 400mg, 28 days @ 2 q.d.s. = £3.70.
Tablets dispersible codeine 8mg + **aspirin** 400mg, 28 days @ 2 q.d.s. = £8.18.

Co-codamol 8/500 (non-proprietary)
Tablets codeine 8mg + **paracetamol** 500mg, 28 days @ 2 q.d.s. = £2.58.
Tablets dispersible codeine 8mg + **paracetamol** 500mg, 28 days @ 2 q.d.s. = £11.54.
Capsules codeine 8mg + **paracetamol** 500mg, 28 days @ 2 q.d.s. = £18.37.

Co-codamol 30/500 (non-proprietary)
Tablets codeine 30mg + **paracetamol** 500mg, 28 days @ 2 q.d.s. = £16.84.
Capsules codeine 30mg + **paracetamol** 500mg, 28 days @ 2 q.d.s. = £18.39.

Kapake® (Galen 028 3833 4974)
Tablets codeine 30mg + **paracetamol** 500mg, 28 days @ 2 q.d.s. = £16.87.
Capsules codeine 30mg + **paracetamol** 500mg, 28 days @ 2 q.d.s. = £16.87.
Sachets codeine 30mg + **paracetamol** 500mg, 28 days @ 2 q.d.s. = £19.11.

Solpadol® (Sanofi-Synthelabo 01483 505515)
Tablets codeine 30mg + **paracetamol** 500mg, 28 days @ 2 q.d.s. = £16.89.
Tablets effervescent codeine 30mg + **paracetamol** 500mg, 28 days @ 2 q.d.s. = £20.27; *contain 18.6mmol* Na^+*/tablet*; avoid in renal impairment or cardiac failure.
Capsules codeine 30mg + **paracetamol** 500mg, 28 days @ 2 q.d.s. = £16.89.

Tylex® (Schwarz 01494 797500)
Capsules codeine 30mg + **paracetamol** 500mg, 28 days @ 2 q.d.s. = £18.39.
Tablets effervescent codeine 30mg + **paracetamol** 500mg, 28 days @ 2 q.d.s. = £20.28; *contain 13.6mmol* Na^+*/tablet*; avoid in renal impairment or cardiac failure.

Co-codamol 60/1000
Kapake® (Galen 028 3833 4974)
Sachets codeine 60mg + **paracetamol** 1g, 28 days @ 1 q.d.s. = £19.11.

1 Beaver W (1966) Mild analgesics: a review of their clinical pharmacology (Part II). *American Journal of Medical Science*. **251**: 576–599.

2 Beaver WT *et al.* (1978) Analgesic studies of codeine and oxycodone in patients with cancer. I. Comparisons of oral with intramuscular codeine and of oral with intramuscular oxycodone. *Journal of Pharmacology and Experimental Therapeutics*. **207**: 92–100.

3 Lurcott G (1999) The effects of the genetic absence and inhibition of CYP2D6 on the metabolism of codeine and its derivatives, hydrocodone and oxycodone. *Anesthesia Progress*. **45**: 154–156.

4 Hanks G and Cherry N (1997) Opioid analgesic therapy. In: D Doyle *et al.* (eds) *Oxford Textbook of Palliative Medicine*. Oxford University Press, Oxford, pp.331–355.

5 Quiding H *et al.* (1993) Analgesic effect and plasma concentrations of codeine and morphine after two dose levels of codeine following oral surgery. *European Journal of Clinical Pharmacology*. **44**: 319–323.

6 Anonymous (1989) Drugs in the management of acute diarrhoea in infants and young children. *Bulletin of the WHO*. **67**: 94–96.

7 Persson K *et al.* (1992) The postoperative pharmacokinetics of codeine. *European Journal of Clinical Pharmacology*. **42**: 663–666.

DEXTROPROPOXYPHENE BNF 4.7.2

Class: Opioid analgesic.

Indications: Mild-to-moderate pain.

Pharmacology

Propoxyphene is a synthetic derivative of **methadone** and its analgesic properties reside in the dextro-isomer, dextropropoxyphene. It is a μ-opioid receptor agonist with affinity similar to that of **codeine**. It is also a weak NMDA-receptor-channel blocker but this is probably clinically irrelevant.[1] Dextropropoxyphene undergoes extensive dose-dependent first-pass hepatic metabolism; systemic availability increases with increasing doses.[2] The principal metabolite, norpropoxyphene, is also analgesic but crosses the blood-brain barrier to a much lesser extent. Both dextropropoxyphene and norpropoxyphene achieve steady-state plasma concentrations 5–7 times greater than those after the first dose. Randomised controlled trials in patients with postsurgical pain, arthritis and musculoskeletal pain collectively show no added benefit when dextropropoxyphene is combined with **paracetamol** compared with **paracetamol** alone.[3] Such reports have led to doubts about the general efficacy of dextropropoxyphene. However, dextropropoxyphene 65mg has been shown to have a definite analgesic effect in several placebo-controlled trials and a dose-response curve has been established, thereby confirming its efficacy (Figure 5.8).[4]

Dextropropoxyphene causes less nausea and vomiting, drowsiness and dry mouth than low-dose **morphine**, particularly during initial treatment.[5] The relative potency of a single dose of dextropropoxyphene is 1/2–2/3 that of **codeine**.[2] Cumulation occurs with multiple doses,[6] and, when given regularly, dextropropoxyphene can be regarded as equipotent with **codeine** and **dihydrocodeine**.

Bio-availability 40% PO.

Onset of action 20–30min.

Time to peak plasma concentation 2–2.5h.

Plasma halflife 6–12h, increasing to >50h in elderly;[7] norpropoxyphene 30–36h.

Duration of action 4–6h, longer in elderly.

Cautions and undesirable effects

For full list, see manufacturer's SPC.

Dextropropoxyphene may enhance the effect of **warfarin**, **carbamazepine** and other CNS depressants, including alcohol. Dextropropoxyphene prolongs the plasma halflife of **alprazolam** by 50% (12h → 18h); it has no effect on the metabolism of **lorazepam** and a clinically unimportant effect on **diazepam**.[8] Also see Strong opioids, p.168.

Dose and use

Dextropropoxyphene is marketed as either the hydrochloride salt or as napsilate; dextropropoxyphene *napsilate* 100mg is equivalent to dextropropoxyphene *hydrochloride* 65mg, the difference relating to the different molecular weights of the two salts. In the UK, it is used almost exclusively in compound tablets with **paracetamol** as **co-proxamol**. The manufacturer's licence is restricted to 2 tablets q.d.s., i.e. 8 tablets in 24h; this is an artificial limit and derives from cases of self-poisoning. Clinically, the dose need be limited only to the total daily dose of **paracetamol**; 12 tablets contain 4g.

Supply

Co-proxamol (non-proprietary)

Tablets dextropropoxyphene hydrochloride 32.5mg + **paracetamol** 325mg, 28 days @ 2 q.d.s. = £2.69.

Doloxene® (Lilly 01256 315000)

Capsules dextropropoxyphene hydrochloride 65mg (as napsilate 100mg), 28 days @ 1 q.d.s. = £9.18 (~~NHS~~).

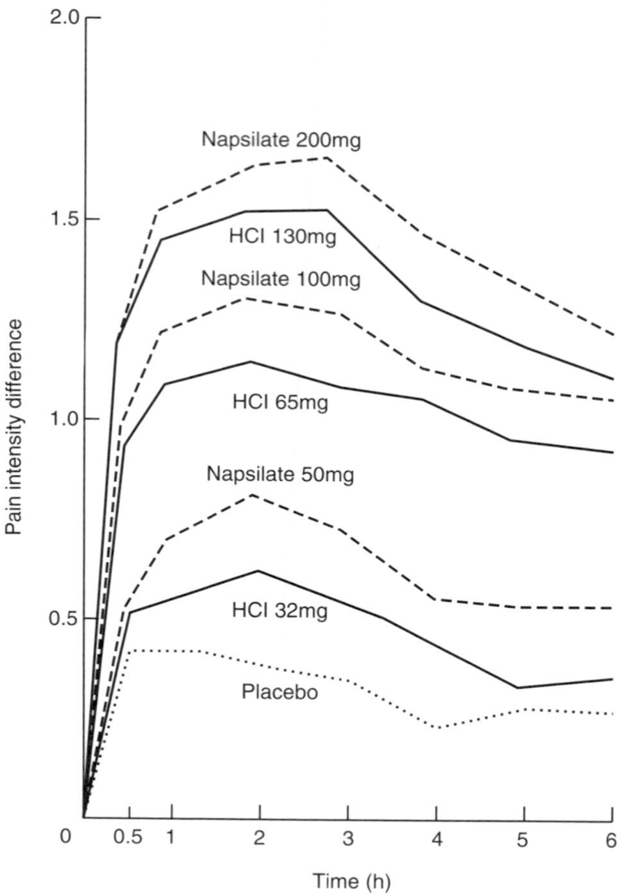

Figure 5.8 Incremental pain relief with increasing doses of dextropropoxyphene hydrochloride and dextropropoxyphene napsilate.[4] Placebos do not have a dose-response curve.

1 Ebert B *et al.* (1998) Dextropropoxyphene acts as a noncompetitive N-methyl D-aspartate antagonist. *Journal of Pain and Symptom Management.* **15**: 269–274.

2 Perrier D and Gibaldi M (1972) Influence of first-pass effect on the systemic availability of propoxyphene. *The Journal of Clinical Pharmacology.* **Nov/Dec**: 449–452.

3 Li-Wan-Po A and Zhang W (1997) Systematic overview of co-proxamol to assess analgesic effects of addition of dextropropoxyphene to paracetamol. *British Medical Journal.* **315**: 1565–1571.

4 Beaver WT (1984) Analgesic efficacy of dextropropoxyphene and dextropropoxyphene-containing combinations: a review. *Human Toxicology.* **3**: 191s–220s.

5 Mercadante S *et al.* (1998) Dextropropoxyphene versus morphine in opioid-naive cancer patients with pain. *Journal of Pain and Symptom Management.* **15**: 76–81.

6 Twycross R (1984) Plasma concentrations of dextropropoxyphene and norpropoxyphene. *Human Toxicology.* **3**: 58s–59s.

7 Crome P *et al.* (1984) Pharmacokinetics of dextropropoxyphene and nordextropropoxyphene in elderly hospital patients after single and multiple doses of distalgesic. Preliminary analysis of results. *Human Toxicology.* **3**: 41s–48s.
8 Abernethy D *et al.* (1985) Interaction of propoxyphene with diazepam, alprazolam and lorazepam. *British Journal of Clinical Pharmacology.* **19**: 51–57.

DIHYDROCODEINE BNF 4.7.2

Class: Opioid analgesic.

Indications: Moderate-to-severe pain.

Pharmacology

Dihydrocodeine is a semisynthetic analogue of **codeine** which also relieves pain and cough, and causes constipation.[1,2] Like **codeine**, dihydrocodeine is a substrate for CYP2D6 and its partial metabolism to dihydromorphine is limited in poor metabolisers and is blocked by CYP2D6 inhibitors such as **fluoxetine**, **paroxetine** and **quinidine**.[3] However, unlike **codeine**, there is no evidence that such inhibition reduces the analgesic effect of dihydrocodeine. By injection 60mg provides significantly more analgesia than 30mg and is comparable to **morphine** 10mg.[4,5] Dihydrocodeine is about twice as potent as **codeine** by injection parenterally but, because its oral bio-availability is low, the two drugs are essentially equipotent by mouth.[6]
Bio-availability 20% PO.
Onset of action 30min.
Time to peak plasma concentration 1.7h.
Plasma halflife 3.5–4.5h.
Duration of action 4h.

Cautions and undesirable effects

For full list, see manufacturer's SPC.
Sedation, dizziness, hallucinations 4%, disturbed dreams 4%, nausea and vomiting, headache, vertigo, constipation. Like **morphine** and **codeine**, dihydrocodeine is more toxic in renal failure, probably because of cumulation of an active glucuronide.[7] Also see Strong opioids, p.168.

Dose and use

- usual starting dose 30mg q6h–q4h
- increase if necessary to 60mg q6h–q4h.

The higher dose is associated with a significant increase in undesirable effects.[8]

Supply

Dihydrocodeine (non-proprietary)
Tablets 30mg, 28 days @ 30mg q.d.s. = £3.92.
Oral solution 10mg/5ml, 28 days @ 30mg q.d.s. = £35.84.
***Injection* CD** 50mg/ml, 1ml amp = £1.98.

DF 118 Forte® (Martindale 01708 386660)
Tablets 40mg, 28 days @ 40mg t.d.s. = £9.67.

Modified-release
DHC Continus® (Napp 01223 424444)
Tablets m/r 60mg, 90mg, 120mg, 28 days @ 60mg b.d. = £6.69.

1 Keats AS *et al.* (1957) Studies of analgesic drugs: dihydrocodeine. *Journal of Pharmacology and Experimental Therapeutics.* **120**: 354–360.
2 Weiss B (1959) Dihydrocodeine. A pharmacologic review. *American Journal of Pharmacy.* **August**: 286–301.

3 Fromm M *et al.* (1995) Dihydrocodeine: A new opioid substrate for the polymorphic CYP2D6 in humans. *Clinical Pharmacology and Therapeutics*. **58:** 374–382.
4 Seed JC *et al.* (1958) A comparison of the analgesic and respiratory effects of dihydrocodeine and morphine in man. *Archives Internationales de Pharmacodynamie et de Therapie*. **116**: 293–339.
5 Palmer RN *et al.* (1966) Incidence of unwanted effects of dihydrocodeine bitartrate in healthy volunteers. *Lancet.* **2**: 620–621.
6 Anonymous (1991) Dihydrocodeine (tartrate). In: C Dollery (ed) *Therapeutic Drugs*. Churchill Livingstone, Edinburgh, pp.D133–136.
7 Barnes J *et al.* (1985) Dihydrocodeine in renal failure: further evidence for an important role in the kidney in the handling of opioid drugs. *British Medical Journal.* **290**: 740–742.
8 McQuay H *et al.* (1993) A multiple dose comparison of ibuprofen and dihydrocodeine after third molar surgery. *British Journal of Oral and Maxillofacial Surgery.* **31**: 95–100.

TRAMADOL — BNF 4.7.2

Class: Opioid analgesic.

Indications: Moderate-to-severe pain.

Pharmacology

Tramadol is a synthetic centrally acting analgesic with both opioid and non-opioid properties.[1,2] It stimulates neuronal serotonin release and inhibits the presynaptic re-uptake of both noradrenaline (norepinephrine) and serotonin. In animal models, tramadol also has an anti-inflammatory effect which is independent of PG inhibition.[3] **Naloxone** only partially reverses the analgesic effect of tramadol.[1] Tramadol is converted in the liver to O-desmethyltramadol (M1) which is itself an active substance, 2–4 times more potent than tramadol. Further biotransformation results in inactive metabolites which are excreted by the kidneys. A comparison of receptor site affinities and mono-amine re-uptake inhibition illustrates the unique combination of properties which underlie the action of tramadol (Table 5.9 and 5.10); it is necessary to invoke synergism to explain its analgesic effect. The importance of M1 is shown by studies in poor metabolisers of sparteine/debrisoquine. Poor metabolisers lack the iso-enzyme, CYP2D6; they comprise 5–10% of the white population in Europe. In such subjects, tramadol has little or no analgesic effect.[4] Tramadol causes much less constipation and respiratory depression than equi-analgesic doses of **morphine**.[5] It has no effect on pressures in the biliary and pancreatic ducts.[6] Its dependence liability is also considerably less,[7] and it is not a CD.[8] By injection, tramadol is 1/10 as potent as **morphine**. By mouth, because of much better bio-availability, it is 1/5 as potent; it can be regarded as double strength **codeine**.

Bio-availability 75% PO; >90% with multiple doses.[9]
Onset of action 30min.
Time to peak plasma concentration 2h; 4–8h m/r.
Plasma halflife 6h; active metabolite 7.4h; these more than double in cirrhosis and severe renal failure.
Duration of action 4–6h.

Table 5.9 Opioid receptor affinities: K_i (μM) values[a,1]

	Mu	*Delta*	*Kappa*
Morphine	0.0003	0.09	0.6
Dextropropoxyphene	0.03	0.38	1.2
Codeine	0.2	5	6
Tramadol	2	58	43

a. the lower the K_i value, the greater the receptor affinity.

Table 5.10 Inhibition of mono-amine uptake: K_i (μM) values[a,1]

	Noradrenaline (norepinephrine)	*Serotonin*
Imipramine	0.0066	0.021
Tramadol	0.78	0.99
Dextropropoxyphene Codeine Morphine	IA[b]	IA[b]

a. the lower the K_i value, the greater the receptor affinity
b. IA = inactive at 10μM.

Cautions
Epilepsy, raised intracranial pressure, severe renal or hepatic impairment. Use with caution in patients taking medication which lowers seizure threshold, notably tricyclic antidepressants and SSRIs. **Carbamazepine** decreases the effect of tramadol. Seizures have been reported in patients receiving tramadol after rapid IV injection.

Undesirable effects
For full list, see manufacturer's SPC.
Also see Strong opioids, p.168.

Dose and use
- usual oral doses are 50–100mg q4h–q6h
- maximum recommended dose 400mg/day; higher doses have been given, e.g. 600mg/day, and sometimes more.

Supply
Tramadol (non-proprietary)
Capsules 50mg, 28 days @ 100mg q.d.s. = £22.15.

Tramake Insts® (Galen 028 3833 4974)
Sachets 50mg, 100mg, 28 days @ 100mg q.d.s. = £33.41; *contain 9.7mmol and 14.6mmol Na^+/sachet respectively*; avoid in renal impairment or cardiac failure.

Zamadol® (ASTA Medica 01223 423434)
Capsules 50mg, 28 days @ 100mg q.d.s. = £32.52.
Injection 50mg/ml, 2ml amp = £1.18.

Zydol® (Pharmacia 01908 661101)
Capsules 50mg, 28 days @ 100mg q.d.s. = £37.88.
Tablets soluble 50mg, 28 days @ 100mg q.d.s. = £34.12.
Injection 50mg/ml, 2ml amp = £1.24.

Modified-release
Zamadol® SR (ASTA Medica 01223 423434)
Capsules m/r 50mg, 100mg, 150mg, 200mg, 28 days @ 200mg b.d. = £30.66.

Dromadol® SR (IVAX 08705 020304)
Tablets m/r 75mg, 100mg, 150mg, 200mg, 28 days @ 200mg b.d. = £29.87.
Dromadol® XL (IVAX 08705 020304)
Tablets m/r 150mg, 200mg, 300mg, 400mg, 28 days @ 400mg o.d. = £34.09.

Zydol SR® (Pharmacia 01908 661101)
Tablets m/r 100mg, 150mg, 200mg, 28 days @ 200mg b.d. = £34.09.
Zydol XL® (Pharmacia 01908 661101)
Tablets m/r 150mg, 200mg, 300mg, 400mg, 28 days @ 400mg o.d. = £37.88.

1 Raffa RB *et al.* (1992) Opioid and nonopioid components independently contribute to the mechanism of action of tramadol, an 'atypical' opioid analgesic. *Journal of Pharmacology and Therapeutics.* **260**: 275–285.
2 Lee C *et al.* (1993) Tramadol: a preliminary review of its pharmacodynamic and pharmacokinetic properties, and therapeutic potential in acute and chronic pain states. *Drugs.* **46**: 313–340.
3 Buccellati C *et al.* (2000) Tramadol anti-inflammatory activity is not related to a direct inhibitory action on prostaglandin endoperoxide synthases. *European Journal of Pain.* **4**: 413–415.
4 Poulsen L *et al.* (1996) The hypoalgesic effect of tramadol in relation to CYP2D6. *Clinical Pharmacology and Therapeutics.* **60**: 636–644.
5 Wilder-Smith C and Bettiga A (1997) The analgesic tramadol has minimal effect on gastro-intestinal motor function. *British Journal of Clinical Pharmacology.* **43**: 71–75.
6 Staritz M *et al.* (1986) Effect of modern analgesic drugs (Tramadol, pentazocine, and buprenorphine) on the bile duct sphincter in man. *Gut.* **27**: 567–569.
7 Preston K *et al.* (1991) Abuse potential and pharmacological comparison of tramadol and morphine. *Drug and Alcohol Dependency.* **27**: 7–18.
8 Radbruch L *et al.* (1996) A risk-benefit assessment of tramadol in the management of pain. *Drug Safety.* **15**: 8–29.
9 Gibson T (1996) Pharmacokinetics, efficacy, and safety of analgesia with a focus on tramadol HCl. *American Journal of Medicine.* **101**: 47s–53s.

STRONG OPIOIDS — BNF 4.7.2

Strong opioids exist to be given, not merely to be withheld; their use is dictated by therapeutic need and response, not by brevity of prognosis.

Morphine is generally the strong opioid of choice for cancer pain management.[1,2] Other strong opioids are used mainly when **morphine** is not readily available or when the patient has intolerable undesirable effects with **morphine**.[3] Differences between opioids relate in part to differences in receptor affinity (Table 5.11). Improved pain relief should not be expected if a patient is switched to another opioid of similar opioid-receptor affinity. However, the incidence or severity of undesirable effects may be significantly altered when, for example, a patient is switched from **morphine** to **fentanyl (transdermal)**.

Table 5.11 Receptor affinity of opioid analgesics and naloxone[4–6]

Drug	*Receptor type*		
	Mu	*Kappa*	*Delta*
Morphine Fentanyl Hydromorphone	A	–	–
Oxycodone	–	A	–
Methadone	A	–	A(?)
Buprenorphine	pA	Ant	A
Pentazocine	pA	A	ant
Pethidine	a	–	–
Naloxone	Ant	Ant	Ant

A = strong agonist; a = weak agonist; Ant = strong antagonist; ant = weak antagonist;
pA = partial agonist; x = negligible activity; – = no activity.

Strong opioids are not the panacea for cancer pain; they are generally best administered with a non-opioid. Further, even combined use does not guarantee success, particularly with neuropathic pain or if the psychosocial dimension of suffering is ignored. Other reasons for poor relief include:

- underdosing (failure to titrate the dose upwards)
- poor patient compliance (patient not taking medication)
- poor alimentary absorption because of vomiting.

Pentazocine should not be used; it is a weak opioid by mouth[7,8] and often causes psychotomimetic effects (dysphoria, depersonalisation, frightening dreams, hallucinations).[9]

Pethidine[10] and **dextromoramide**[11] have short durations of action and are not recommended for round-the-clock prophylactic analgesia. Some centres use SL **dextromoramide** in patients taking regular **morphine** as additonal analgesia before a painful procedure but, because of its variable absorption, it may not be equally effective for all patients.[12] However, at other centres, such procedures are timed to coincide with the peak plasma concentration after a regular or p.r.n. dose of **morphine** or are undertaken after an individually titrated dose of **transmucosal fentanyl**.

Undesirable effects

For full list, see manufacturer's SPC.

Strong opioids tend to cause the same range of undesirable effects (Box 5.E), although to a varying degree. It is necessary to develop strategies to deal with the undesirable effects of **morphine** and other strong opioids, particularly nausea and vomiting, and constipation.[13]

Box 5.E Undesirable effects of opioid analgesics

Common initial
Nausea and vomiting
Drowsiness
Unsteadiness
Delirium (acute confusional state)

Common ongoing
Constipation
Nausea and vomiting

Occasional
Dry mouth
Sweating
Pruritus
Hallucinations
Myoclonus

Rare
Respiratory depression
Psychological dependence

Respiratory depression

Pain is a physiological antagonist to the central depressant effects of opioids.

Strong opioids do not cause clinically important respiratory depression in patients in pain.[14] **Naloxone**, a specific opioid antagonist, is rarely needed in palliative care. In contrast to post-operative patients, cancer patients with pain:

- have generally been receiving a weak opioid for some time, i.e. are not opioid naïve
- take medication by mouth (slower absorption, lower peak concentration)
- titrate the dose upwards step by step (less likelihood of an excessive dose being given).

The relationship of the therapeutic dose to the lethal dose of a strong opioid (the therapeutic ratio) is greater than commonly supposed. For example, patients who take a double dose of **morphine** at bedtime are no more likely to die during the night than those who do not.[15]

Tolerance and dependence

Tolerance to strong opioids is not a practical problem.[16,17] Psychological dependence (addiction) to **morphine** is rare in patients.[18,19] Caution in this respect should be reserved for patients with a present or past history of substance abuse (Box 5.F); even then strong opioids should be used when there is clinical need.[20,21] Physical dependence does not prevent a reduction in the dose of **morphine** if the patient's pain ameliorates, e.g. as a result of radiotherapy or a nerve block.[22]

Box 5.F Contract for controlled substance prescriptions with addicts[a]

Controlled substance medications (i.e. narcotics, tranquilizers and barbiturates) are very useful, but have high potential for misuse and are therefore closely controlled by the local, state, and federal government. They are intended to relieve pain, to improve function and/or ability to work, not simply to feel good. Because my physician is prescribing such medication for me to help manage my condition, I agree to the following conditions:

1 I am responsible for my controlled substance medications. If the prescription of medication is lost, misplaced, or stolen, or if I use it up sooner than prescribed, I understand that it will not be replaced.
2 I will not request or accept controlled substance medication from any other physicians or individual while I am receiving such medication from Dr.________________. Besides being illegal to do so, it may endanger my health. The only exception is if it is prescribed while I am admitted in a hospital.
3 Refills of controlled substance medication:
   a Will be made only during Dr. __________________ regular office hours, in person, once each month during a scheduled office visit. Refills, will not be made at night, on holidays, or weekends.
   b Will not be made if I "run out early". I am responsible for taking the medication in the dose prescribed and for keeping track of the amount remaining.
   c Will not be made as an "emergency", such as on Friday afternoon because I suddenly realize I will "run out tomorrow". I will call at least seventy-two hours ahead if I need assistance with a controlled substance medication prescription.
4 I will bring in the containers of all medications prescribed by Dr. ________________ each time I see him even if there is no medication remaining. These will be in the original containers from the pharmacy for each medication.
5 I understand that if I violate any of the above conditions, my controlled substances prescription and/or treatment with Dr. ________________ may be ended immediately. If the violation involves obtaining controlled substances from another individual, as described above, I may also be reported to my physician, medical facilities, and other authorities.
6 I understand that the main treatment goal is to improve my ability to function and/or work. In consideration of that goal and the fact that I am being given potent medication to help me reach that goal, I agree to help myself by the following better health habits: exercise, weight control, and the non-use of tobacco and alcohol. I understand that only through following a healthier life-style can I hope to have the most successful outcome to my treatment.

I have been fully informed by Dr. _____________ and his staff regarding psychological dependence (addiction) of a controlled substance, which I understand is rare. I know that some persons may develop a tolerance, which is the need to increase the dose of the medication to achieve the same effect of pain control, and I do know that I will become physically dependent on the medication. This will occur if I am on the medication for several weeks, and, when I stop the medication, I must do so slowly and under medical supervision or I may have withdrawal symptoms.

I have read this contract and it has been explained to my by Dr. ________________ and/or his staff. In addition, I fully understand the consequences of violating said contract.

________________________	________	________________________	________
Patient's Signature	Date	Witness	Date

a. reproduced with permission from Hansen 1999.[23] ©Southern Medical Association.

Opioid switching

Some patients need to be switched from **morphine** (or other strong opioid) to an alternative, about 20% according to a recently published prospective survey.[24] Changes from **morphine** to **fentanyl (transdermal)** (or *vice versa*) are included in this figure. Higher figures have been published elsewhere, e.g. 44%.[25] The lower figure better reflects clinical experience in the UK (Twycross R, unpublished data). The main reasons for switching opioids are:

- poor compliance (→ **transdermal fentanyl**)
- intractable constipation (→ **transdermal fentanyl**)
- poor response to **morphine** plus an NSAID (→ **methadone**)[26]
- neurotoxicity (cognitive failure/delirium, hallucinations, myoclonus, hyperalgesia, allodynia).

Hydromorphone, **oxycodone** and **methadone** have all been substituted successfully for morphine in cases of neurotoxicity.[27–29]

When converting from an alternative strong opioid to oral **morphine**, the initial dose depends on the relative potency of the two drugs (Table 5.12). For most drugs at typical doses, these approximate conversion ratios are safe for switching in both directions, except perhaps for **hydromorphone**. Some sources suggest a conversion ratio of about 5:1 if switching from **morphine** to **hydromorphone** but only 4:1 if switching from **hydromorphone** to **morphine**.[30,31] *These differ considerably from the manufacturer's recommendation of 7.5:1.*[32,33]

Table 5.12 Approximate oral analgesic equivalence to morphine[a]

Analgesic	*Potency ratio with morphine*	*Duration of action (hours)*[b]
Codeine Dihydrocodeine Dextropropoxyphene	1/10	3–6
Pethidine	1/8	2–4
Tramadol	1/5[c]	4–6
Dipipanone (in Diconal UK)	1/2	4–6
Papaveretum	2/3[d]	3–5
Oxycodone	1.5–2[c]	3–4
Dextromoramide	[2][e]	2–3
Levorphanol (not UK)	5	4–6
Methadone	5–10[f]	8–12
Hydromorphone	7.5[g]	4–5
Buprenorphine (*sublingual*)	60	6–8
Fentanyl (*transdermal*)	100–150	72

a. multiply dose of opioid by its potency ratio to determine the equivalent dose of morphine sulphate/hydrochloride
b. dependent in part on severity of pain and on dose; often longer lasting in very elderly and those with renal dysfunction
c. tramadol and oxycodone are both relatively more potent by mouth because of high bio-availability; parenteral potency ratios with morphine are 1/10 and 3/4 respectively
d. papaveretum (strong opium) is standardised to contain 50% morphine base; potency expressed in relation to morphine sulphate
e. dextromoramide: a single 5mg dose is equivalent to morphine 15mg in terms of peak effect but is shorter acting; overall potency ratio adjusted accordingly
f. methadone: a single 5mg dose is equivalent to morphine 7.5mg. Has a variable long plasma halflife and broad-spectrum receptor affinity results in a much higher than expected potency ratio when given repeatedly[37]
g. manufacturer's recommended ratio.

Switching at high doses

The recommended equivalent doses of the strong opioids are an approximate guide only; they cannot be exact for everybody.[30,31,34] They are based on typical **morphine** doses. As the dose of **morphine** escalates, e.g. >2g/24h, the recommended equivalent doses will become progressively more erroneous. Any error may well be compounded by high concentrations of morphine's main metabolite, M3G which is said to neutralise the analgesic effect of **morphine** by a non-opioidergic neuro-excitatory mechanism.[35,36] Thus, when converting at high dose levels it is best to give 1/2–1/4 of the calculated equivalent dose. A separate strategy is necessary for **methadone**.

1 World Health Organization (1986) *Cancer pain relief.* WHO, Geneva.

2 Hanks G *et al.* (2001) Morphine and alternative opioids in cancer pain: the EAPC recommendations. *British Journal of Cancer.* **84**: 587–593.

3 Cherny N (1996) Opioid analgesics: comparative features and prescribing guidelines. *Drugs.* **51**: 713–737.

4 Hill RG (1992) Multiple opioid receptors and their ligands. *Frontiers of Pain.* **4**: 1–4.

5 Corbett AD *et al.* (1993) Selectivity of ligands for opioid receptors. In: A Herz (ed) *Opioids.* Springer-Verlag, London, pp.657–672.

6 Ross F and Smith M (1997) The intrinsic antinociceptive effects of oxycodone appear to be kappa-opioid receptor mediated. In: *Eighth World Congress on Pain.* Vancouver, IASP Press, Seattle.

7 Hoskin P and Hanks G (1991) Opioid agonist-antagonist drugs in acute and chronic pain states. *Drugs.* **41**: 326–344.

8 Twycross R (1994) Pentazocine. In: *Pain Relief in Advanced Cancer.* Churchill Livingstone, Edinburgh, pp.247–248.

9 Woods A *et al.* (1974) Medicines evaluation and monitoring group: central nervous system effects of pentazocine. *British Medical Journal.* **1**: 305–307.

10 Twycross R (1994) Pethidine. In: *Pain Relief in Advanced Cancer.* Churchill Livingstone, Edinburgh, pp.286–290.

11 Twycross R (1994) Dextromoramide. In: *Pain Relief in Advanced Cancer.* Churchill Livingstone, Edinburgh, pp.290–291.

12 Jones T *et al.* (1996) Dextromoramide pharmacokinetics following sublingual administration. *Palliative Medicine.* **10**: 313–317.

13 Cherny N *et al.* (2001) Strategies to manage the adverse effects of oral morphine: an evidence-based report. *Journal of Clinical Oncology.* **19**: 2542–2554.

14 Borgbjerg FM *et al.* (1996) Experimental pain stimulates respiration and attenuates morphine-induced respiratory depression: a controlled study in human volunteers. *Pain.* **64**: 123–128.

15 Regnard CFB and Badger C (1987) Opioids, sleep and the time of death. *Palliative Medicine.* **1**: 107–110.

16 Collin E *et al.* (1993) Is disease progression the major factor in morphine 'tolerance' in cancer pain management? *Pain.* **55**: 319–326.

17 Portenoy RK (1994) Tolerance to opioid analgesics: clinical aspects. *Cancer Surveys.* **21**: 49–65.

18 Passik S and Portenoy R (1998) Substance abuse issues in palliative care. In: A Berger (ed) *Principles and Practice of Supportive Oncology.* Lippincott-Raven, Philadelphia, pp.513–529.

19 Joranson D *et al.* (2000) Trends in medical use and abuse of opioid analgesics. *Journal of the American Medical Association.* **283**: 1710–1714.

20 Passik S *et al.* (1998) Substance abuse issues in cancer patients. Part 1: prevalence and diagnosis. *Oncology.* **12**: 517–521.

21 Passik S *et al.* (1998) Substance abuse issues in cancer patients. Part 2: evaluation and treatment. *Oncology.* **12**: 729–734.

22 Twycross RG and Wald SJ (1976) Longterm use of diamorphine in advanced cancer. In: JJ Bonica and D Albe-Fessard (eds) *Advances in Pain Research and Therapy,* Vol 1. Raven Press, New York, pp.653–661.

23 Hansen H (1999) Treatment of chronic pain with antiepileptic drugs. *Southern Medical Journal.* **92**: 642–649.

24 Sarhill N *et al.* (2001) Parenteral opioid rotation in advanced cancer: A prospective study. Abstracts of the MASCC/ISOO 13th International Symposium Supportive Care in Cancer, Copenhagen, Denmark, June 14–16. *Supportive Care in Cancer.* **9**: 307.

25 Cherny NJ *et al.* (1995) Opioid pharmacotherapy in the management of cancer pain: a survey of strategies used by pain physicians for the selection of analgesic drugs and routes of administration. *Cancer.* **76**: 1283–1293.
26 Morley J and Makin M (1998) The use of methadone in cancer pain poorly responsive to other opioids. *Pain Reviews.* **5**: 51–58.
27 Ashby M *et al.* (1999) Opioid substitution to reduce adverse effects in cancer pain management. *Medical Journal of Australia.* **170**: 68–71.
28 Sjogren P *et al.* (1994) Disappearance of morphine-induced hyperalgesia after discontinuing or substituting morphine with other opioid antagonists. *Pain.* **59**: 313–316.
29 Hagen N and Wanson R (1997) Strychnine-like multifocal myoclonus and seizures in extremely high-dose opioid administration: treatment strategies. *Journal of Pain and Symptom Management.* **14**: 51–58.
30 Anderson R *et al.* (2001) Accuracy in equianalgesic dosing: conversion dilemmas. *Journal of Pain and Symptom Management.* **21**: 397–406.
31 Pereira J *et al.* (2001) Equianalgesic dose ratios for opioids: a critical review and proposals for long-term dosing. *Journal of Pain and Symptom Management.* **22**: 672–687.
32 McDonald C and Miller A (1997) A comparative potency study of a controlled release tablet formulation of hydromorphone with controlled release morphine in patients with cancer pain. *European Journal of Palliative Care. Abstracts of the Fifth Congress.*
33 Moriarty M *et al.* (1999) A randomised crossover comparison of controlled release hydromorphone tablets with controlled release morphine tablets in patients with cancer pain. *Journal of Clinical Research.* **2**: 1–8.
34 Pasternak G (2001) Incomplete cross tolerance and multiple mu opioid peptide receptors. *Trends in Pharmacological Sciences.* **22**: 67–70.
35 Smith MT (2000) Neuroexcitatory effects of morphine and hydromorphone: evidence implicating the 3-glucuronide metabolites. *Clinical and Experimental Pharmacology and Physiology.* **27**: 524–528.
36 Gong Q-L *et al.* (1992) Morphine 3-glucuronide may functionally antagonize M6G induced antinociception and ventilatory depression in the rat. *Pain.* **48**: 249–255.
37 Bruera E *et al.* (1996) Opioid rotation in patients with cancer pain. *Cancer.* **78**: 852–857.

MORPHINE — BNF 4.7.2

Class: Opioid analgesic.

Indications: Moderate-to-severe pain, diarrhoea, cough, †dyspnoea.

Contra-indications: None, if titrated carefully against a patient's pain.

Pharmacology

Morphine is the main pharmacologically active constituent of opium. Its effects are mediated by specific opioid receptors both within the CNS and peripherally. Under normal circumstances, its main peripheral action is on smooth muscle. However, in the presence of inflammation, normally silent peripheral receptors become activated.[1] The liver is the principal site of morphine metabolism.[2] Metabolism also occurs in other organs,[3] including the CNS.[4] Glucuronidation is rarely impaired except in severe hepatic failure,[5] and morphine is well tolerated in patients with mild-to-moderate hepatic impairment.[6] However, with impairment severe enough to prolong the prothrombin time, the plasma halflife of morphine may be increased[3] and the dose of morphine may need to be reduced or given less often, i.e. q6h–q8h. The major metabolites of morphine are morphine-3-glucuronide (M3G) and morphine-6-glucuronide (M6G);[7] M6G binds to opioid receptors whereas M3G does not. M6G contributes substantially to the analgesic effect of morphine, and can cause nausea and vomiting, sedation and respiratory depression.[8,9] In renal failure, the plasma halflife of M6G increases from 2.5h up to 7.5h, and is likely to lead to cumulative toxicity unless the frequency of administration and/or the dose of morphine is reduced. When given regularly, the oral to SC potency ratio of morphine is between 1:2 and 1:3, the same ratio holds true for IM and IV injections.[5,10]

Bio-availability 35% PO, ranging from 15–64%; 25% PR.
Peak effect 30–60min IM; 5–90min SC.
Time to peak plasma concentration 15–60min PO; 10–20min IM/SC; 1–6h m/r.
Plasma halflife 1.5–4.5h PO; 1.5h IV.
Duration of action 3–6h; 12h m/r (MST Continus®, Zomorph®); 24h m/r (MXL®); 24h m/r PR.

Undesirable effects

For full list, see manufacturer's SPC.
See Table 5.13. Also see Strong opioids, p.168.

Dose and use

Oral morphine

Morphine should generally be given together with a non-opioid.

Morphine is administered as tablets ('normal-release') or aqueous solutions. An increasing range of m/r preparations is available: tablets, capsules, suspensions and rectal tampons (non-dissolving suppository). There are no generic m/r morphine tablets. Because the pharmacokinetic profiles differ,[12–14] it is best to keep individual patients on the same brand. Most are administered b.d., some o.d. Patients can be started on either an ordinary (normal-release) or a m/r preparation (Box 5.G). The time to peak plasma concentration is significantly shorter with an aqueous solution of morphine compared with a normal-release tablet (0.5h vs 1.5h, data on file, Boehringer Ingelheim) suggesting that morphine solutions are a better option than tablets for p.r.n. use.

Traditionally, to make things easier for patients, morphine q4h has been given on waking, 1000h, 1400h, 1800h with a double dose at bedtime. Although clinically this seems satisfactory, a recent non-blinded study concluded that patients who take a single dose at bedtime plus a regular 0200h dose need significantly fewer p.r.n. doses during the night and have less pain on waking in the morning.[15] However, pending confirmation from a double-blind trial, the traditional approach is still recommended.

When adjusting the dose of morphine, generally increase by 33–50%. Two-thirds of patients never need more than 30mg q4h (or m/r morphine 100mg q12h); the rest need up to 200mg q4h (or m/r morphine 600mg q12h), and occasionally more. Instructions must be clear: extra p.r.n. morphine does not mean that the next regular dose is omitted. It is easier for the patient if the p.r.n. dose is the same as the q4h dose but some centres recommend 1/4–1/2 of the q4h dose.[16] *The p.r.n. dose must be increased when the regular dose is increased.* A laxative should be prescribed routinely unless there is a strong reason for not doing so, e.g. the patient has an ileostomy (see Opioid-induced constipation, p.19). An anti-emetic should be supplied for p.r.n. use during the first week or prescribed regularly if the patient has had nausea with a weak opioid, e.g. **haloperidol** 1.5mg stat & o.n.

Suppositories and enemas continue to be necessary in about 1/3 of patients. *Constipation may be more difficult to manage than the pain.* Warn patients about the possibility of initial drowsiness. If swallowing is difficult or vomiting persists, give 1/3 of the oral dose as CSCI **diamorphine** (or 1/2 the oral dose of morphine as CSCI morphine). Alternatively, morphine may be given PR (same dose as PO).

Initial dose titration with IV morphine

Initial dose titration with small boluses of IV morphine provides a method of rapidly determining morphine-responsiveness, e.g. in 30–40min (Box 5.H).[17] This approach is ideal in countries where patients travel long distances and cannot readily return for monitoring. IV *patient-controlled analgesia* (PCA) can be used but is more costly, requires inpatient admission and takes >10h to achieve relief.[18]

Buccal morphine

Morphine is slowly absorbed through the buccal mucosa.[19] In the past it was successfully used by this route in moribund patients cared for at home.

Rectal morphine

Morphine is absorbed from suppositories.[20] From the lower and middle rectum, it will enter the systemic circulation by-passing the liver. From the upper rectum, it will undergo hepatic first-pass metabolism after it enters the portal circulation. However, there are extensive anastomoses between the rectal veins which make it impossible to predict how much will enter the portal circulation.[21,22] Despite the uncertainty, in practice the same dose is given PR as PO. Although not licensed for this route, m/r morphine tablets have been used PR to provide emergency

Table 5.13 Potential intolerable effects of morphine

Type	*Effects*	*Initial action*	*Comment*
For general undesirable effects of opioid analgesics, see Box 5.E, p.169.			
Gastric stasis	Epigastric fullness, flatulence, anorexia, hiccup, persistent nausea	Metoclopramide 10–20mg q4h	If the problem persists, change to an alternative opioid
Sedation	Intolerable persistent sedation	Reduce dose of morphine; consider methylphenidate 10mg o.d.–b.d.	Sedation may be caused by other factors; stimulant rarely appropriate
Cognitive failure	Agitated delirium with hallucinations	Prescribe haloperidol 3–5mg stat & p.rn.; reduce dose of morphine and, if no improvement, switch to an alternative opioid	Some patients develop intractable delirium with one opioid but not with an alternative opioid
Myoclonus	Multifocal twitching ± jerking of limbs	Prescribe diazepam/midazolam 5mg stat & p.r.n.; reduce dose of morphine but increase again if pain recurs	Unusual with typical oral doses; more common with high dose IV and spinal morphine
Hyperexcitability	Abdominal muscle spasms, symmetrical jerking of legs; whole-body allodynia, hyperalgesia (manifests as excruciating pain)	Prescribe diazepam/midazolam 5mg stat & p.r.n.; reduce dose of morphine; consider changing to an alternative opioid	A rare syndrome in patients receiving intrathecal or high dose IV morphine; occasionally seen with typical oral and SC doses
Vestibular stimulation	Movement-induced nausea and vomiting	Prescribe cyclizine *or* dimenhydrinate *or* promethazine 25–50mg q8h–q6h	If intractable, try an alternative opioid or levomepromazine (methotrimeprazine)
Pruritus	Whole-body itch with systemic morphine; localised to upper body or face/nose with spinal morphine	Ondansetron 8mg IV stat and 8mg PO b.d. for 3–5 days	This is a central phenomenon and does not respond to H_1-antihistamines; centrally-acting opioid antagonists also relieve the itch but antagonise analgesia[11]
Histamine release	Bronchoconstriction → dyspnoea	Prescribe IV/IM antihistamine (e.g. chlorphenamine 5–10mg) and a bronchodilator; change to a chemically distinct opioid immediately e.g. methadone	Rare

Box 5.G Starting a patient on morphine PO

Oral morphine is indicated in patients with pain which does not respond to the optimised combined use of a non-opioid and a weak opioid.

The starting dose of morphine is calculated to give a greater analgesic effect than the medication already in use:
- if the patient was previously receiving a weak opioid, give 10mg q4h or m/r 20–30mg q12h
- if changing from an alternative strong opioid (e.g. fentanyl, methadone) a much higher dose of morphine may be needed
- if the patient is frail and elderly, a lower dose helps to reduce initial drowsiness, confusion and unsteadiness, e.g. 5mg q4h
- because of cumulation of an active metabolite, a lower and/or less frequent regular dose may be preferable in renal failure, e.g. 5–10mg q6h.

If the patient takes two or more p.r.n. doses in 24h, the regular dose should be increased by 30–50% every 2–3 days.

Upward titration of the dose of morphine stops when either the pain is relieved or intolerable undesirable effects supervene. In the latter case, it is generally necessary to consider alternative measures. The aim is to have the patient free of pain and mentally alert.

Because of poor absorption, m/r morphine may not be satisfactory in patients troubled by frequent vomiting or those with diarrhoea or an ileostomy. M/r morphine should be used with caution if there is renal impairment.

Scheme 1: ordinary (normal-release) morphine tablets or solution
- morphine given q4h 'by the clock' with p.r.n. doses of equal amount
- after 1–2 days, recalculate q4h dose based on total used in previous 24h (regular + p.r.n. use)
- continue q4h and p.r.n. doses
- increase the regular dose until there is adequate relief throughout each 4h period, taking p.r.n. use into account
- *a double dose at bedtime obviates the need to wake the patient for treatment during the night.*

Scheme 2: ordinary (normal-release) morphine and modified-release (m/r) morphine
- begin as for Scheme 1
- when the q4h dose is stable, replace with m/r morphine q12h, or o.d. if a 24h preparation is prescribed
- the q12h dose will be *three times* the previous q4h dose; an o.d. dose will be *six times* the previous q4h dose, rounded to a convenient number of tablets or capsules
- continue to provide ordinary morphine tablets or solution for p.r.n. use; give the equivalent of a q4h dose, i.e. 1/6 of the total daily dose.

Scheme 3: m/r morphine and ordinary (normal-release) morphine
- starting dose generally m/r morphine 20–30mg b.d.
- use ordinary morphine tablets or solution for p.r.n. medication; give about 1/6 of the daily dose
- increase the dose of m/r morphine every 2–3 days until there is adequate relief throughout each 12h period, taking p.r.n. use into account.

analgesia in moribund patients while organising a more reliable method of delivering analgesia, e.g. CSCI.[23]

M/r morphine suppositories for o.d. use are now available in the UK and make PR administration more feasible.[24] The suppository is a non-dissolving hydrogel suppository that releases morphine over 24h. It is indicated for the treatment of severe pain in patients with advanced cancer unable to take oral medication. The oral:rectal dose conversion is 1:1, i.e. the

Box 5.H Dose titration with IV morphine (Calicut, India)[17]

Prerequisites
Pain, i.e. ⩾5/10 on a numerical scale.
Likelihood of a partial or complete response to morphine.[a]

Method
Obtain venous access with a butterfly cannula.
Give metoclopramide 10mg IV routinely.
Dilute the contents of 15mg morphine ampoule in a 10ml syringe.[b]
Inject 1.5mg every 10min until the patient is pain-free or complains of undue sedation.
If patients experience nausea, give additional metoclopramide 5mg IV.

Results
Dose required (with approximate percentages):

1.5–4.5mg (40%)	10.5–15mg (15%)
6–9mg (40%)	>15mg (5%).

Complete relief in 80%; none in 1%.
Drop outs 2%.
Undesirable effects: sedation 32%; other 3%.

Ongoing treatment
Prescribe a dose of PO morphine q4h which is similar to the IV requirement, rounded to the nearest 5mg, i.e. relief with morphine 3–6mg IV → 5mg PO etc; the minimum dose is 5mg q4h.
Instruct patients to take p.r.n. doses and to adjust the dose the next day according to need.

a. most patients will already be taking a NSAID
b. ampoule strength is determined by local availability.

total daily oral morphine dose is given as a Moraxen® suppository PR o.d. Up to 2 suppositories at a time may be inserted to provide the required dose. Peak plasma concentrations are achieved within 5h of administration, and the halflife following removal is 2–3h. After about 24h suppositories should be expelled, either by a normal bowel movement, or by the use of a laxative suppository prior to insertion of the next dose. Used suppositories should be disposed of by flushing down the toilet. If a Moraxen® suppository is lost by defaecation before 24h, a new one should be inserted immediately to maintain pain relief. Specific contra-indications to this formulation and route of administration are painful anorectal conditions and neutropenia ($<0.5 \times 10^9$/L). Caution is advised with mucus-producing rectal tumours.

Spinal morphine
If given epidurally (ED) or intrathecally (IT), a much lower dose of morphine has a much greater analgesic effect because of the proximity to the opioid receptors in the dorsal horn of the spinal cord. The ED dose is about 1/10 and the IT dose 1/100 of the dose of PO morphine. Undesirable effects are correspondingly reduced. In the UK, <5% of cancer patients needing morphine receive it spinally (data on file).

The main indications for spinal morphine are:
- intractable pain despite the appropriate combined use of standard and adjuvant analgesics
- intolerable undesirable effects with systemic opioids.

To increase the effect of spinal analgesia in neuropathic pain, morphine is often combined with **bupivacaine**, and sometimes **clonidine**.

Topical morphine
Nociceptive afferent nerve fibres contain peripheral opioid receptors which are silent except in the presence of local inflammation.[1,25] This property is exploited in joint surgery where morphine is given intra-articularly at the end of the operation.[26] Topical morphine has also been used successfully to relieve otherwise intractable pain associated with cutaneous ulceration,

often sacral decubitus.[27–29] It is often given as a 0.1% (1mg/ml) gel, using Intrasite®. A higher dose may be necessary, e.g. 0.3–0.5%, in other situations:

- oral mucositis
- vaginal inflammation associated with a fistula
- rectal ulceration.[28]

The amount of gel applied varies according to the size and the site of the ulcer but is typically 5–10ml applied b.d.–t.d.s. The topical morphine is kept in place with:

- a non-absorbable pad or dressing, e.g. Opsite®
- gauze coated with petroleum jelly.

Supply

Unless indicated otherwise, all preparations are **CD**.

Normal-release oral preparations
Sevredol® (Napp 01223 424444)
Tablets 10mg, 20mg, 50mg; 10mg and 100mg dose = £0.11 and £1.08 respectively.
***Oral solution* PoM** 10mg/5ml, 10mg dose = £0.08.
Concentrated oral solution 100mg/5ml, 100mg dose = £0.87.

Oramorph® (Boehringer Ingelheim 01344 424600)
***Oral solution* PoM** 10mg/5ml, 10mg dose = £0.09.
Oral solution unit dose vials 10mg (**PoM**), 30mg, 100mg/5ml; 10mg and 100mg dose = £0.13 and £1.24 respectively.
Concentrated oral solution 100mg/5ml, 100mg dose = £0.91.

Modified-release oral preparations
Morcap® SR (Faulding DBL 01926 820820)
Capsules m/r 20mg, 50mg, 100mg, 28 days @ 100mg b.d. = £46.76.

MST Continus® (Napp 01223 424444)
Tablets m/r 5mg, 10mg, 15mg, 30mg, 60mg, 100mg, 200mg, 28 days @ 100mg b.d. = £49.62.
Oral suspension (sachet of m/r granules to mix with water) 20mg, 30mg, 60mg, 100mg, 200mg sachets, 28 days @ 100mg b.d. = £176.60.

Zomorph® (Link 01403 272451)
Capsules m/r 10mg, 30mg, 60mg, 100mg, 200mg, 28 days @ 100mg b.d. = £29.77.
Can be administered as a suspension or, if preferred, they can be added to hot liquids, e.g. soup. After 15min in water at 50°C, only 9% of the morphine is released (but 42% by 30min).

MXL® (Napp 01223 424444)
Capsules m/r 30mg, 60mg, 90mg, 120mg, 150mg, 200mg, 28 days @ 200mg o.d. = £49.62.

Normal-release rectal preparations
Morphine hydrochloride or sulphate (non-proprietary)
Suppositories 10mg, 15mg, 20mg, 30mg; 10mg dose = £0.51.

Modified-release rectal preparations
Moraxen® (Schwarz 01494 797500)
Rectal tampons (non-dissolving suppositories m/r) 35mg, 50mg, 75mg, 100mg, 28 days @ 100mg o.d. = £168.

Parenteral preparations
Morphine sulphate (non-proprietary)
Injection 10mg, 15mg, 20mg, 30mg/ml, 1ml and 2ml amp = £0.72–£1.59.

1 Krajnik M *et al.* (1998) Opioids affect inflammation and the immune system. *Pain Reviews.* **5**: 147–154.

2 Hasselstrom J *et al.* (1986) The metabolism and bioavailability of morphine in patients with severe liver cirrhosis. *British Journal of Clinical Pharmacology.* **29**: 289–297.

3 Mazoit J-X *et al.* (1987) Pharmacokinetics of unchanged morphine in normal and cirrhotic subjects. *Anesthesia and Analgesia.* **66**: 293–298.

4 Sandouk P *et al.* (1991) Presence of morphine metabolites in human cerebrospinal fluid after intracerebroventricular administration of morphine. *European Journal of Drug Metabolism and Pharmacology.* **16**: 166–171.
5 Max MB *et al.* (1992) *Principles of Analgesic Use in the Treatment of Acute Pain and Cancer Pain* (3e). American Pain Society, Skokie, Illinois, p.12.
6 Regnard CFB and Twycross RG (1984) Metabolism of narcotics (letter). *British Medical Journal.* **288**: 860.
7 McQuay HJ *et al.* (1990) Oral morphine in cancer pain: influences on morphine and metabolite concentration. *Clinical Pharmacology and Therapeutics.* **48**: 236–244.
8 Osborne RJ *et al.* (1986) Morphine intoxication in renal failure: the role of morphine-6-glucuronide. *British Medical Journal.* **292**: 1548–1549.
9 Thompson P *et al.* (1992) Mophine-6-glucuronide: a metabolite of morphine with greater emetic potency than morphine in the ferret. *British Journal of Pharmacology.* **106**: 3–8.
10 Hanks G *et al.* (2001) Morphine and alternative opioids in cancer pain: the EAPC recommendations. *British Journal of Cancer.* **84**: 587–593.
11 Jones E and Bergasa N (1999) The pruritus of cholestasis. *Hepatology.* **29**: 1003–1006.
12 Bloomfield S *et al.* (1993) Analgesic efficacy and potency of two oral controlled-release morphine preparations. *Clinical Pharmacology and Therapeutics.* **53**: 469–478.
13 Gourlay G *et al.* (1993) A comparison of Kapanol (a new sustained-release morphine formulation), MST Continus and morphine solution in cancer patients: pharmacokinetic aspects. *Presented at the Seventh World Congress on Pain*, IASP Press, Seattle.
14 West R and Maccarrone C (1993) Single dose pharmacokinetics of a new oral sustained-release morphine formulation, Kapanol capsules. *Presented at the Seventh World Congress on Pain*, IASP Press, Seattle.
15 Todd J *et al.* (2001) An assessment of the efficacy and tolerability of a 'double dose' of immediate-release morphine at bedtime. *Presented at the Seventh Congress of EAPC, Palermo, Italy.*
16 Donnelly S *et al.* (2002) Morphine in cancer pain management: a practical guide. *Supportive Care in Cancer.* **10**: 13–35.
17 Kumar K *et al.* (2000) Intravenous morphine for emergency treatment of cancer pain. *Palliative Medicine.* **14**: 183–188.
18 Radbruch L *et al.* (1999) Intravenous titration with morphine for severe cancer pain: report of 28 cases. *Clinical Journal of Pain.* **15**: 173–178.
19 Coluzzi P (1998) Sublingual morphine: efficacy reviewed. *Journal of Pain and Symptom Management.* **16**: 184–192.
20 deBoer AG *et al.* (1982) Rectal drug administration: clinical pharmacokinetic considerations. *Clinical Pharmacokinetics.* **7**: 285–311.
21 Johnson AG and Lux G (1988) *Progress in the Treatment of Gastrointestinal Motility Disorder. The role of cisapride.* Excerpta Medica, Amsterdam.
22 Ripamonti C and Bruera E (1991) Rectal, buccal and sublingual narcotics for the management of cancer pain. *Journal of Palliative Care.* **7**: 30–35.
23 Wilkinson T *et al.* (1992) Pharmacokinetics and efficacy of rectal versus oral sustained-release morphine in cancer patients. *Cancer Chemotherapy and Pharmacology.* **31**: 251–254.
24 Bruera E *et al.* (1999) Twice-daily versus once-daily morphine sulphate controlled-release suppositories for the treatment of cancer pain. *Supportive Care in Cancer.* **7**: 280–283.
25 Krajnik M and Zylicz Z (1997) Topical opioids – fact or fiction? *Progress in Palliative Care.* **5**: 101–106.
26 Likar R *et al.* (1999) Dose-dependency of intra-articular morphine analgesia. *British Journal of Anaesthesia.* **83**: 241–244.
27 Back NI and Finlay I (1995) Analgesic effect of topical opioids on painful skin ulcers. *Journal of Pain and Symptom Management.* **10**: 493.
28 Krajnik M *et al.* (1999) Potential uses of topical opioids in palliative care – report of 6 cases. *Pain.* **80**: 121–125.
29 Twillman R *et al.* (1999) Treatment of painful skin ulcers with topical opioids. *Journal of Pain and Symptom Management.* **17**: 288–292.

DIAMORPHINE BNF 4.7.2

Class: Strong opioid analgesic.

Indications: As for **morphine**; used in the UK instead of parenteral **morphine**.

Pharmacology

Diamorphine (di-acetylmorphine, heroin) is generally considered to be a pro-drug without intrinsic activity.[1] *In vivo*, it is rapidly de-acetylated (plasma halflife 3min) to 6-mono-acetylmorphine
(6-MAM) (plasma halflife 20min) and then to **morphine** itself.[2] However, some mice (CXBX strain) are relatively insensitive to **morphine** but respond to both 6-MAM and morphine-6-glucuronide,[3] suggesting that 6-MAM may act at a specific subset of μ-opioid receptors. IM diamorphine is more than twice as potent as **morphine**.[4–6] The greater potency of parenteral diamorphine could be because 6-MAM is more potent than morphine[7] or because diamorphine and 6-MAM cross the blood-brain barrier more readily than **morphine**. However, by mouth the two opioids are almost equipotent.[8]

Diamorphine IM has a slightly faster onset of action than **morphine** IM.[4,9] This probably relates to the greater lipid solubility of diamorphine, permitting more rapid absorption from the site of injection. On the other hand, **morphine** acts more quickly IV.[10] The explanation for this apparent paradox probably lies in the need for diamorphine to be converted into an active metabolite and differences in plasma protein binding (diamorphine 40%, **morphine** 20%). In terms of analgesic efficacy and effect on mood, diamorphine has no clinical advantage over **morphine** by oral or SC/IM routes.[5,6,8] Diamorphine hydrochloride is much more soluble than **morphine** sulphate/hydrochloride and is the strong opioid of choice for parenteral use in the UK because large amounts can be given in very small volumes (Table 5.14). Diamorphine, like **morphine**, can be given by many different routes, including spinally. In contrast to **morphine**, because of its greater lipid solubility, diamorphine can also be given intranasally using a nasal dosing device.[11]

Bio-availability probably zero; unknown percentage available as 6-MAM.
Onset of action 5–10min SC.
Time to peak plasma concentration 1.5–2h PO as 6-MAM and morphine.
Plasma halflife 3min IV; metabolised to active metabolites.
Duration of action 4h.

Table 5.14 Solubility of selected opioids[12]

Preparation	*Amount of water needed to dissolve 1g at 25°C (ml)*
Morphine	5000
Morphine hydrochloride	24
Morphine sulphate	21
Diamorphine hydrochloride	1.6[a]
Hydromorphone	3

a. 1g of diamorphine hydrochloride dissolved in 1.6ml has a volume of 2.4ml.

Undesirable effects

For full list, see manufacturer's SPC.
Also see Strong opioids, p.168.

Dose and use

The following conversion ratios are approximate but serve as a general guide:

- PO **morphine** to SC diamorphine, give 1/3 of the PO dose
- PO diamorphine to SC diamorphine, give 1/2 of the PO dose.

Supply

Diamorphine hydrochloride is available for medicinal use only in the UK.
Unless indicated otherwise, all preparations are **CD**.

Diamorphine (non-proprietary)
Tablets 10mg, 10mg dose = £0.12.
Injection 5mg amp = £1.18; 10mg amp = £1.36; 30mg amp = £1.62; 100mg amp = £4.50; 500mg amp = £20.68.

1 Inturrisi CE *et al.* (1984) The pharmacokinetics of heroin in patients with chronic pain. *New England Journal of Medicine.* **310**: 1213–1217.
2 Barrett DA *et al.* (1992) The effect of temperature and pH on the deacetylation of diamorphine in aqueous solution and in human plasma. *Journal of Pharmacy and Pharmacology.* **44**: 606–608.
3 Rossi G *et al.* (1996) Novel receptor mechanisms for heroin and morphine-6B-glucuronide analgesia. *Neuroscience Letters.* **216**: 1–4.
4 Reichle CW *et al.* (1962) Comparative analgesic potency of heroin and morphine in post-operative patients. *Journal of Pharmacology and Experimental Therapeutics.* **136**: 43–46.
5 Beaver WT *et al.* (1981) Comparison of the analgesic effect of intramuscular heroin and morphine in patients with cancer pain. *Clinical Pharmacology and Therapeutics.* **29**: 232.
6 Kaiko RF *et al.* (1981) Analgesic and mood effects of heroin and morphine in cancer patients with postoperative pain. *New England Journal of Medicine.* **304**: 1501–1505.
7 Wright CI and Barbour FA (1935) The respiratory effects of morphine, codeine and related substances. *Journal of Pharmacology and Experimental Therapeutics.* **54**: 25–33.
8 Twycross RG (1977) Choice of strong analgesic in terminal cancer: diamorphine or morphine? *Pain.* **3**: 93–104.
9 Dundee JW *et al.* (1966) Studies of drugs given before anaesthesia XI: diamorphine (heroin) and morphine. *British Journal of Anaesthesia.* **38**: 610–619.
10 Morrison L *et al.* (1991) Comparison of speed of onset of analgesic effect of diamorphine and morphine. *British Journal of Anaesthesia.* **66**: 656–659.
11 Kendall J *et al.* (2001) Multicentre randomised controlled trial of nasal diamorphine for analgesia in children and teenagers with clinical fractures. *British Medical Journal.* **322**: 261–265.
12 Hanks GW and Hoskin PJ (1987) Opioid analgesics in the management of pain in patients with cancer: a review. *Palliative Medicine.* **1**: 1–25.

*ALFENTANIL — BNF 15.1.4.3

Class: Opioid analgesic.

Indications: Intra-operative analgesia; †an alternative in cases of intolerance to other strong opioids, particularly in renal failure.[1]

Pharmacology

Alfentanil is a synthetic derivative of **fentanyl** with distinct properties, e.g. a more rapid onset of action, a shorter duration of action, and a potency approximately 1/4 that of **fentanyl** but 10 times more than **diamorphine**.[1,2] Alfentanil is less lipophilic than **fentanyl**.[3] Alfentanil is metabolised in the liver by cytochrome CYP3A4 to inactive compounds. Dose reductions may be necessary in patients with severe liver impairment but not in renal failure. Although analgesic tolerance has been reported in animals,[4] tolerance does not appear to be a problem clinically. As with all fentanils, there is little point in spinal administration because of the rapid clearance into the systemic circulation.[5,6] Alfentanil is available only as an injection and has been used successfully by short-term CSCI to provide pain relief during dressing changes in a trauma patient.[7]

Onset of action <2min IV; <5min IM.
Time to peak plasma concentration 15min IM.
Plasma halflife 100min (see Table 5.15).
Duration of action 10min IV; 1h IM.

Table 5.15 Pharmacokinetics of single IV doses of fentanyl and alfentanil[8]

	Fentanyl	*Alfentanil*
Onset of action (min)	1.5	0.75
Plasma halflife (min)	220	100
Duration of action (min)	30–60	10

Cautions
As for **morphine** (see p.173).

Undesirable effects
For full list, see manufacturer's SPC.
Also see Strong opioids, p.168.

Dose and use
SC
For procedural pain in patients already receiving regular strong opioids, give as a series of 1mg SC/IV doses at 5min intervals. Once the effective dose is determined, give this as a single SC dose. (Note: there are no published data on the use of alfentanil in this way.)
Episodic (breakthrough) pain
Conventionally, p.r.n. SC doses are approximately 1/6 of the total 24h dose.
CSCI
Used mostly for patients in renal failure in whom there is evidence of **morphine** neuro-excitability. The following are approximate dose conversion ratios:
- SC **diamorphine** to SC alfentanil, give 1/10 of the 24h dose[9]
- PO **morphine** to SC alfentanil, give 1/30 of the 24h dose.

Supply
Unless indicated otherwise, all preparations are **CD**.

Rapifen® (Janssen-Cilag 01494 567567)
Injection 500microgram/ml, 2ml amp = £0.72; 10ml amp = £3.31.
Injection 5mg/ml, 1ml amp = £2.65.

1 Kirkham SR and Pugh R (1995) Opioid analgesia in uraemic patients. *Lancet.* **345**: 1185.
2 Larijani G and Goldberg M (1987) Alfentanil hydrochloride: a new short acting narcotic analgesic for surgical procedures. *Clinical Pharmacy.* **6**: 275–282.
3 Bernards C (1999) Clinical implications of physicochemical properties of opioids. In: C Stein (ed) *Opioids in Pain Control: basic and clinical aspects.* Cambridge University Press, Cambridge, pp.166–187.
4 Kissin I *et al.* (2000) Acute tolerance to continuously infused alfentanil: the role of cholecystokinin and N-methyl-D-aspartate-nitric oxide systems. *Anesthesia and Analgesia.* **91**: 110–116.
5 Burm A *et al.* (1994) Pharmacokinetics of alfentanil after epidural administration. Investigation of systemic absorption kinetics with a stable isotope method. *Anesthesiology.* **81**: 308–315.
6 Ummenhofer W *et al.* (2000) Comparative spinal distribution and clearance kinetics of intrathecally administered morphine, fentanyl, alfentanil, and sufentanil. *Anesthesiology.* **92**: 739–953.
7 Gallagher G *et al.* (2001) Target-controlled alfentanil analgesia for dressing change following extensive reconstructive surgery for trauma. *Journal of Pain and Symptom Management.* **21**: 1–2.
8 Scholz J *et al.* (1996) Clinical pharmacokinetics of alfentanil, fentanyl and sufentanil. An update. *Clinical Pharmacokinetics.* **31**: 275–292.

9 Dickman A *et al.* (2002) *The Syringe Driver: Continuous Subcutaneous Infusions in Palliative Care.* Oxford University Press, Oxford.

BUPRENORPHINE BNF 4.7.2

Class: Opioid analgesic.

Indications: Moderate-to-severe cancer pain and severe non-malignant pain not responding to non-opoids; an alternative in cases of intolerance to other strong opioids.

Contra-indications: Buprenorphine TD should not be used when there is need for rapid titration of opioid medication for moderate-to-severe pain.

Pharmacology

Buprenorphine is a potent partial μ-opioid receptor agonist, κ-opioid receptor *antagonist* and a weak δ-opioid receptor agonist.[1,2] It is an alternative to oral **morphine** in the low-to-middle part of **morphine**'s dose range. Subjective and physiological effects are generally similar to **morphine**. Buprenorphine is metabolised in the liver principally to inactive norbuprenorphine (mediated by CYP3A4). Buprenorphine and norbuprenorphine also undergo conjugation with glucuronic acid. Buprenorphine is safe to use in patients with renal impairment; no dose adjustment is necessary in patients with mild-to-moderate hepatic impairment. Buprenorphine has high lipid solubility and is available as a *sublingual* tablet and as a transdermal patch. Ingestion markedly reduces bio-availability.[3] Vomiting is more common after SL administration than after IM injection or transdermal application. Buprenorphine has either no effect or a smaller effect than **morphine** on pressure within the biliary and pancreatic ducts.[4,5] Buprenorphine does slow intestinal transit, but probably less so than **morphine**.[6] In low doses, buprenorphine and **morphine** (or alternative μ-opioid receptor agonist) are additive in their effects; at very high doses of buprenorphine (>10mg/24h?), antagonism could theoretically occur. However, with typical doses, it is possible to switch either way between buprenorphine and **morphine** (or other μ-opioid receptor agonist) without loss of analgesia.[7] **Naloxone** does not reverse the effect of buprenorphine when used in standard doses. However, respiratory depression is not seen with clinically recommended doses. In the event of respiratory depression following massive self-poisoning, IV **doxapram** (a non-specific respiratory stimulant) can be given, or IV **naloxone** *4mg*, stat and by CIVI. The analgesic ceiling dose for buprenorphine is about 8–10mg/24h,[2,8] equivalent to about **morphine** 480–600mg/24h PO. The ceiling dose for effects other than analgesia is 16–32mg/24h.[2] 400microgram SL is equivalent to 300microgram IM. Buprenorphine TD is approximately half as potent as **fentanyl** TD.

Bio-availability 50% SL; 15% PO.

Onset of action 30min SL; 15min IM; peak effect 3h; about 12–24h TD, *longer for lowest patch strength* (peak effect 2–3 days).

Time to peak plasma concentration 3–5h SL; 2–5h IM; about 60h TD.

Plasma halflife 2.5–3h IV, SL; 30–36h TD.

Duration of action 6–9h SL, IM; 3 days TD.

Undesirable effects

For full list, see manufacturer's SPC.

Also see Strong opioids, p.168.

Dose and use

If previously receiving a weak opioid, a patient should start on 200microgram SL q8h with the advice that, 'If it is not more effective than your previous tablets, take a further 200microgram after 1h, and 400microgram q8h after that'. With daily doses of over 3mg, patients may prefer to take fewer tablets q6h. The potency ratio of buprenorphine to **morphine** is debatable. We suggest that, when switching from buprenorphine SL to **morphine** PO, the daily dose of buprenorphine is multiplied by 60 (for level transfer), or by 100 (if previous poor pain control) to give an appropriate starting total daily dose of **morphine** with subsequent titration according to response. However, some centres adopt a lower transfer factor, e.g. 30–40.

TD buprenorphine is available in three strengths for the relief of *chronic* pain. These deliver approximately 800, 1200 and 1600microgram/24h respectively. Buprenorphine 52.5microgram/h is approximately equivalent to **fentanyl** TD 25microgram/h. For general advice and recommended starting doses, see manufacturer's SPC. Continue to prescribe oral **morphine**, or alternative opioid, for 12h after applying the first TD patch; use buprenorphine 200microgram SL for breakthrough pain. For patients who have not been receiving a strong opioid, the lowest patch strength should be prescribed.

Supply

Unless indicated otherwise, all preparations are **CD**.

Temgesic® (Schering-Plough 01707 363636)
Tablets SL 200microgram, 400microgram, 28 days @ 200microgram t.d.s. = £9.63.
Injection 300microgram/ml, 1ml amp = £0.53.

Transtec® (Napp Pharmaceuticals 01223 424444)
Patches (for 3 days) 35microgram/h, 1 = £5.79; 52.5microgram/h, 1 = £8.69; 70microgram/h, 1 = £11.59.

1 Rothman R (1995) Buprenorphine: a review of the binding literature. In: A Cowan and J Lewis (eds) *Buprenorphine: combatting drug abuse with a unique opioid.* Wiley-Liss, New York, pp.19–29.
2 Budd K (2002) Buprenorphine: a review. *Evidence Based Medicine in Practice (April 2002)*. Hayward Medical Communications, Newmarket.
3 McQuay H and Moore R (1995) Buprenorphine kinetics in humans. In: A Cowan and J Lewis (eds) *Buprenorphine: combatting drug abuse with a unique opioid.* Wiley-Liss, New York, pp.137–147.
4 Pausawasdi S *et al.* (1984) The effect of buprenorphine and morphine on intraluminal pressure of the common bile duct. *Journal of the Medical Association of Thailand.* **67**: 329–333.
5 Staritz M *et al.* (1986) Effect of modern analgesic drugs (tramadol, pentazocine, and buprenorphine) on the bile duct sphincter in man. *Gut.* **27**: 567–569.
6 Anonymous (1979) Buprenorphine injection (Temgesic). *Drug and Therapeutics Bulletin.* **17**: 17–19.
7 Atkinson R *et al.* (1990) The efficacy in sequential use of buprenorphine and morphine in advanced cancer pain. In: D Doyle (ed). *Opioids in the Treatment of Cancer Pain*. Royal Society of Medicine Services, London, pp.81–87.
8 Lewis J (1995) Clinical pharmacology of buprenorphine in relation to its use as an analgesic. In: A Cowan and J Lewis (eds) *Buprenorphine: combatting drug abuse with a unique opioid.* Wiley-Liss, New York, pp.151–163.

FENTANYL (TRANSDERMAL) BNF 4.7.2

Class: Opioid analgesic.

Indications: Severe chronic pain, including †AIDS,[1] †morphine intolerance (see Table 5.13, p.175). Also see Box 5.1, p.186.

Contra-indications: The need for rapid titration of strong opioid medication for severe pain.

Pharmacology

Transdermal (TD) fentanyl is a self-adhesive skin patch with a rate-limiting membrane which allows a standardised amount of fentanyl to cross each hour from the patch into the skin. It is used in the management of chronic severe pain,[2–4] particularly in cancer.[5–12] Fentanyl (like **morphine**) is a strong μ-opioid receptor agonist. Because of its high lipophilicity, fentanyl (unlike **morphine**) is sequestrated in body fats, including epidural fat and the white matter of the CNS.[13,14] This means that fentanyl given by any route (including spinally), after systemic redistribution, acts supraspinally mainly in the thalamus (white matter). Any effect in the dorsal horn (grey matter) is probably minimal.[13] This may account for the clinical observation that patients with poor pain relief despite using very high doses (e.g. 600microgram/h TD) sometimes obtain good relief with relatively smaller doses of **morphine** or **diamorphine**, e.g. 10–20mg SC.[15] On the other hand, the lipophilic nature of fentanyl probably accounts for its reduced tendency to cause constipation (Figure 5.9).[16]

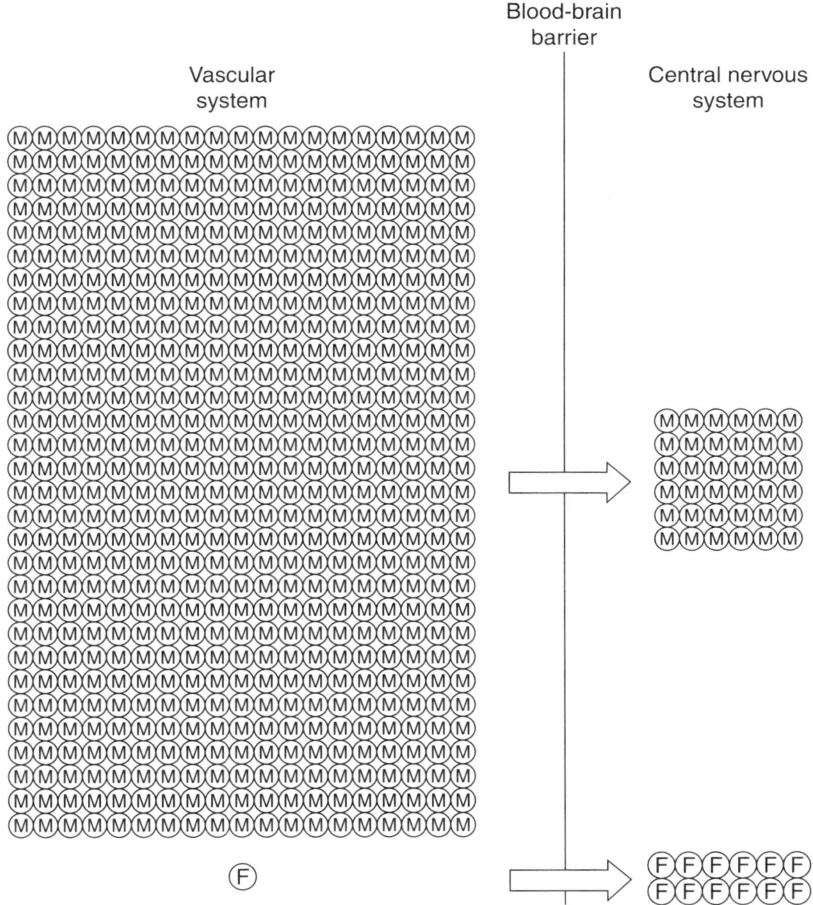

Figure 5.9 Distribution of equipotent doses of morphine and fentanyl in the vascular and central nervous systems based on animal data.[16] Converting from oral or parenteral morphine to transdermal or parenteral fentanyl will result in a massive decrease in opioid molecules outside the CNS. This will result in less constipation and could, in physically-dependent subjects, precipitate peripherally-mediated withdrawal symptoms.

With the TD patch, steady-state plasma concentrations of fentanyl are achieved after 36–48h.[1] Time to reach a minimal effective plasma concentration ranges from 3–23h.[17] After removal of a patch, the elimination plasma halflife is 13–22h.[18] Elimination principally involves biotransformation in the liver by cytochrome P450 3A4 to inactive norfentanyl which undergoes urinary excretion. Less than 7% is excreted unchanged. If effective analgesia does not last for 3 days, the correct response is to increase the patch strength. Even so, a small percentage of patients do best if the patch is changed every 2 days.[19] The manufacturer recommends a conversion ratio for **morphine** and fentanyl of 150:1 but some centres use a conversion ratio of 100:1 when deciding the initial patch strength.[20]

TD fentanyl is less constipating than **morphine**.[5,19,21,22] Thus, when converting from **morphine** to fentanyl, the dose of laxative should be halved and subsequently adjusted according to need. Some patients experience withdrawal symptoms when changed from **morphine**

PO to TD fentanyl despite satisfactory pain relief, e.g. colic, diarrhoea and nausea together with sweating and restlessness. This phenomenon is probably also accounted for by the differences between the two opioids in relation to their relative impact on peripheral and central μ-opioid receptors. Such symptoms are easily treatable by using rescue doses of **morphine** until they resolve after a few days. TD fentanyl can be continued until the death of the patient, and the dose varied as necessary. It is important to give adequate rescue doses of an alternative strong opioid (see Table 5.12, p.171) or use **transmucosal fentanyl** instead.
Bio-availability 92%.
Onset of action 12h.
Time to peak plasma concentration 36–48h.
Plasma halflife 17h.
Duration of action 72h; for some patients, 48h.[23]

Cautions

The rate of absorption of fentanyl from the patch may be increased in febrile patients, or if the skin under the patch becomes vasodilated because of an external heat source such as an electric blanket or heat pad.

Undesirable effects

For full list, see manufacturer's SPC.
Less constipating than equivalent doses of **morphine**,[5,19,21,22] and may be less emetogenic. Also see Strong opioids, p.168.

Dose and use

The use of TD fentanyl patches is summarised in Box 5.1. TD fentanyl is sometimes a good first-choice strong opioid, e.g. in patients with severe dysphagia (e.g. head and neck cancer), renal failure and social circumstances which make the use of (divertable) tablets undesirable. Convenient p.r.n. doses are shown in Table 5.16.

Box 5.1 Guidelines for the use of transdermal fentanyl patches

1 Transdermal (TD) fentanyl is an alternative strong opioid which can be used in place of both PO morphine and CSCI morphine/diamorphine in the management of cancer pain.

2 Indications for using TD fentanyl include:
- intolerable undesirable effects with morphine, e.g. nausea and vomiting, constipation, hallucinations
- renal failure (no active metabolite)
- dysphagia
- 'tablet phobia' or poor compliance with oral medication.

3 TD fentanyl is *contra-indicated* in patients who need rapid titration of their medication for severe uncontrolled pain.
Pain not relieved by morphine will *not* be relieved by fentanyl. If in doubt, seek specialist advice before prescribing TD fentanyl.

4 TD fentanyl patches are available in 4 strengths: 25, 50, 75 and 100microgram/h *for 3 days*:
- patients with inadequate relief from codeine, dextropropoxyphene or dihydrocodeine ⩾240 mg/day should start on 25microgram/h
- patients on oral morphine: *divide 24h dose in mg by 3* and choose nearest patch strength in microgram/h
- patients on CSCI diamorphine: choose nearest patch strength in microgram/h to mg/24h of diamorphine.

Note: the latter two doses are higher than the manufacturer's recommendations.

5 An alternative method of deciding the initial patch strength is to use a potency ratio of 100 (as in Germany) and to round down to the nearest convenient patch size. [Example: morphine daily dose 120mg ÷ 100 = fentanyl daily dose 1.2mg, i.e. patch strength 50microgram/h.]

continued

Box 5.1 Continued

6 Apply the patch to *dry, non-inflamed, non-irradiated, hairless skin* on the upper arm or trunk; body hair may be clipped but not shaved. May need micropore to ensure adherence.

7 Systemic analgesic concentrations are generally reached within 12h; so if converting from:
- 4-hourly oral morphine, give regular doses for the first 12h after applying the patch
- 12-hourly m/r morphine, apply the patch and the final m/r dose at the same time
- 24-hourly m/r morphine, apply the patch 12h after the final m/r dose
- a syringe driver, continue the syringe driver for about 12h after applying the patch.

8 Steady-state plasma concentrations of fentanyl are achieved after 36–48h; the patient should use p.r.n. doses liberally during the first 3 days, particularly during the first 24h. Rescue doses should be approximately half the fentanyl patch strength given as normal-release morphine in mg. [Example: with fentanyl 50microgram/h, use morphine 20–30mg p.r.n.]

9 After 48h, if a patient continues to need 2 or more rescue doses of morphine a day, the patch strength should be increased by 25microgram/h. When using the manufacturer's recommended starting doses, about 50% of patients need to increase the patch strength after the first 3 days.

10 About 10% of patients experience opioid withdrawal symptoms when changed from morphine to TD fentanyl. These manifest with symptoms like gastric flu and lasts for a few days; p.r.n. doses of morphine can be used to relieve troublesome symptoms.

11 Fentanyl is less constipating than morphine; halve the dose of laxatives when starting fentanyl and titrate according to need. Some patients develop diarrhoea; if troublesome, use rescue doses of morphine to control it, and completely stop laxatives.

12 Fentanyl probably causes less nausea and vomiting than morphine but, if necessary, prescribe haloperidol 1.5mg stat & o.n.

13 In febrile patients, the rate of absorption of fentanyl increases, and occasionally causes toxicity, principally drowsiness. Absorption may also be enhanced by an external heat source over the patch, e.g. electric blanket or hot-water bottle; patients should be warned about this. Patients may shower with a patch but should not soak in a hot bath.

14 Remove patches after 72h; change the position of the new patches so as to rest the underlying skin for 3–6 days.

15 A reservoir of fentanyl cumulates in the skin under the patch, and significant blood levels persist for 24h, sometimes more, after removing the patch. This only matters, of course, if TD fentanyl is discontinued.

16 In moribund patients, continue TD fentanyl and give additional diamorphine p.r.n. Rescue doses of SC diamorphine can be based on the 'rule of 5', i.e. divide the patch strength by 5 and give as mg of diamorphine. [Example: with fentanyl 100microgram/h, use diamorphine 20mg p.r.n.] If $\geqslant$2 p.r.n. doses are required/24h, give diamorphine by CSCI, starting with a dose equal to the sum of the p.r.n. doses over the preceding 24h. The p.r.n. dose may need to be adjusted taking into account the total opioid dose (i.e. fentanyl TD and diamorphine CSCI).

17 TD fentanyl is unsatisfactory in $<$5% of patients, generally because of failure to remain adherent or allergy to the silicone adhesive.

18 Used patches still contain fentanyl; after removal, fold the patch with the adhesive side inwards and discard in a sharps container (hospital) or dustbin (home); wash hands. Ultimately any unused patches should be returned to a pharmacy.

Some centres use TD fentanyl in opioid-naïve patients, i.e. skip the traditional step 2 of the WHO analgesic ladder.[24] However, fentanyl 25microgram/h (600microgram/24h), equivalent to

morphine 60mg PO, is more than some patients need. It is therefore recommended that, as a general rule, a patient's approximate opioid requirement is determined by first using a weak opioid or **morphine** PO before introducing TD fentanyl.

Table 5.16 Rescue medication for patients receiving transdermal fentanyl[a]

Patch strength (microgram/h)	*PO morphine (mg)*	*SC morphine (mg)*	*SC diamorphine (mg)*
25	15	10	5
50	30	15	10
75	40	20	15
100	60	30	20

a. doses rounded to a convenient quantity in terms of tablets or injections.

Box 5.J Fentanyl patch chart: nursing record

Nottingham City Hospital NHS Trust
HAYWARD HOUSE
Fentanyl Patch Chart

Patient Name:
Date of birth:
Hospital No:

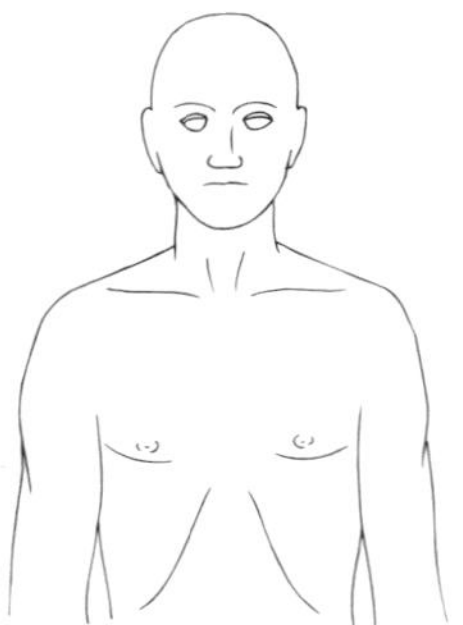

Mark the site of application of the patch with the date that it was applied.

Apply to dry, flat, non-hairy skin on the torso or upper arm. Press firmly in place with the hand for 30 seconds to ensure good contact. Rotate sites.

Information

- fentanyl patches need to be prescribed on the inpatient prescription chart. Sign as usual and also document on this chart
- a nurse should check that each patch is still in place at 1000h and 2200h and sign overleaf. Comments should be made if a problem is found, stating action taken (e.g. patch lifted so needed to be secured with Tegaderm)
- fentanyl patches should be replaced every 72 hours. After removal, fold patches in half with the adhesive side inwards and discard in a 'sharps' bin, witnessed by a second nurse and signed for.

continued

Box 5.J Continued

Date & time patch applied	Strength & number of patches Site	Signature	B.d. observations 1000h	Sign	2200h	Sign	Removal and destruction Date/Time/Sign Comments
Example					*23/2* ✓	*AS*	*26/2/98*
23/2/98	*25mcg/h × 1*	*S Thorp*	*24/2* ✓	*ST*	*24/2* ✓	*MB*	*1000h*
1000h	*Left arm*		*25/2* ✓	*ST*	*25/2* ✓	*MB*	*S Thorp*
			26/2 ✓	*AS*			*A Smith*

Moving from 25microgram/h to 50microgram/h (a dose increase of 100%) may result in a marked (but temporary) increase in undesirable effects.[25] However, if patients have been taking several rescue doses per day of morphine (or other strong opioid) for breakthrough pain, increasing from 25microgram/h to 50microgram/h is likely to be well tolerated. Adjusting the patch strength on a *daily* basis during the initial period of dose titration is *not* recommended.[26] With inpatients, a fentanyl patch chart is helpful (Box 5.J).

Supply

Unless indicated otherwise, all preparations are **CD**.

Durogesic® (Janssen-Cilag 01494 567567)
Patches (for 3 days) 25microgram/h, 1 = £5.79; 50microgram/h, 1 = £10.82; 75microgram/h, 1 = £15.09; 100microgram/h, 1 = £18.59.

1 Newshan G and Lefkowitz M (2001) Transdermal fentanyl for chronic pain in AIDS: a pilot study. *Journal of Pain and Symptom Management*. **21**: 69–77.

2 Simpson R *et al.* (1997) Transdermal fentanyl as treatment for chronic low back pain. *Journal of Pain and Symptom Management*. **14**: 218–224.

3 Milligan K and Campbell C (1999) Transdermal fentanyl in patients with chronic, nonmalignant pain: a case study series. *Advances in Therapy*. **16**: 73–77.

4 Allan L *et al.* (2001) Randomised crossover trial of transdermal fentanyl and sustained release oral morphine for treating chronic non-cancer pain. *British Medical Journal*. **322**: 1154–1158.

5 Ahmedzai S and Brooks D (1997) Transdermal fentanyl versus sustained-release oral morphine in cancer pain: preference, efficacy and quality of life. *Journal of Pain and Symptom Management.* **13**: 254–261.

6 Wong J-N *et al.* (1997) Comparison of oral controlled-release morphine with transdermal fentanyl in terminal cancer pain. *Acta Anaesthesiologica Singapore.* **35**: 25–32.

7 Yeo W *et al.* (1997) Transdermal fentanyl for severe cancer-related pain. *Palliative Medicine.* **11**: 233–239.

8 Sloan P *et al.* (1998) A clinical evaluation of transdermal therapeutic system fentanyl for the treatment of cancer pain. *Journal of Pain and Symptom Management.* **16**: 102–111.

9 Kongsgaard U and Poulain P (1998) Transdermal fentanyl for pain control in adults with chronic cancer pain. *European Journal of Pain.* **2**: 53–62.

10 Nugent M *et al.* (2001) Long-term observations of patients receiving transdermal fentanyl after a randomized trial. *Journal of Pain and Symptom Management.* **21**: 385–391.

11 Payne R *et al.* (1998) Quality of life and cancer pain: satisfaction and side effects with transdermal fentanyl versus oral morphine. *Journal of Clinical Oncology.* **16**: 1588–1593.

12 Radbruch L *et al.* (2001) Transdermal fentanyl for the management of cancer pain: a survey of 1005 patients. *Palliative Medicine.* **15**: 309–321.

13 Bernards C (1999) Clinical implications of physicochemical properties of opioids. In: C Stein (ed) *Opioids in Pain Control: basic and clinical aspects.* Cambridge University Press, Cambridge, pp.166–187.

14 Ummenhofer W *et al.* (2000) Comparative spinal distribution and clearance kinetics of intrathecally administered morphine, fentanyl, alfentanil, and sufentanil. *Anesthesiology.* **92**: 739–953.

15 Zylicz Z (2001) Personal communication.

16 Herz A and Teschemacher H-J (1971) Activities and sites of antinociceptive action of morphine-like analgesics and kinetics of distribution following intravenous, intracerebral and intraventricular application. *Advances in Drug Research.* **6**: 79–119.

17 Gourlay GK *et al.* (1989) The transdermal administration of fentanyl in the treatment of post-operative pain: pharmacokinetics and pharmacodynamic effects. *Pain.* **37**: 193–202.

18 Portenoy RK *et al.* (1993) Transdermal fentanyl for cancer pain. *Anesthesiology.* **78**: 36–43.

19 Donner B *et al.* (1998) Long-term treatment of cancer pain with transdermal fentanyl. *Journal of Pain and Symptom Management.* **15**: 168–175.

20 Donner B *et al.* (1996) Direct conversion from oral morphine to transdermal fentanyl: a multicenter study in patients with cancer pain. *Pain.* **64**: 527–534.

21 Grond S *et al.* (1997) Transdermal fentanyl in the long-term treatment of cancer pain: a prospective study of 50 patients with advanced cancer of the gastrointestinal tract or the head and neck region. *Pain.* **69**: 191–198.

22 Megens A *et al.* (1998) Comparison of the analgesic and intestinal effects of fentanyl and morphine in rats. *Journal of Pain and Symptom Management.* **15**: 253–258.

23 Smith J and Ellershaw J (1999) Improvement in pain control by change of fentanyl patch after 48 hours compared with 72 hours. *Poster EAPC Congress, Geneva.* PO1/1376.

24 Vielvoye-Kerkmeer A *et al.* (2000) Transdermal fentanyl in opioid-naive cancer pain patients: an open trial using transdermal fentanyl for the treatment of chronic cancer pain in opioid-naive patients and a group using codeine. *Journal of Pain and Symptom Management.* **19**: 185–192.

25 Mercadante S *et al.* (2001) Clinical problems with transdermal fentanyl titration from 25 to 50mcg/hr. *Journal of Pain and Symptom Management.* **21**: 448–449.

26 Korte W *et al.* (1996) Day-to-day titration to initiate transdermal fentanyl in patients with cancer pain: short and long term experiences in a prospective study of 39 patients. *Journal of Pain and Symptom Management.* **11**: 139–146.

FENTANYL (TRANSMUCOSAL) BNF 4.7.2

Class: Opioid analgesic.

Indications: Episodic (breakthrough) pain in patients on regular strong opioid therapy.

Pharmacology

Oral transmucosal fentanyl citrate (OTFC) is a 'lozenge on a stick' containing fentanyl in a hard sweet matrix.[1] Fentanyl (like **morphine**) is a strong μ-opioid receptor agonist. Because of its high lipophilicity, fentanyl (unlike **morphine**) is sequestrated in body fats, including epidural fat and the white matter of the CNS.[2,3] This means that fentanyl given by any route (including spinally), after systemic redistribution, acts supraspinally mainly in the thalamus (white matter). Any effect in the dorsal horn (grey matter) is probably minimal.[2] This may account for the clinical observation that patients with poor pain relief despite using very high doses (e.g. 600microgram/h TD) may obtain good relief with relatively smaller doses of **morphine** or **diamorphine** (e.g. 10–20mg SC).[4]

With OTFC, about 25% of the dose is absorbed rapidly through the buccal mucosa into the systemic circulation leading to onset of pain relief within 5–10min.[5] The remainder is swallowed and absorbed more slowly. It is subject to intestinal and hepatic first-pass metabolism and only 1/3 of this amount (25% of the total dose) is available systemically. Peak plasma concentration increases linearly with increasing doses, 200–1600microgram.[6] Elimination principally involves biotransformation in the liver by cytochrome CYP3A4 to inactive norfentanyl which undergoes urinary excretion. Less than 7% is excreted unchanged.

The optimal dose is determined by titration, and cannot be predicted by a patient's regular dose of opioid.[7,8] Pain relief is achieved more quickly than with **morphine** PO and it is generally well tolerated.[9,10] About 25% of patients fail to obtain relief at the highest dose, i.e. 1600microgram, or have unacceptable undesirable effects. OTFC has been used successfully over extended periods (mean 3 months) without loss of efficacy.[11] As a cheaper alternative, when only small doses are required, some centres prefer to use the parenteral formulation for transmucosal administration (0.5–2ml of 50microgram/ml).[12]

Bio-availability 50%, divided equally between transbuccal and gastro-intestinal absorption.
Onset of action 5–10min.
Time to peak plasma concentration 20–40min.
Plasma halflife 6h.[6]
Duration of action 1–3.5h, longer with higher doses.[5]

Undesirable effects

For full list, see manufacturer's SPC.
Drowsiness, dizziness, nausea.[11] Occasional mouth ulceration. Also see Strong opioids, p.168.

Dose and use

In order to achieve maximum mucosal exposure to the fentanyl, the lozenge should be placed in a cheek and moved constantly up and down, and changed at intervals from one cheek to the other. It should not be chewed. The aim is to consume the lozenge within 15min. If necessary, moisten the mouth beforehand with water:

- starting dose 200microgram
- if 15min after consuming the lozenge there is inadequate analgesia, use a second 200microgram lozenge
- not more than two lozenges should be used for any one episode of pain
- continue with 200microgram for a further 3 episodes of pain, allowing a second lozenge when necessary
- if on review, the episodic pain is not controlled satisfactorily with 200microgram, increase to 400microgram
- use a second 400microgram lozenge if necessary
- titrate upwards until a dose is found which provides adequate analgesia with little or no undesirable effects.

The lozenge should be removed from the mouth once the pain is relieved; partly consumed lozenges should be dissolved under hot running water and the handle discarded in a waste container out of reach of children. Once a satisfactory dose is found, the manufacturer recommends that no more than 4 doses per day should be used. If more is required, consider increasing the dose of the regular strong opioid. The dose of OTFC may subsequently need to be retitrated.

Fentanyl solution

Some centres use the parenteral formulation of fentanyl for transmucosal use. Using a 1ml graduated oral syringe:

- starting dose 25–50microgram (0.5–1ml of 50microgram/ml)
- increase if necessary to 50–100microgram; many patients do not need more than this
- doses >100microgram are impractical because 2ml is the maximum volume that can be reliably kept in the mouth for transmucosal absorption.[13]

Supply

Unless indicated otherwise, all preparations are **CD**.

Actiq® (Elan 01438 765100)
Lozenge with oromucosal applicator 200, 400, 600, 800, 1200 and 1600microgram, 1 lozenge *of any dose* = £6.48.

Sublimaze® (Janssen-Cilag 01494 567567)
Injection 50microgram/ml, 2ml = £0.24.

1 Chandler S (1999) Oral transmucosal fentanyl citrate: a new treatment for breakthrough pain. *American Journal of Hospice and Palliative Care*. **16 (2)**: 489–491.

2 Bernards C (1999) Clinical implications of physicochemical properties of opioids. In: C Stein (ed) *Opioids in Pain Control: basic and clinical aspects*. Cambridge University Press, Cambridge, pp.166–187.

3 Ummenhofer W *et al.* (2000) Comparative spinal distribution and clearance kinetics of intrathecally administered morphine, fentanyl, alfentanil, and sufentanil. *Anesthesiology*. **92**: 739–953.

4 Zylicz Z (2001) Personal communication.

5 Lichtor J *et al.* (1999) The relative potency of oral transmucosal fentanyl citrate compared with intravenous morphine in the treatment of moderate to severe postoperative pain. *Anesthesia and Analgesia*. **89**: 732–738.

6 Streisand J *et al.* (1998) Dose proportionality and pharmacokinetics of oral transmucosal fentanyl citrate. *Anesthesiology*. **88**: 305–309.

7 Christie J *et al.* (1998) Dose-titration, multicenter study of oral transmucosal fentanyl citrate for the treatment of breakthrough pain in cancer patients using transdermal fentanyl for persistent pain. *Journal of Clinical Oncology*. **16**: 3238–3248.

8 Portenoy R *et al.* (1999) Oral transmucosal fentanyl citrate (OTFC) for the treatment of breakthrough pain in cancer patients: a controlled use titration study. *Pain*. **79**: 303–312.

9 Farrar J *et al.* (1998) Oral transmucosal fentanyl citrate: randomized, double-blinded, placebo-controlled trial for treatment of breakthrough pain in cancer patients. *Journal of the National Cancer Institute*. **90**: 611–616.

10 Coluzzi P *et al.* (2001) Breakthrough cancer pain: a randomized trial comparing oral transmucosal fentanyl citrate (OTFC) and morphine sulfate immediate release (MSIR). *Pain*. **91**: 123–130.

11 Payne R *et al.* (2001) Long-term safety of oral transmucosal fentanyl citrate for breakthrough cancer pain. *Journal of Pain and Symptom Management*. **22**: 575–583.

12 Gardner-Nix J (2001) Oral transmucosal fentanyl and sufentanil for incident pain. *Journal of Pain and Symptom Management*. **22**: 627–630.

13 Zeppetella G (2001) Sublingual fentanyl citrate for cancer-related breakthrough pain: a pilot study. *Palliative Medicine*. **15:** 323–328.

HYDROMORPHONE — BNF 4.7.2

Class: Opioid analgesic.

Indications: Severe pain in cancer; †an alternative in cases of intolerance to other strong opioids.

Pharmacology

Hydromorphone is an analogue of **morphine** with similar pharmacokinetic and pharmacodynamic properties.[1] According to the manufacturer, hydromorphone PO and SC/IM is about 7.5 times more potent than **morphine**.[2,3] However, others suggest that when switching from **morphine** to hydromorphone, the conversion ratio is approximately 5:1 and when switching from hydromorphone to **morphine** a ratio of 4:1 should be used.[4,5] Hydromorphone provides useful analgesia for about 4h. As with **morphine**, there is wide interpatient variation in bio-availability. The SPC for hydromorphone lists hepatic impairment as a contra-indication. There are no pharmacokinetic data to justify this but at some point hepatic impairment will lead to an increased plasma hydromorphone concentration. The main metabolite is hydromorphone-3-glucuronide (H3G); hydromorphone-6-glucuronide (H6G) is not formed.[6,7] Two minor metabolites, dihydro-isomorphine and dihydromorphine, are pharmacologically active; they are metabolised to 6-glucuronides. Hydromorphone clearance is unchanged in renal impairment but metabolites will accumulate. Typical opioid hyperexcitability (see Table 5.13, p.175) has been reported in patients with renal failure taking hydromorphone.[6,7] Normal H3G to hydromorphone plasma ratio is 27:1 but in renal failure it is 100:1.[8] By the spinal route in opioid-naïve subjects, hydromorphone causes less pruritus than **morphine** (11% vs 44%).[9]

Bio-availability 37–62% PO.[5]

Onset of action 15min SC/IM; 30min PO.

Time to peak plasma concentration 1h PO.

Plasma halflife 2.5h early phase, with a prolonged late phase.

Duration of action 4–5h; m/r 12h.

Undesirable effects

For full list, see manufacturer's SPC.

Also see Strong opioids, p.168.

Dose and use

Hydromorphone is used in the same way as **morphine**; either q4h or q12h if using a m/r preparation. The standard capsule size reflects the potency ratio of hydromorphone to morphine (× 7.5); hence hydromorphone 1.3mg = morphine 10mg. Hydromorphone is also available in high potency ampoules containing 10mg/ml, 20mg/ml and 50mg/ml to facilitate use by CSCI (unlicensed in UK). When converting from PO to SC, divide the dose of hydromorphone by 6.

Supply

Unless indicated otherwise, all preparations are **CD**.

Palladone® (Napp 01223 424444)
Capsules 1.3mg, 2.6mg; 1.3mg dose = £0.15.

Palladone® SR (Napp 01223 424444)
Caspules m/r 2mg, 4mg, 8mg, 16mg, 24mg, 28 days @ 2mg, 8mg and 24mg b.d. = £18.73, £50.07 and £142.70 respectively.

Hydromorphone hydrochloride
Injection 10mg/ml; 20mg/ml; 50mg/ml. (Unlicensed, available as a special order from Martindale 01708 386660; see Special orders and named patient supplies, p.349.)

1 Sarhill N *et al.* (2001) Hydromorphone: pharmacology and clinical applications in cancer patients. *Supportive Care in Cancer.* **9**: 84–96.

2 McDonald C and Miller A (1997) A comparative potency study of a controlled release tablet formulation of hydromorphone with controlled release morphine in patients with cancer pain. *European Journal of Palliative Care. Abstracts of the Fifth Congress.*

3 Moriarty M *et al.* (1999) A randomised crossover comparison of controlled release hydromorphone tablets with controlled release morphine tablets in patients with cancer pain. *Journal of Clinical Research.* **2**: 1–8.

4 Anderson R *et al.* (2001) Accuracy in equianalgesic dosing: conversion dilemmas. *Journal of Pain and Symptom Management.* **21**: 397–406.

5 Pereira J *et al.* (2001) Equianalgesic dose ratios for opioids: a critical review and proposals for long-term dosing. *Journal of Pain and Symptom Management.* **22**: 672–687.
6 Babul N and Darke AC (1992) Putative role of hydromorphone metabolites in myoclonus. *Pain.* **51**: 260–261.
7 Davis M and Wilcock A (2001) Modified-release opioids. *European Journal of Palliative Care.* **8**: 142–146.
8 Babul N *et al.* (1995) Hydromorphone metabolite accumulation in renal failure. *Journal of Pain and Symptom Management.* **10**: 184–186.
9 Chaplan SR *et al.* (1992) Morphine and hydromorphone epidural analgesia. *Anesthesiology.* **77**: 1090–1094.

*METHADONE — BNF 4.7.2

Class: Opioid analgesic.

Indications: Severe pain, cough, †an alternative in cases of intolerance to other strong opioids, †**morphine** poorly-responsive pain, †pain relief in severe renal failure.[1,2]

Pharmacology

Methadone is a synthetic strong opioid with mixed properties.[3] Thus, it is a μ-opioid receptor agonist, possibly a δ-opioid receptor agonist,[4] an NMDA-receptor-channel blocker,[5,6] and a presynaptic blocker of serotonin re-uptake.[7] Methadone is a racemic mixture; L-methadone is responsible for almost all the analgesic effect, whereas D-methadone is a useful antitussive. Methadone is a basic and lipophilic drug which is absorbed well from all routes of administration. There is a high volume of distribution with only about 1% of the drug in the blood. Methadone accumulates in tissues when given repeatedly, creating an extensive reservoir.[8] Protein binding (principally to a glycoprotein) is 60–90%;[9] this is double that of **morphine**. Both volume of distribution and protein binding contribute to the long plasma halflife, and cumulation is a potential problem. Methadone is metabolised chiefly in the liver to several metabolites.[10] About half of the drug and its metabolites are excreted by the intestines and half by the kidneys; most of the latter unchanged.[11] Renal and hepatic impairment do not affect methadone clearance.[12,13]

In single doses, methadone PO is about 1/2 as potent as IM,[14] and IM a single dose of methadone is marginally more potent than **morphine**. With repeated doses, methadone is several times more potent. It is also longer acting; with chronic administration, analgesia lasts 6–12h and sometimes more. Some patients who obtain only poor relief with **morphine** but severe undesirable effects (drowsiness, delirium, nausea and vomiting) obtain good relief with relatively low-dose methadone with few or no undesirable effects. Methadone may be particularly beneficial for neuropathic pain because of its NMDA antagonism (see **ketamine**, p.289). Methadone is also useful in patients with chronic renal failure who have developed excessive drowsiness ± delirium with **morphine** because of cumulation of morphine-6-glucuronide.[2] However, for moribund patients, **alfentanil** is probably a better choice. Methadone can also be used as a strong opioid analgesic in former narcotic addicts who are being maintained on methadone.[15]
Bio-availability 80% (range 40–100%) PO.
Onset of action 30min; 15min IM.
Time to peak plasma concentration 4h PO; 1h IM.
Plasma halflife 8–75h;[16] longer in older patients; acidifying the urine results in a shorter halflife (20h) and raising the pH with sodium bicarbonate a longer halflife (>40h).[17]
Duration of action 4–5h PO and 3–5h IM single dose; 6–12h repeated doses.

Cautions

The lipid-solubility and long halflife of methadone means that cumulation to a significant extent is bound to occur, particulary in elderly patients; p.r.n. dose titration is generally necessary to avoid this potential hazard (see below).[18] MAOIs may prolong and enhance the respiratory depressant effects of methadone. **Carbamazepine**, **phenobarbital**, **phenytoin** and **rifampicin** increase the metabolism of methadone; **amitriptyline** and **cimetidine** decrease its metabolism. Methadone increases plasma **zidovudine** concentration.

Undesirable effects

For full list, see manufacturer's SPC.

Local erythema and induration when given by CSCI.[19] Rarely, methadone may cause myoclonus.[20] Also see Strong opioids, p.168.

Dose and use

Dose titration is different from **morphine**.[2,21–25] Most centres in the UK use the guidelines proposed by Morley and Makin (Box 5.K). For 2–3 days patients are advised to take a dose *q3h p.r.n.*; after which patients can be converted to either a b.d. or t.d.s regimen.[2] An alternative approach is given in Box 5.L. Maintenance doses vary considerably; most are ≤80mg/24h.[24]

Box 5.K Calculating the starting dose of methadone: scheme 1 (Morley & Makin)[2]

Stop morphine abruptly; i.e. do *not* reduce progressively over several days.

Prescribe a dose of methadone that is 1/10 of the 24h PO morphine dose *up to a maximum of 30mg.*

Allow the patient to take the prescribed dose *q3h p.r.n.*

On day 6, the amount of methadone taken over the previous two days is noted and converted into a regular q12h dose, with provision for a similar or smaller dose q3h p.r.n.

If p.r.n. medication is still needed, increase the dose of methadone by 1/2–1/3 every 4–6 days. [Example: 10mg b.d. → 15mg b.d.; 30mg b.d → 40mg b.d.]

Box 5.L Calculating the starting dose of methadone: scheme 2 (Nauck)[25]

Stop morphine abruptly; i.e. do *not* reduce progressively over several days.

Initially prescribe methadone 5–10mg PO q4h *and* q1h p.r.n. *whatever the dose of morphine.*

After 12–24h, if frequent p.r.n. doses are still needed and the pain is not easing, increase methadone to 10–15mg q4h and q1h p.r.n.

After 72h, reduce regular methadone to q8h *and* q3h p.r.n.
Subsequently, increase the dose of methadone every 4–5 days if still needing multiple p.r.n. doses.

Methadone is sometimes given by CSCI; it causes significant local inflammation in many patients necessitating site rotation and possibly other measures.[26] Methadone can also be given IV.[27] When converting from PO to SC/IV, it is advisable to reduce the dose of methadone by 50%. This allows for the wide variability in PO bio-availability (40–100%). Subsequent upward adjustments in the dose can be made every few days if necessary. However, if the patient is moribund, death is likely to occur relatively quickly, i.e. before the impact of reducing the dose has time to manifest in the patient with high oral bio-availability.

Supply

Unless indicated otherwise, all preparations are **CD**.

Methadone (non-proprietary)
Tablets 5mg, 28 days @ 30mg b.d = £19.96.
Oral solution 1mg/ml, 28 days @ 30mg b.d = £25.50.
Injection 10mg/ml, 1ml amp = £0.86; 2ml amp = £1.45; 3.5ml amp = £1.78; 5ml amp = £1.92.

Methadose® (from Rosemont 0113 244 1999)
Oral concentrate 10mg/ml, 20mg/ml, 28 days @ 30mg b.d = £14.31. (*The oral concentrate should be dispensed only after dilution to the required strength using Methadose® Diluent.*)

1 Gannon C (1997) The use of methadone in the care of the dying. *European Journal of Palliative Care*. **4**: 152–158.
2 Morley J and Makin M (1998) The use of methadone in cancer pain poorly responsive to other opioids. *Pain Reviews*. **5**: 51–58.
3 Watanabe S (2001) Methadone the renaissance. *Journal of Palliative Care*. **17**: 117–120.
4 Raynor K *et al.* (1994) Pharmacological characterization of the cloned kappa-, delta-, and mu-opioid receptors. *Molecular Pharmacology*. **45**: 330–334.
5 Ebert B *et al.* (1995) Ketobemidone, methadone and pethidine are non-competitive N-methyl-D-aspartate (NMDA) antagonists in the rat cortex and spinal cord. *Neuroscience Letter*. **187**: 165–168.
6 Gorman A *et al.* (1997) The d- and l-isomers of methadone bind to the non-competitive site on the N-methyl-D-aspartate (NMDA) receptor in rat forebrain and spinal cord. *Neuroscience Letters*. **223**: 5–8.
7 Codd E *et al.* (1995) Serotonin and norepinephrine uptake inhibiting activity of centrally acting analgesics: structural determinants and role in antinociception. *Journal of Pharmacology and Experimental Therapeutics*. **274**: 1263–1270.
8 Robinson AE and Williams FM (1971) The distribution of methadone in man. *Journal of Pharmacy and Pharmacology*. **23**: 353–358.
9 Eap CB *et al.* (1990) Binding of D-methadone, L-methadone and DL-methadone to proteins in plasma of healthy volunteers: role of variants of X1-acid glycoprotein. *Clinical Pharmacology and Therapeutics*. **47**: 338–346.
10 Fainsinger R *et al.* (1993) Methadone in the management of cancer pain: clinical review. *Pain*. **52**: 137–147.
11 Inturrisi CE and Verebely K (1972) The levels of methadone in the plasma in methadone maintenance. *Clinical Pharmacology and Therapeutics*. **13**: 633–637.
12 Kreek MJ *et al.* (1980) Methadone use in patients with chronic renal disease. *Drug Alcohol Dependence*. **5**: 197–205.
13 Novick DM *et al.* (1981) Methadone disposition in patients with chronic liver disease. *Clinical Pharmacology and Therapeutics*. **30**: 353–362.
14 Beaver WT *et al.* (1967) A clinical comparison of the analgesic effects of methadone and morphine administered intramuscularly, and of orally and parenterally administered methadone. *Clinical Pharmacology and Therapeutics*. **8**: 415–426.
15 Manfredi P *et al.* (2001) Methadone analgesia in cancer pain patients on chronic methadone maintenance therapy. *Journal of Pain and Symptom Management*. **21**: 169–174.
16 Sawe J (1986) High dose morphine and methadone in cancer patients: clinical pharmacokinetic consideration of oral treatment. *Clinical Pharmacology*. **11**: 87–106.
17 Nilsson MI *et al.* (1982) Pharmacokinetics of methadone during maintenance treatment: adaptive changes during the induction phase. *European Journal of Clinical Pharmacology*. **22**: 343–349.
18 Hendra T *et al.* (1996) Fatal methadone overdose. *British Medical Journal*. **313**: 481–482.
19 Bruera E *et al.* (1991) Local toxicity with subcutaneous methadone. Experience of two centers. *Pain*. **45**: 141–143.
20 Sarhill N *et al.* (2001) Methadone-induced myoclonus in advanced cancer. *American Journal of Hospice and Palliative Care*. **18 (1)**: 51–53.
21 Ripamonti C *et al.* (1997) An update on the clinical use of methadone cancer pain. *Pain*. **70**: 109–115.
22 Hagen N and Wasylenko E (1999) Methadone: outpatient titration and monitoring strategies in cancer patients. *Journal of Pain and Symptom Management*. **18**: 369–375.
23 Mercadante S *et al.* (1999) Rapid switching from morphine to methadone in cancer patients with poor response to morphine. *Journal of Clinical Oncology*. **17**: 3307–3312.
24 Scholes C *et al.* (1999) Methadone titration in opioid-resistant cancer pain. *European Journal of Cancer Care*. **8**: 26–29.
25 Nauck F *et al.* (2001) A German model for methadone conversion. *American Journal of Hospice and Palliative Care*. **18 (3)**: 200–202.
26 Mathew P and Storey P (1999) Subcutaneous methadone in terminally ill patients: manageable local toxicity. *Journal of Pain and Symptom Management*. **18**: 49–52.
27 Fitzgibbon D and Ready L (1997) Intravenous high-dose methadone administered by patient controlled analgesia and continuous infusion for the treatment of cancer pain refractory to high-dose morphine. *Pain*. **73**: 259–261.

OXYCODONE BNF 4.7.2

Class: Opioid analgesic.

Indications: Moderate-to-severe pain in patients with cancer, postoperative pain, †an alternative in cases of intolerance to other strong opioids.

Pharmacology

Oxycodone is a strong opioid with similar properties to **morphine**.[1–4] Animal studies with selective opioid antagonists suggest that oxycodone and **morphine** produce analgesia through different populations of opioid receptors. Thus, naloxonazine (a selective μ-opioid receptor antagonist) completely blocks morphine-induced antinociception in rats but does not attenuate the effect of oxycodone.[5] In contrast, norbinaltorphimine (a selective κ-opioid receptor antagonist) completely blocks oxycodone-induced antinociception but does not attentuate the effect of morphine. Oxycodone is partly metabolised to **oxymorphone**, a strong opioid analgesic which by injection is 10 times more potent than **morphine**. The biotransformation is mediated by cytochrome CYP2D6. After blocking this by quinidine, the effects of oxycodone in volunteers are unchanged, indicating that oxycodone is an analgesic in its own right, and that the contribution by **oxymorphone** is small.[6,7] Parenterally oxycodone is about 3/4 as potent as **morphine**.[8] However, its oral bio-availability is much higher than **morphine**. This means that oxycodone by mouth is about 1.5–2 times more potent than oral **morphine**.[9,10] The SPC for oxycodone lists hepatic impairment as a contra-indication. There are no pharmacokinetic data to justify this but, in moderate hepatic impairment, oxycodone and noroxycodone concentrations increase (but the oxymorphone concentration decreases). In renal impairment the clearance of oxycodone, noroxycodone and conjugated oxymorphone are reduced. Oxycodone plasma concentration increases by 50% and the halflife lengthens by 1h.[8] Oxycodone is given q4h–q6h.

Bio-availability 75% PO, ranging from 60–87%.[11,12]
Onset of action 20–30min PO.
Time to peak plasma concentration 1–1.5h; 3h m/r.
Plasma halflife 3.5h; 4.5h in renal failure.
Duration of action 4–6h; 12h m/r.

Undesirable effects

For full list, see manufacturer's SPC.

Essentially the same as **morphine**, but in one study constipation was more common and vomiting less common with oxycodone.[13] Also see Strong opioids, p.168.

Dose and use

Oral

Normal-release oxycodone is used in the same way as **morphine** but q6h rather than q4h. Because oxycodone is more expensive, it should generally be reserved for patients who cannot tolerate **morphine**. M/r preparations are biphasic in their release of oxycodone, i.e. an initial relatively fast release leading to early onset of analgesia and a slow release to provide a 12h duration of action.

Rectal

Oxycodone *pectinate* 30mg suppositories are available in the UK and Canada. Oxycodone *pectinate* is a primitive m/r formulation which converts a q4h drug into a q8h suppository; effectively superseded by CSCI **diamorphine/morphine**, or by m/r **morphine** rectal tampon. If used, start with a convenient dose PR, approximately 1/2 that of the previous PO **morphine**. Oxycodone *hydrochloride* 5mg suppositories are available in the USA; these are equivalent to **morphine** 10mg and are given q4h.

Supply

Unless indicated otherwise, all preparations are **CD**.

OxyNorm® (Napp 01223 424444)
Capsules 5mg, 10mg, 20mg, 5mg dose = £0.19.
Oral solution 1mg/ml, 5mg dose = £0.19.
Concentrated oral solution 10mg/ml, 5mg dose = £0.19.

Modified-release
OxyContin® (Napp 01223 424444)
Tablets m/r 10mg, 20mg, 40mg, 80mg, 28 days @ 10mg, 20mg and 80mg b.d. = £21.43, £42.86 and £171.46 respectively.

Oxycodone pectinate
Suppositories m/r 30mg. (Unlicensed available as a special order from BCM specials 0800 952 1010; see Special orders and named patient supplies, p.349.)

1 Glare PA and Walsh TD (1993) Dose-ranging study of oxycodone for chronic pain in advanced cancer. *Journal of Clinical Oncology*. **11**: 973–978.
2 Poyhia R *et al.* (1993) Oxycodone: an alternative to morphine for cancer pain. A review. *Journal of Pain and Symptom Management*. **8**: 63–67.
3 Shah S and Hardy J (2001) Oxycodone: a review of the literature. *European Journal of Palliative Care*. **8**: 93–96.
4 Davis M *et al.* (2002) Normal-release and controlled-release oxycodone: pharmacokinetics, pharmacodynamics, finances, fad, fatality and facts. *Supportive Care in Cancer*. In press.
5 Ross F and Smith M (1997) The intrinsic antinociceptive effects of oxycodone appear to be kappa-opioid receptor mediated. *Pain*. **73**: 151–157.
6 Heiskanen T *et al.* (1998) Effects of blocking CYP2D6 on oxycodone. *Clinical Pharmacology and Therapeutics*. **64**: 603–611.
7 Smith M *et al.* (2001) Oxycodone has a distinctly different pharmacology from morphine. *European Journal of Pain*. **15 (suppl A)**: 135–136.
8 Kaiko R *et al.* (1996) Clinical pharmacokinetics of controlled-release oxycodone in renal impairment. *Clinical Pharmacology and Therapeutics*. **59**: 130.
9 Heiskanen T *et al.* (1996) Double-blind, randomised, repeated dose, crossover comparison of controlled-release oxycodone and controlled-release morphine in cancer pain I: pharmacodynamic profile. In: *Abstracts of Eighth World Congress on Pain*. IASP Press, Seattle, pp.17–18.
10 Kaiko R *et al.* (1996) Analgesic onset and potency of oral controlled-release (CR) oxycodone and controlled-release morphine. *Clinical Pharmacology and Therapeutics*. **59**: 130.
11 Leow K *et al.* (1992) Single-dose and steady-state pharmacokinetics and pharmacodynamics of oxycodone in patients with cancer. *Clinical Pharmacology and Therapeutics*. **52**: 487–495.
12 Poyhia R *et al.* (1992) The pharmacokinetics and metabolism of oxycodone after intramuscular and oral administration to healthy subjects. *British Journal of Clinical Pharmacology*. **33**: 617–621.
13 Heiskanen T and Kalso E (1997) Controlled-release oxycodone and morphine in cancer related pain. *Pain*. **73**: 37–45.

OPIOID ANTAGONISTS BNF 4.10 & 15.1.7

Several opioid antagonists are available. **Nalorphine**[1] and **nalbuphine**[2,3] are mixed opioid agonist-antagonists, whereas **naloxone**, **naltrexone**, **nalmefene** (not UK) and **methylnaltrexone** (not UK) are pure antagonists, i.e. have a high degree of affinity for opioid receptors but no intrinsic activity.

Naloxone is used principally to reverse life-threatening respiratory depression; **naltrexone** is used to prevent relapse in former opioid-dependent patients who have remained opioid-free for at least 7 days. Both are used in the management of pruritus associated with cholestasis.[4] Pruritus in cholestasis is a central phenomenon caused by increased opioidergic tone secondary to an increase in plasma enkephalin concentration.[5,6] Opioid antagonists are effective in counterbalancing the increased tone, and thereby relieve the pruritus.[7–10] Unfortunately, an opioid-like withdrawal syndrome may be precipitated.[5,11] This can be avoided by using small incremental doses of an opioid antagonist. The opioid system is also involved but, in uraemic pruritus, there is no increase in opioidergic tone (and therefore no danger of a withdrawal syndrome). Instead, in uraemia, an imbalance between the μ-opioid receptors (pruritus-inducible) and κ-opioid receptors (pruritus-suppressive) develops which predisposes to the development of pruritus.[12] Data from two trials of **naltrexone** is uraemic pruritus give conflicting results; benefit was seen in the trial in patients with very severe pruritus[13] but not in those with moderately severe pruritus.[14]

Methylnaltrexone is a quaternary compound which does not readily cross the blood-brain barrier. It is therefore a peripheral opioid receptor antagonist. It is used to correct opioid-induced constipation.[15]

1 Martindale (1996) *Martindale: The Extra Pharmacopoeia* (31e). Royal Pharmaceutical Society, London, p.986.
2 Lewis JR (1980) Evaluation of new analgesics. Butorphanol and nalbuphine. *Journal of the American Medical Association.* **243**: 1465–1467.
3 Cohen SE *et al.* (1992) Nalbuphine is better than naloxone for treatment of side effects after epidural morphine. *Anesthesia and Analgesia.* **75**: 747–752.
4 Jones E and Bergasa N (1999) The pruritus of cholestasis. *Hepatology.* **29**: 1003–1006.
5 Thornton J and Losowksy M (1988) Opioid peptides and primary biliary cirrhosis. *British Medical Journal.* **297**: 1501–1504.
6 Swain M *et al.* (1992) Endogenous opioids accumulate in plasma in a rat model of acute cholestasis. *Gastroenterology.* **103**: 630–635.
7 Bergasa N *et al.* (1992) A controlled trial of naloxone infusions for the pruritus of chronic cholestasis. *Gastroenterology.* **102**: 544–549.
8 Bergasa N *et al.* (1995) Effects of naloxone infusions in patients with the pruritus of cholestasis. *Annals of Internal Medicine.* **123**: 161–167.
9 Bergasa N *et al.* (1998) Open-label trial of oral nalmefene therapy for the pruritus of cholestasis. *Hepatology.* **27**: 679–684.
10 Bergasa N *et al.* (1999) Oral nalmefene therapy reduces scratching activity due to the pruritus of cholestasis: a controlled study. *Journal of the American Academy of Dermatology.* **41**: 431–434.
11 Jones E and Dekker R (2000) Florid opioid withdrawal-like reaction precipitated by naltrexone in a patient with chronic cholestasis. *Gastroenterology.* **118**: 431–432.
12 Kumagai H *et al.* (2000) Endogenous opioid system in uraemic patients. *British Journal of Clinical Pharmacology.* Abstracts of the Joint Meeting of the Seventh World Conference on Clinical Pharmacology and IUPHAR – Division of Clinical Pharmacology and the Fourth Congress of the European Association for Clinical Pharmacology and Therapeutics (EACPT): 282.
13 Peer G *et al.* (1996) Randomised crossover trial of naltrexone in uraemic patients. *Lancet.* **348**: 1552–1554.
14 Pauli-Magnus C *et al.* (2000) Naltrexone does not relieve uremic pruritus. *Journal of the American Society of Nephrology.* **11**: 514–519.
15 Yuan C-S *et al.* (2000) Methylnaltrexone for reversal of constipation due to chronic methadone use. *Journal of the American Medical Association.* **283**: 367–372.

NALOXONE — BNF 15.1.7

Class: Opioid antagonist.

Indications: Reversal of opioid-induced respiratory depression.

Pharmacology

Naloxone is a pure and potent opioid antagonist. It has a high affinity for opioid receptors and reverses the effect of opioid analgesics by displacement in a dose-related manner. Partial antagonism may be obtained by using small doses. Activity after oral administration is low; it is only 1/15 as potent by mouth as by injection. Naloxone is rapidly metabolised by the liver, primarily to naloxone glucuronide which is excreted by the kidneys. The most important clinical property of naloxone is reversal of opioid-induced respiratory depression (and other opioid effects) caused by either an overdose of an opioid (including **codeine** and **dextropropoxyphene**) or an exaggerated response to conventional doses. Naloxone also reverses the opioid effects of **pentazocine** and other mixed agonist-antagonists; antagonism of **buprenorphine** is less complete because of the latter's high receptor affinity. *Naloxone is not effective against respiratory depression caused by non-opioids such as barbiturates.* Naloxone has also been shown to be of benefit in patients with chronic idiopathic constipation,[1] septic shock,[2] morphine-induced peripheral vasodilation,[3] ischaemic central neurological deficits[4,5] and poststroke central pain.[6]

Postoperative pain studies indicate that low-dose naloxone reduces the undesirable effects of **morphine**.[7,8] Naloxone 400microgram/70kg/24h CIVI, reduced **morphine** requirements and halved the incidence of nausea and vomiting (about 80% to 40%) and of pruritus (50% to 25%).[7] Whether this benefit from naloxone can be utilised in palliative care is not yet clear. These findings can be explained if the μ- δ- and κ-opioid receptors respond to ligands in a bimodal way.[9] If this is the case, opioid receptors would have an excitatory as well as an inhibitory mode. Excitation would produce hyperalgesia (and possibly tolerance), whereas inhibition would produce typical opioid analgesic and other effects. This theory can also be used to explain why high doses of morphine sometimes cause hyperalgesia.[10]

Bio-availability 6% PO.

Onset of action 1–2min IV; 2–5min SC/IM.

Plasma halflife 30–80min.

Duration of action 30min–4h, situation dependent.

Cautions

Naloxone should *not* be used for drowsiness and/or delirium which is not life-threatening because of the danger of totally reversing the opioid analgesia and precipitating severe/agonising pain and a major physical withdrawal syndrome.

Undesirable effects

For full list, see manufacturer's SPC.

Nausea and vomiting. Occasionally severe hypertension, pulmonary oedema, tachycardia, arrhythmias, cardiac arrest;[11] doses as small as 100–400microgram of naloxone have been implicated.[12] The mechanism of these sporadic events may be related to the centrally-mediated catecholamine responses to opioid reversal.[13]

Dose and use

Naloxone is best given IV but, if not practical, may be given IM or SC. After IV injection, antagonism lasts for 15–90min. The BNF contains two entries for naloxone. One relates to overdosage by addicts and recommends *800microgram–2mg* IV every 2–3min up to a total of 10mg if necessary, with the possibility of an ongoing IV infusion. The other relates to reversal of respiratory depression caused by the medicinal use of opioids. In this circumstance, *100–200microgram* IV should be given, with increments of *100microgram* every 2min until respiratory function is satisfactory. Further IM doses should be given after 1–2h if there is concern that further absorption of the opioid will result in delayed respiratory depression. Even lower doses have been recommended (Box 5.M). *It is important to titrate dose against respiratory function and not the level of consciousness because total antagonism will cause a return of severe pain with hyperalgesia and, if physically dependent, severe physical withdrawal symptoms and marked agitation.*

Box 5.M Naloxone for iatrogenic opioid overdose (based on the recommendations of the American Pain Society)[14]

If respiratory rate ≥8/min and the patient easily rousable and not cyanosed, adopt a policy of 'wait and see'; consider reducing or omitting the next regular dose of morphine.

If respiratory rate <8/min, patient barely rousable/unconscious and/or cyanosed:

- dilute a standard ampoule containing naloxone 40microgram to 10ml with saline for injection
- administer 0.5ml (20microgram) IV every 2min until the patient's respiratory status is satisfactory
- further boluses may be necessary because naloxone is shorter acting than morphine (and other opioids).

Supply

Naloxone (non-proprietary)
Injection 400microgram/ml, 1ml amp = £6.92.

Narcan® (Bristol-Myers Squibb 020 8572 7422)
Injection 400microgram/ml, 1ml amp = £4.54.

1 Kreek MJ *et al.* (1983) Naloxone, a specific opioid antagonist, reverses chronic idiopathic constipation. *Lancet.* **i**: 261–262.
2 Peters WP *et al.* (1981) Pressor effect of naloxone in septic shock. *Lancet.* **i**: 529–532.
3 Cohen RA and Coffman JD (1980) Naloxone reversal of morphine-induced peripheral vasodilatation. *Clinical Pharmacology and Therapeutics.* **28**: 541–544.
4 Baskin DS and Hosobuchi Y (1981) Naloxone reversal of ischaemic neurological deficits in man. *Lancet.* **ii**: 272–275.
5 Bousigue J-Y *et al.* (1982) Naloxone reversal of neurological deficit. *Lancet.* **ii**: 618–619.
6 Ray D and Tai Y (1988) Infusions of naloxone in thalamic pain. *British Medical Journal.* **296**: 969–970.
7 Gan T *et al.* (1997) Opioid-sparing effects of a low-dose infusion of naloxone in patient-administered morphine sulfate. *Anesthesiology.* **87**: 1075–1081.
8 Joshi G *et al.* (1999) Effects of prophylactic nalmefene on the incidence of morphine-related side effects in patients receiving intravenous patient-controlled analgesia. *Anesthesiology.* **90**: 1007–1011.
9 Crain S and Shen K (2000) Antagonists of excitatory opioid receptor functions enhance morphine's analgesic potency and attenuate opioid tolerance/dependence liability. *Pain.* **84**: 121–131.
10 Sjogren P *et al.* (1994) Disappearance of morphine-induced hyperalgesia after discontinuing or substituting morphine with other opioid antagonists. *Pain.* **59**: 313–316.
11 Partridge BL and Ward CF (1986) Pulmonary oedema following low-dose naloxone administration. *Anesthesiology.* **65**: 709–710.
12 Pallasch TJ and Gill CJ (1981) Naloxone associated morbidity and mortality. *Oral Surgery.* **52**: 602–603.
13 Smith G and Pinnock C (1985) Editorial: naloxone – paradox or panacea? *British Journal of Anaesthesia.* **57**: 547–549.
14 Max MB *et al.* (1992) *Principles of Analgesic Use in the Treatment of Acute Pain and Cancer Pain* (3e). American Pain Society, Skokie, Illinois, p.12.

NALTREXONE — BNF 4.10

Class: Opioid antagonist.

Indications: Prevention of relapse in detoxified opioid addicts; †pruritus associated with cholestasis[1,2] and, possibly, chronic renal failure.[3,4]

Contra-indications: Patients currently dependent on opioids; acute hepatitis or liver failure.

Pharmacology

Naltrexone is a specific opioid antagonist with actions similar to those of **naloxone**.[3–5] It is more potent and has a longer duration of action. It reversibly blocks the pharmacological effects of opioids and is used in the treatment of opioid-dependence as an aid to maintaining abstinence following opioid withdrawal. Naltrexone is well absorbed from the gastro-intestinal tract but undergoes extensive first-pass metabolism.[6,7] It is extensively metabolised in the liver and the major metabolite, 6-β-naltrexol, may also possess weak antagonist activity. Naltrexone and its metabolites are excreted mainly in the urine. Less than 1% of an oral dose of naltrexone is excreted unchanged.[8]

Bio-availability 5–40% PO.
Onset of action no data.
Time to peak plasma concentration 1h.
Plasma halflife 4h; 13h for 6-β-naltrexol; secondary terminal halflife 4 days.
Duration of action 1–3 days.

Cautions

Opioid withdrawal-like syndrome in patients with cholestatic pruritus. Hepatic and renal impairment. Occasional hepatotoxicity.[9]

Undesirable effects

For full list, see manufacturer's SPC.
Very common (<10%): in detoxified opioid addicts – insomnia, anxiety, nervousness, intestinal colic, nausea and vomiting, low energy, joint and muscle pain, headaches.

Dose and use

Cholestatic pruritus

- starting dose 12.5mg b.d. (some centres start with *1mg* o.d.)
- increase after 3–5 days to 25mg b.d./50mg o.d.
- escalate slowly over several weeks
- the effective dose range is 50–300mg o.d.

Uraemic pruritus

- starting dose 50mg o.d.[3,4]
- although no published evidence to support dose titration, consider increasing to 100mg o.d. after 1 week if starting dose ineffective.

Supply

Nalorex® (Bristol-Myers Squibb 020 8572 7422)
Tablets 50mg scored, 28 days @ 50mg o.d. = £42.51.

1 Carson K *et al.* (1996) Pilot study of the use of naltrexone to treat the severe pruritus of cholestatic liver disease. *American Journal of Gastroenterology.* **91**: 1022–1023.
2 Wolfhagen F *et al.* (1997) Oral naltrexone treatment for cholestatic pruritus: A double-blind, placebo-controlled study. *Gastroenterology.* **113**: 1264–1269.
3 Peer G *et al.* (1996) Randomised crossover trial of naltrexone in uraemic patients. *Lancet.* **348**: 1552–1554.
4 Pauli-Magnus C *et al.* (2000) Naltrexone does not relieve uremic pruritus. *Journal of the American Society of Nephrology.* **11**: 514–519.
5 Verebey K *et al.* (1976) Naltrexone: disposition, metabolism and effects after acute and chronic dosing. *Clinical Pharmacology and Therapeutics.* **20**: 315–328.
6 Gonzalez J and Brogden R (1988) Naltrexone: a review of its pharmacodynamic and pharmacokinetic properties and therapeutic efficacy in the management of opioid dependence. *Drugs.* **35**: 192–213.
7 Crabtree B (1984) Review of naltrexone: a long-acting opiate antagonist. *Clinical Pharmacy.* **3**: 273–280.
8 Wall M *et al.* (1981) Metabolism and disposition of naltrexone in man after oral and intravenous administration. *Drug Metabolism and Disposition.* **9**: 369–375.
9 Meyer M *et al.* (1984) Bioequivalence, dose-proportionality, and pharmacokinetics of naltrexone after oral administration. *Journal of Clinical Psychiatry.* **45**: 15–19.
10 Wall M *et al.* (1984) Naltrexone disposition in man after subcutaneous administration. *Drug Metabolism and Disposition.* **12**: 677–682.
11 Mitchell J (1986) Naltrexone and hepatotoxicity. *Lancet.* **i**: 1215.

6: INFECTIONS

The BNF Section 5 contains a comprehensive account of antibiotic use and many hospitals have antibiotic policies which govern local practice. Information presented here is limited to common situations in palliative care, or which demand decisive immediate action. When in doubt, obtain advice from a microbiologist.

CANDIDAL INFECTION — BNF 5.2

Oropharyngeal candidiasis is a common fungal infection in debilitated patients. In AIDS patients, oesophageal candidiasis is also common. Risk factors include:

- dry mouth
- topical antibiotics
- in AIDS, CD4+ cell count below 200cells/mm^3.

Invasive fungal disease is a complication of cytotoxic chemotherapy; its treatment is not dealt with here.[1]

General strategy

A systemically administered imidazole antifungal antibiotic, e.g. **ketoconazole** or **fluconazole**, is the treatment of choice, particularly in AIDS.[2,3] Topical oral **nystatin** is preferred at some centres because of the emergence of resistance to the imidazole antifungals. However, treatment q.d.s., particularly with concurrent *denture removal and cleaning* (necessary with topical agents) is more demanding in terms of time which, in hospital, means nurses' time. There is little to choose between **nystatin** and **ketoconazole** in relation to cost. However, particularly in AIDS, relapse is more common with **ketoconazole** (and **clotrimazole**) than with the more expensive **fluconazole** and **itraconazole**.[4]

The absorption of **ketoconazole** is markedly reduced in hypochlorhydric states. Systemic absorption is therefore a concern in patients with AIDS-related hypochlorhydria and in those receiving an antacid, H_2-receptor antagonist (e.g. **cimetidine**, **ranitidine**), a PPI (e.g. **lansoprazole**, **omeprazole**), **sucralfate**, or **didanosine** (a nucleoside reverse transcriptase inhibitor used in AIDS).[5] In hypochlorhydria, absorption from **itraconazole** capsules is variable but from the oral solution absorption is reliable and bio-availability higher.

Fluconazole achieves a higher clinical and mycological response rate than **ketoconazole** in AIDS patients.[2,3] A striking feature of **fluconazole** is the speed of response. Even with the most intractable forms of AIDS-associated *Candida*, a response is generally seen in <10 days with 50mg/day or <5 days with 100–200mg/day.[6,7] In cases of **fluconazole** resistance, **itraconazole** is recommended.[8] Response rates in HIV+ patients are 97% for **itraconazole** solution and 87% for **fluconazole**.[9]

Ketoconazole, **miconazole** and **itraconazole** have an inhibitory effect on cytochrome P450-mediated enzymes (see p.331). This results in inhibition of adrenal steroid synthesis (cortisol, testosterone, oestrogens and progesterone) and of the metabolism of certain drugs. **Fluconazole** has minimal effect in this respect.

Cautions

Serious drug interactions: when prescribing an imidazole antifungal (**fluconazole, itraconazole, ketoconazole** or **miconazole**), avoid concurrent administration with **astemizole, terfenadine** and **cisapride** (see Cytochrome P450, p.331).

Dose and use

In oropharyngeal and oesophageal candidiasis, higher doses for a longer period are generally necessary in AIDS.

Topical agents

- **nystatin** q.d.s.–q4h
  - suspension (100 000units/ml) 1–5ml
  - pastilles (100 000units)
  - popsicles (locally prepared) 5ml of nystatin suspension mixed with blackcurrant or other fruit juice concentrate and frozen in an ice tray with small rounded cups.

Patients must remove their dentures before each dose and clean them before re-insertion; failure to do this leads to treatment failure. At night dentures should be soaked in water containing 5ml of **nystatin** 100 000units/ml or in dilute **sodium hypochlorite** solution (Milton®). Most patients respond to a 10-day course but some need continuous treatment.

Systemic agents

These are more convenient than **nystatin** and obviate the need for denture removal at each administration. *Even so, it is important to remove and clean the underside of the dentures every day to remove any adherent infected debris.* Regimens include:

- **ketoconazole** 200mg tablet o.d. for 5 days; take after food to reduce gastric irritation. Most patients respond but 1/3 relapse and need retreatment.[10] *Liver damage has been reported in some patients treated for >10 days*
- **fluconazole** 150mg capsule stat; response and relapse rates similar to **ketoconazole** but it is more expensive. Immunosuppressed patients may need 100–200mg o.d. indefinitely; at some centres extended courses of 50mg o.d. are given for patients with a major risk factor
- **miconazole** 120mg/5ml gel q.d.s. is administered by teaspoon and the patient spreads it around the mouth with the tongue. However, the effect is mainly systemic. It is more expensive and less convenient than **ketoconazole** o.d.

Supply

Nystatin (non-proprietary)
Oral suspension 100 000units/ml, 7 days @ 1ml q.d.s.= £2.05.

Nystan® (Bristol-Myers Squibb 020 8572 7422)
Pastilles 100 000units, 7 days @ 1 q.d.s.= £3.24.
Oral suspension 100 000units/ml, 7 days @ 1ml q.d.s.= £2.05.

Ketoconazole
Nizoral® (Janssen-Cilag 01494 567567)
Tablets 200mg, 5 days @ 200mg o.d.= £2.62.

Fluconazole
Diflucan® (Pfizer 01304 616161)
Capsules 50mg, 150mg, 200mg, single dose 150mg = £7.12; 7 days @ 50mg o.d.= £16.61.
Oral suspension 50mg, 200mg/5ml, single dose 150mg = £7.12; 7 days @ 50mg o.d.= £16.61.

Miconazole
Daktarin® (Janssen-Cilag 01494 567567)
Oral gel (sugar-free) 120mg/5ml, 15g, 80g tube, 7 days @ 5ml q.d.s. = £10.50.

Itraconazole
Sporanox® (Janssen-Cilag 01494 567567)
Capsules 100mg, 15 days @ 100mg o.d. = £15.72.
Oral solution 10mg/ml, 14 days @ 100mg b.d. = £97.59.

1 Leather H and Wingard J (2001) Infections following hematopoietic stem cell transplantation. *Infectious Diseases of Clinics of North America.* **15**: 483–520.
2 DeWit S *et al.* (1989) Comparison of fluconazole and ketoconazole for oropharyngeal candidiasis in AIDS. *Lancet.* **1**: 746–748.
3 Greenspan D (1994) Treatment of oropharyngeal candidiasis in HIV-positive patients. *Journal of the American Academy of Dermatology.* **31**: S51–S55.
4 Vazquez J (1999) Options for the management of mucosal candidiasis in patients with AIDS and HIV infection. *Pharmacotherapy.* **19**: 76–87.
5 Piscitelli S *et al.* (1996) Drug interactions in patients infected with human immuno-deficiency virus. *Clinical Infectious Diseases.* **23**: 685–693.
6 Hay R (1990) Overview of studies of fluconazole in oropharyngeal candidiasis. *Review of Infectious Diseases.* **2**: S334–S337.
7 Darouiche R (1998) Oropharyngeal and esophageal candidiasis in immunocompromised patients: treatment issues. *Clinical Infectious Diseases.* **26**: 259–274.
8 Martin M (1999) The use of fluconazole and itraconazole in the treatment of *Candida albicans* infections: a review. *Journal of Antimicrobial Chemotherapy.* **44**: 429–437.
9 Graybill J *et al.* (1998) Randomized trial of itraconazole oral solution for oropharyngeal candidiasis in HIV/AIDS patients. *American Journal of Medicine.* **104**: 33–39.
10 Regnard C (1994) Single dose fluconazole versus five day ketoconazole in oral candidiasis. *Palliative Medicine.* **8**: 72–73.

METRONIDAZOLE BNF 5.1.11 + 13.10.1

Class: Antibiotic.

Indications: Anaerobic infections, malodour caused by anaerobic infection, pseudo-membranous colitis (see *Clostridium difficile* enteritis, p.212).

Pharmacology

Metronidazole is highly active against anaerobic bacteria and protozoa. Although it has no activity against aerobic organisms *in vitro*, in mixed infections *in vivo* both aerobes and anaerobes appear susceptible. Unlike most other antibiotics, resistance to metronidazole among anaerobes is uncommon. Metronidazole can be applied topically to malodourous fungating cancers and decubitus ulcers but is more expensive by this route.[1,2] The malodour is due to volatile fatty acids produced by anaerobic bacteria. **Tinidazole** is similar to metronidazole with a longer duration of action; it causes less gastro-intestinal disturbance but costs more.[3]
Bio-availability 100% PO; 60–80% PR; 20% PV.
Onset of action 20–60min PO; 5–12h PR.
Time to peak plasma concentration 1–2h PO; 3h PR.
Plasma halflife 6–11h.
Duration of action 8–12h.

Cautions

Metronidazole precipitates a **disulfiram**-like reaction with alcohol in 2–24% of patients.[4,5] Metabolites of metronidazole, like **disulfiram**, inhibit alcohol dehydrogenase, xanthine oxidase and aldehyde dehydrogenase. Inhibition of alcohol dehydrogenase leads to activation of microsomal enzyme oxidative pathways, generating ketones and lactate which may cause acidosis.[6] Xanthine oxidase inhibition can lead to noradrenaline (norepinephrine) excess.[6] Accumulation of acetaldehyde is probably responsible for most of the symptoms, e.g. flushing of the face and neck, headaches, epigastric discomfort, nausea and vomiting, and a fall in blood pressure. Patients should be warned that if they drink alcohol when taking metronidazole they may have an unpleasant reaction. However, generally this is little more than a moderate food aversion; the occasional patient may vomit profusely. The risk of a reaction with metronidazole PV is small because absorption is low.[7]

Undesirable effects

For full list, see manufacturer's SPC.

Nausea and vomiting, unpleasant taste, furred tongue, gastro-intestinal disturbance. May cause darkening of urine; anaphylaxis has been reported. For patients unable to tolerate metronidazole, the more expensive **tinidazole** can be substituted.

Dose and use

Anaerobic infections

Metronidazole 400mg PO t.d.s. for 2 weeks; 400mg PO b.d. in elderly debilitated patients. Tablets should be taken with or after food but suspensions are taken on an empty stomach, i.e. 1h a.c. If malodour or other symptoms and signs of infection recur, retreat and after 2 weeks continue indefinitely with 200mg b.d.

Ascending cholangitis (associated with a stent in the bile duct)

Metronidazole 400mg PO q8h and **cefuroxime** 1500mg IV q8h. Generally taken by mouth, but if the patient is not able to retain oral preparations may need to be given IV (with **cefuroxime**). Rectal administration is another option but causes proctitis; use by this route is best limited to 2–3 days.

Fungating tumours

Metronidazole applied topically as a gel, using a crushed 200mg tablet in Aquagel® or KY® jelly,[8] or by applying liberal amounts of a commercially-produced gel.[1,2,9,10] The dose from a crushed tablet is several times greater than that from commercial preparations. The higher dose may have an observable impact (reduced odour) within 24h compared with several days for commercial preparations.[8]

Clostridium difficile enteritis (see p.212)

Supply

Metronidazole (non-proprietary)
Tablets 200mg, 400mg, 500mg, 7 days @ 400mg t.d.s. = £0.87.
Oral suspension 200mg/5ml, 7 days @ 400mg t.d.s. = £16.13.
IV infusion 5mg/ml, 100ml = £3.83.

Flagyl® (Hawgreen 01462 441831)
Tablets 200mg, 400mg, 7 days @ 400mg t.d.s. = £8.25.
Oral suspension 200mg/5ml, 7 days @ 400mg t.d.s. = £20.35.
Suppositories 500mg, 1g, 3 days @ 1g t.d.s + 4 days 1g b.d. = £34.00.

Flagyl® (Aventis Pharma 01732 584000)
IV infusion 5mg/ml, 100ml = £3.41, *contains 13.6mmol Na^+/100ml bag.*

Topical preparations
Anabact® (CHS 01603 735200)
Gel 0.75% 15g = £4.47; 30g = £7.89.

Metrotop® (SSL 01565 624000)
Gel 0.8% 15g = £4.73; 30g = £8.36; use tube once only.

Crushed tablets cost about £0.15 per topical application compared with £5–£8 for a proprietary gel.

1 Newman V *et al.* (1989) The use of metronidazole gel to control the smell of malodorous lesions. *Palliative Medicine.* **3**: 303–305.
2 Editorial (1990) Management of smelly tumours. *Lancet.* **335**: 141–142.
3 Carmine A *et al.* (1982) Tinidazole in anaerobic infections: a review of its antibacterial activity, pharmacological properties and therapeutic efficacy. *Drugs.* **24**: 85–117.
4 deMattos H (1968) Relations between alcoholism and the gastrointestinal system. Experience using metronidazole. *Hospital (Rio J).* **74**: 1669–1676.
5 Penick S *et al.* (1969) Metronidazole in the treatment of alcoholism. *American Journal of Psychiatry.* **125**: 1063–1066.
6 Harries D *et al.* (1990) Metronidazole and alcohol: potential problems. *Scottish Medical Journal.* **35**: 179–180.
7 Plosker G (1987) Possible interaction between ethanol and vaginally administered metronidazole. *Clinical Pharmacology.* **6**: 189–193.

8 Twycross R and Wilcock A (2001) *Symptom Management in Advanced Cancer* (3e). Radcliffe Medical Press, Oxford.

9 Ashford R *et al.* (1984) Double-blind trial of metronidazole in malodorous ulcerating tumours. *Lancet.* **i**: 1232–1233.

10 Thomas S and Hay N (1991) The antimicrobial properties of two metronidazole medicated dressings used to treat malodorous wounds. *Pharmaceutical Journal.* **246**: 264–266.

URINARY TRACT INFECTIONS — BNF 5.1.13

Urinary tract infections (UTIs) are more common in women than in men. *Escherichia coli* is the most common cause of UTI. Less common causes include *Proteus* and *Klebsiella spp. Pseudomonas aeruginosa* infections are generally associated with functional or anatomical abnormalities of the renal tract. *Staphylococcus epidermidis* and *Enterococcus faecalis* infection may complicate catheterisation or instrumentation. Whenever possible a specimen of urine should be collected for culture and sensitivity testing before starting antibiotic therapy.

Treatment strategy

Initially use **Multistix 8SG** to decide whether a patient has a UTI. Each stick costs <£0.20 (compare £20 for a MSU) and the result is available immediately (Box 6.A). If a UTI is suspected clinically and supported by the Multistix 8SG results:

- send a MSU for culture and sensitivity
- start empirical treatment with **trimethoprim** 200mg PO b.d. *or* IV **cefuroxime** and/or IV **gentamicin** if systemically unwell (see BNF for dose regimens).

Recommendations vary in relation to duration of antibiotic treatment from 3 days for an uncomplicated UTI in a woman to 10 days for children, men, and women with fever and/or loin pain.

Box 6.A Using Multistix 8SG to diagnose urinary tract infections

Multistix 8SG measure urinary pH and specific gravity, and the presence and amount of:

- glucose
- ketone
- blood
- protein
- nitrate, a bacterial metabolite
- leucocytes, produced by inflammation/infection.

How to do the test

- take a mid-stream specimen of urine (MSU)
- dip the strip into the urine and remove immediately
- after 60sec read nitrate result
- after 2min read the leucocyte result

} the colours on the strips should be compared to the bottle colours.

Late readings are of no value.

Significance of the results

Leucocyte and nitrate positive	infection is probable; send MSU
Nitrate only *or* leucocyte only positive	infection possible; MSU advisable
Leucocyte and nitrate negative	infection is unlikely; no need to send MSU unless definite urinary tract symptoms.

In *catheterised patients* bacterial colonisation is normal and is not necessarily harmful; it should not be investigated unless symptomatic. For patients who are about to be decatheterised, antibiotics for 48h before removal significantly reduces the risk of post-catheter bacteriuria.[1] In debilitated patients, and in those who find it difficult to take tablets, a single dose of **trimethoprim** 300mg is a useful compromise option; [2] the cure rate is 74% at 1 week and 71% at 6 weeks.[3]

Alternative approaches

These include the use of urinary antiseptics (**methenamine hippurate**, **nitrofurantoin** and **cranberry juice**).

Supply

Trimethoprim (non-proprietary)
Tablets 100mg, 200mg, 10 days @ 200mg b.d. = £0.96.

Monotrim® (Solvay 023 8046 7000)
Tablets 100mg, 200mg, 10 days @ 200mg b.d. = £1.75.
Oral suspension 50mg/5ml, 7 days @ 200mg b.d. = £7.08.

Trimopan® (APS 01323 501111)
Oral suspension 50mg/5ml, 7 days @ 200mg b.d. = £7.08.

Also see **nitrofurantoin**, p.244, **methenamine hippurate**, p.244, **cranberry juice**, p.245.

1 Hustinx W *et al.* (1991) Impact of concurrent antimicrobial therapy on catheter-associated urinary tract infection. *Journal of Hospital Infection.* **18**: 45–56.
2 Bailey R and Abbott G (1978) Treatment of urinary tract infection with a single dose of trimethoprim-sulfamethoxazole. *Canadian Medical Association Journal.* **118**: 551–552.
3 Brumfitt W *et al.* (1982) Comparative trial of trimethoprim and co-trimoxazole in recurrent urinary infections. *Infection.* **10**: 280–284.

ACUTE INFLAMMATORY EPISODES IN A LYMPHOEDEMATOUS LIMB

Acute inflammatory episodes (AIE), often called cellulitis, are common in lymphoedema.[1] AIE are frequently associated with fever, flu-like symptoms or even greater constitutional upset (Box 6.B).

Box 6.B Acute inflammatory episodes

Clinical features

Mild: pain, increased swelling, erythema (well-defined or blotchy).

Severe: extensive erythema with well-defined margins, increased swelling, blistering and weeping skin; often accompanied by fever, nausea and vomiting, pain and, when the leg is affected, difficulty in walking.

Diagnosis

Based on pattern recognition and clinical judgement.

Present history: date of onset, precipitating factor (e.g. insect bite or trauma), treatment received to date.

Past history: details of previous AIE, precipitating factors, antibiotics taken.

Examination: include the sites of lymphatic drainage to and from the inflamed area.

Preventive measures

Patients should be educated about:

- why they are susceptible to AIE, i.e. skin less robust, stagnant fluid, reduced immunity
- the consequence of AIE, i.e. increased swelling, more fibrosis, reduced response to treatment
- the importance of daily skin care, i.e. to improve and maintain the integrity of the skin
- reducing risk, e.g. protect hands when gardening, cleanse cuts, treat fungal infections (*Tinea pedis* is common) with an appropriate antifungal agent
- prophylaxis with antibiotics.

Treatment strategy

In AIE it is often difficult to isolate the pathogen responsible. However, *Streptococcus* is the most likely infective agent. All AIE should be treated promptly with antibiotics to prevent increased morbidity associated with increased swelling and accelerated fibrosis. In the UK, there is no standard regimen for AIE. The following is current practice at Sir Michael Sobell House.[2]

No systemic upset

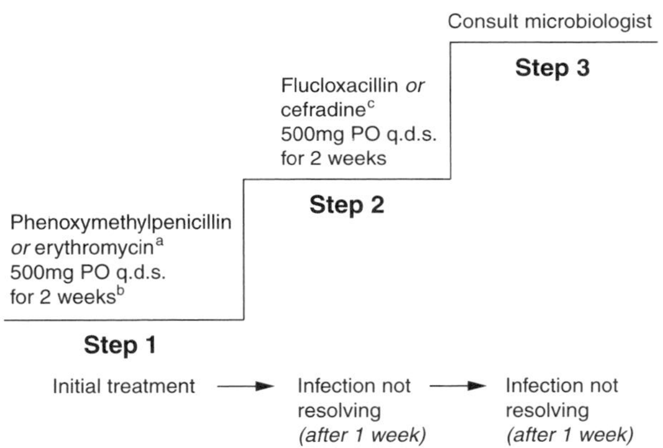

a. alternatives for patients with a history of penicillin allergy (rash); if a history of penicillin anaphylaxis, do not use cefradine but jump from step 1 to step 3

b. some centres use co-amoxiclav 625mg t.d.s. instead. This is active against both *Streptococci* and *Staphylococci* but causes more rashes and diarrhoea, and is more expensive.

Systemic upset

Bed rest is crucial and may necessitate inpatient admission. Blood cultures, aspirates of bullae and surface swabs (if the skin is broken) should be taken to guide treatment in case the infection does not resolve. Meanwhile, prescribe IV antibiotics for 1 week followed by PO antibiotics for 1 week, i.e. 2 weeks in total.

Week 1

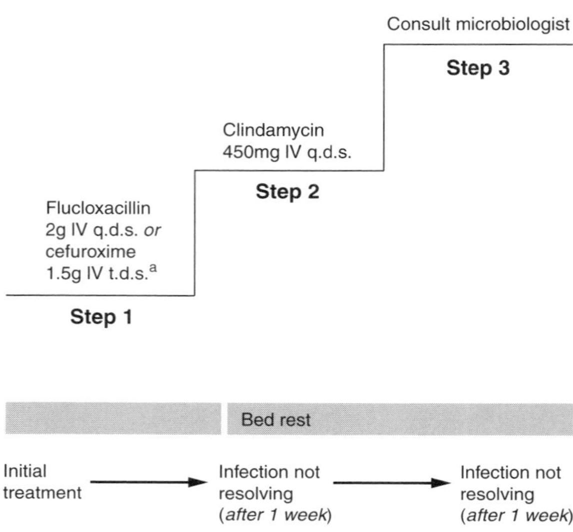

a. alternative for patients with a history of penicillin allergy (rash); if a history of penicillin anaphylaxis, proceed to step 2.

Week 2 If the infection is resolving, continue with PO medication for a second week:

- **flucloxacillin** injections are replaced by capsules 500mg PO q.d.s.
- **cefuroxime** injections are replaced by **cefradine** 1g PO b.d.
- **clindamycin** injections are replaced by capsules 300mg PO q.d.s.

Antibiotic prophylaxis

If an AIE recurs within a year, prescribe **phenoxymethylpenicillin** *500mg o.d. for one year* or **cefradine** 500mg o.d. if a history of penicillin rash. If there is a history of penicillin anaphylaxis, prescribe **clindamycin** 150mg o.d. instead.

Total care

- AIE are painful; analgesics should be prescribed regularly and p.r.n.
- compression garments should not be worn until limb is comfortable
- daily skin hygiene should be continued; washing and gentle drying
- emollients should not be used in the affected area if there is an open wound
- the affected limb should be elevated in a comfortable position, supported on pillows.[3]

Supply

Phenoxymethylpenicillin (non-proprietary)
Tablets 250mg, 14 days @ 500mg q.d.s. = £7.12.
Oral solution 250mg/5ml, 14 days @ 500mg q.d.s. = £12.77.

Erythromycin (non-proprietary)
Tablets e/c 250mg, 14 days @ 500mg q.d.s. = £12.32.
Oral suspension **erythromycin** (as **ethyl succinate**) 250mg, 500mg/5ml, 14 days @ 500mg q.d.s. = £8.37.

Erymax® (Elan 01438 765100)
Capsules (containing e/c pellets) 250mg, 14 days @ 500mg q.d.s. = £21.65.

Erythrocin® (Abbott 01628 773355)
Tablets **erythromycin** (as **stearate**) 250mg, 500mg, 14 days @ 500mg q.d.s. = £15.29.

Flucloxacillin (non-proprietary)
Capsules 250mg, 500mg, 14 days @ 500mg q.d.s. = £9.46.
Oral solution 125mg/5ml, 14 days @ 500mg q.d.s. = £36.18.
Injection 250mg, 500mg, 1g, 7 days @ 2g q.d.s. = £228.48.

Floxapen® (GSK 0800 221441)
Capsules 250mg, 500mg, 14 days @ 500mg q.d.s. = £27.22.
Oral solution 125mg/5ml, 250mg/5ml, 14 days @ 500mg q.d.s. = £39.03.
Injection 250mg, 500mg, 1g vial, 7 days @ 2g q.d.s. = £218.40.

Cefradine (non-proprietary)
Capsules 250mg, 500mg, 14 days @ 500mg q.d.s. = £18.87.

Velosef® (Bristol-Myers Squibb 020 8572 7422)
Capsules 250mg, 500mg, 14 days @ 500mg q.d.s. = £19.60.
Oral solution 250mg/5ml, 14 days @ 500mg q.d.s. = £23.63.

Co-amoxiclav (non-proprietary)
Tablets 250/125 (amoxicillin 250mg/clavulanic acid 125mg), 14 days @ 1 t.d.s. = £19.46.
Tablets 500/125 (amoxicillin 500mg/clavulanic acid 125mg), 14 days @ 1 t.d.s. = £31.44.

Augmentin® (GSK 0800 221441)
Tablets 375mg (amoxicillin 250mg/clavulanic acid 125mg), 14 days @ 1 t.d.s. = £19.58.
Tablets 625mg (amoxicillin 500mg/clavulanic acid 125mg), 14 days @ 1 t.d.s. = £31.46.
Tablets dispersible 250/125 (amoxicillin 250mg/clavulanic acid 125mg), 14 days @ 1 t.d.s. = £21.98.

Cefuroxime
Zinacef® (GSK 0800 221441)
Injection 250mg, 750mg, 7 days @ 1.5g t.d.s. = £106.05.

Clindamycin
Dalacin C® (Pharmacia 01908 661101)
Capsules 75mg, 150mg, 14 days @ 300mg q.d.s. = £50.96.
Injection 150mg/ml, 2ml, 4ml amp, 7 days @ 450mg q.d.s. = £275.24.

---

1 Mortimer P (2000) Acute inflammatory episodes. In: R Twycross *et al.* (eds) *Lymphoedema.* Radcliffe Medical Press, Oxford, pp.130–139.
2 Twycross R and Wilcock A (2001) *Symptom Management in Advanced Cancer* (3e). Radcliffe Medical Press, Oxford.
3 Twycross R *et al.* (2000) *Lymphoedema.* Radcliffe Medical Press, Oxford.

ASCENDING CHOLANGITIS

Ascending cholangitis may occur in patients with a partially obstructed or stented common bile duct. It often causes severe systemic disturbance and should be treated promptly with antibiotics.

Management strategy

Ascending cholangitis should be treated with a combination of an appropriate **cephalosporin** and **metronidazole**:

- **cefuroxime** 1500mg IV q8h for 48h
- **metronidazole** 400mg PO q8h (tablets with or after food; suspension on an empty stomach, i.e. 1h a.c.).

If oral administration is unreliable because of nausea and vomiting, **metronidazole** should be given PR (1g q8h) or IV (500mg q8h). Prolonged rectal use causes proctitis; use by this route is best limited to 2–3 days. **Cefuroxime** can be given IM if IV administration difficult, but 1500mg means an injection of 6ml.

Supply

Cefuroxime
Zinacef® (GSK 0800 221441)
Injection 250mg, 750mg, 2 days @ 1.5g t.d.s. = £30.30.

Also see **metronidazole**, p.205.

CLOSTRIDIUM DIFFICILE ENTERITIS

Pseudomembranous colitis is an uncommon complication of antibiotic therapy (Box 6.C). Symptoms generally begin within 1 week of starting antibiotic therapy or shortly after stopping, but may occur up to 1 month later. It is caused by colonisation of the bowel by *Clostridium difficile* and the production of toxins A and B which cause mucosal damage.

Box 6.C Pseudomembranous colitis

Clinical features
Explosive foul-smelling watery diarrhoea + mucus ± blood
Abdominal pain
Tenderness
Fever

Causal antibiotics

Most prevalent	*Highest incidence*
Ampicillin	Clindamycin
Amoxicillin	Lincomycin
Cephalosporins	
Ciprofloxacin	

Environmental control measures

Spread of *Clostridium difficile* is by the ingestion of spores which can be isolated from the environment around symptomatic patients. Environmental controls ('universal precautions') will prevent the spread of outbreaks:

- patients should be isolated while they have diarrhoea
- carers should use gloves and aprons, and thoroughly wash their hands after patient contact using either soap or alcohol-based products.

Treatment strategy

Clostridium difficile is strongly anaerobic and difficult to culture. Faecal tests to detect *Clostridium difficile* toxins can be used to confirm the diagnosis. If in doubt, endoscopy and rectal biopsy are of value, although a trial of therapy is more practical. **Metronidazole** is the treatment of choice. It is as effective as **vancomycin**[1,2] which is much more expensive and should be given only after seeking specialist advice. **Vancomycin** is generally reserved for patients with an ileus or those who are severely ill. About 20% of patients relapse, most within 3 weeks. This may be caused by germination of residual spores within the colon, re-infection with *Clostridium difficile* or further antibiotic treatment. Mild relapses often resolve spontaneously; repeat treatment with **metronidazole** is still recommended.[3,4] Repeated relapses require prolonged treatment with a slowly decreasing dose of **vancomycin**.[5] *Relapse due to resistance of Clostridium difficile to antibiotic treatment is extremely rare.*

Dose and use

- **metronidazole** 400mg PO t.d.s. for 10 days
- **vancomycin** 125mg PO q.d.s. for 10 days.

Supply

Vancomycin (non-proprietary)
Capsules 125mg, 250mg, 10 days @ 125mg q.d.s. = £94.61.
Injection (powder for reconstitution) 500mg, 1g vial = £6.67 and £13.41 respectively.

Vancocin® (Lilly 01256 315000)
Capsules 125mg, 250mg, 10 days @ 125mg q.d.s. = £126.16.
Injection (powder for reconstitution) 500mg, 1g vial = £8.66 and £17.32 respectively.

Vancomycin *injection can be used to prepare an oral solution as a cheaper alternative to the capsules; add 10ml WFI to a 500mg vial and give 2.5ml q.d.s. with added flavouring (10 day course = £66.70).*

Also see **metronidazole**, p.205.

1 Cherry R *et al.* (1982) Metronidazole: an alternate therapy for antibiotic-associated colitis. *Gastroenterology.* **82**: 849–851.
2 Teasley D *et al.* (1983) Prospective randomized trial of metronidazole versus vancomycin for Clostridium difficile-associated diarrhoea and colitis. *Lancet.* **ii**: 1043–1046.
3 Joint Working Group Report (1994) The prevention and management of Clostridium difficile infection. Department of Health, Public Health Laboratory Service, London.
4 Tabaqchali S and Jumaa P (1995) Diagnosis and management of Clostridium difficile infections. *British Medical Journal.* **310**: 1375–1380.
5 Anonymous (1995) Antibiotic-induced diarrhoea. *Drug and Therapeutics Bulletin.* **33**: 23–24.

7: ENDOCRINE SYSTEM AND IMMUNOMODULATION

BISPHOSPHONATES — BNF 6.6.2

Indications: Hypercalcaemia, bone pain, prophylactic use to reduce the incidence of pain and pathological fracture *in breast cancer and myeloma.*

Pharmacology

The bisphosphonates are stable analogues of naturally occurring pyrophosphate compounds which adsorb strongly to hydroxyapatite crystals in bone mineral, inhibiting their growth and dissolution. They have no impact on the effect of parathyroid-related protein (PTHrP) or on renal tubular re-absorption of calcium. Bisphosphonates are rapidly taken up by the skeleton, particularly at sites of bone resorption and where the mineral is more exposed, and they remain there for weeks or months. In patients with breast cancer and multiple myeloma, administration of bisphosphonates, generally in addition to systemic anticancer therapy, reduces the incidence of skeletal complications, e.g. hypercalcaemia, fracture and bone pain.[1,2] However, approximately eight patients would need to be treated for a year with **pamidronate** in order to prevent one additional skeletal complication and the cost-effectiveness of this has been questioned.[1,2] Their potential to treat and inhibit the development of bone metastases is being investigated.[3,4] Bisphosphonates inhibit osteoclast function and induce apoptosis (programmed cell death) by acting as analogues of pyrophosphate, interfering with cell metabolic pathways (**ibandronate, pamidronate, zoledronic acid**) and/or forming cytotoxic ATP analogues (**clodronate**).[5,6] These cellular effects also extend to macrophages, reducing the production of pro-inflammatory cytokines, and may help explain the reduction in bone pain seen in some patients following bisphosphonates.[7] Several regimens have been recommended for metastatic bone pain when more conventional methods have been exhausted.[7–11]

Hitherto, the two most widely used bisphosphonates have been **pamidronate** and **clodronate**. On account of its greater efficacy, **pamidronate** is generally preferred. However, **pamidronate** will soon be superseded by the third-generation bisphosphonates, e.g. **zoledronic acid** and **ibandronate**, which have greater potency and a shorter administration time.[12] Bisphosphonates are expensive and some recommended regimens are very costly. They are generally given IV, at least initially, because of poor alimentary absorption. For pharmacokinetic details, see Table 7.1.

Table 7.1 Bisphosphonates and the treatment of hypercalcaemia[14–16]

	Zoledronic acid	*Disodium pamidronate*	*Sodium clodronate*
Initial IV dose	4mg	30–90mg	(a) 1500mg (b) 300–600mg daily for 5 days
Onset of effect	<3 days	<3 days	<2 days
Maximum effect	4–7 days	5–7 days	3–5 days
Duration of effect	5 weeks	3 weeks	(a) 2 weeks (b) 3 weeks
Restores normocalcaemia	90%	70%	40–80%
Mechanism of action			
inhibits osteoclasts	+	+	+
stimulates osteoblasts	–	+	–
Initial PO treatment	Ineffective	Ineffective	Effective
Maintenance	IV infusion every 4–8 weeks	IV infusion every 3–4 weeks	Tablets generally prevent relapse

Cautions

Serious drug interactions: symptomatic hypocalcaemia may occur if an aminoglycoside antibiotic is given concurrently with long-term oral **clodronate** therapy.[13]

Renal impairment.

Undesirable effects

For full list, see manufacturer's SPC.
Very common: transient pyrexia and influenza-like symptoms (not **clodronate**), hypocalcaemia, hypophosphataemia. Oral preparations may cause dyspepsia, abdominal pain, diarrhoea or constipation.
Common: headache, nausea, vomiting, lymphocytopenia, transient bone pain, arthralgia, myalgia, generalised pain, hypomagnaesaemia.

Dose and use

Hypercalcaemia

For **zoledronic acid**, see monograph, p.218.
The dose of **disodium pamidronate** depends on the initial corrected plasma calcium concentration (Box 7.A and Table 7.2):
- maximum recommended dose is 90mg IV/treatment
- infusion rate should not exceed *1mg/min*
- concentration should not exceed *60mg/250ml*
- repeat after 1 week if initial response inadequate
- repeat every 3–4 weeks according to plasma calcium concentration.

Box 7.A Correcting plasma calcium concentrations (Oxford Radcliffe Hospital Trust)

Corrected calcium (mmol/L) = measured calcium + (0.022 × (42 – albumin g/L))
e.g. measured calcium = 2.45; albumin = 32
corrected calcium = 2.45 + (0.022 × 10) = 2.67mmol/L

Table 7.2 IV pamidronate for hypercalcaemia[a]

Corrected plasma calcium concentration (mmol/l)	*Dose (mg)*
<3	15–30
3–3.5	30–60
3.5–4	60–90
>4	90

a. manufacturer's recommendations.

Metastatic bone pain

Several regimens have been recommended for when more conventional methods have been exhausted:

- **disodium pamidronate** 90mg IV (50% of patients respond, usually within 7–14 days); if helpful repeat 60–90 mg every 3–4 weeks for as long as benefit is maintained[7]
- **disodium pamidronate** 120mg IV, repeated p.r.n. every 2–4 months[8]
- **disodium pamidronate** 90–120mg IV or **clodronate** 600–1500mg IV, repeated p.r.n. In patients not responding to a first treatment, a second can be tried. If still no response, discontinue[11]
- **sodium clodronate** 1.5g IV initially; plus maintenance therapy 1600mg PO o.d.[9,10]

One prophylactic regimen recommends **disodium pamidronate** 90mg IV every 4 weeks in patients with one or more osteolytic bone metastases ≥1cm in diameter; *very costly.*[1]

Supply

Disodium pamidronate (non-proprietary)
Injection 15mg/5ml vial = £27.50; 30mg/10ml vial = £55; 60mg/10ml vial = £110; 90mg/10ml vial = £165.

Aredia Dry Powder® (Novartis 01276 698370)
Injection (powder for reconstitution) 15mg vial = £29.82; 30mg vial = £59.66; 90mg vial = £170.45.

Sodium clodronate
Bonefos® (Boehringer Ingelheim 01344 424600)
Capsules 400mg, 28 days @ 800mg b.d. = £162.55.
Tablets 800mg, 28 days @ 800mg b.d. = £170.23.
Injection 300mg/5ml, for dilution and use as an infusion, 5ml amp = £13.78; 1.5g infusion = £68.90.

Loron® (Roche 01707 366000)
Capsules 400mg, 28 days @ 800mg b.d. = £162.55.

Loron 520® (Roche 01707 366000)
Tablets 520mg, 28 days @ 1040mg o.d. = £162.57.
1 Loron 520® tablet is equivalent to 2 Loron® capsules in terms of efficacy.

1 Hortobagyi GN *et al.* (1996) Efficacy of pamidronate in reducing skeletal complications in patients with breast cancer and lytic bone metastases. *New England Journal of Medicine.* **335**: 1785–1791.

2 Hillner B *et al.* (2000) Pamidronate in prevention of bone complications in metastatic breast cancer: a cost-effectiveness analysis. *Journal of Clinical Oncology.* **18**: 72.

3 Coleman R (2000) Optimising the treatment of bone metastases by Aredia and Zometa. *Breast Cancer.* **7**: 361–369.

4 Tassone P *et al.* (2000) Growth inhibition and synergistic induction of apoptosis by zoledronate and dexamethasone in human myeloma cell lines. *Leukemia.* **14**: 841–844.

5 Fleisch H (1998) Bisphosphonates: mechanisms of action. *Endocrine Reviews.* **19**: 80–100.

6 Russell R *et al.* (1999) Bisphosphonates: pharmacology, mechanisms of action and clinical uses. *Osteoporosis International.* **9 (suppl 2)**: S66–S80.

7 Crosby V *et al.* (1998) A randomized controlled trial of intravenous clodronate. *Journal of Pain and Symptom Management.* **15**: 266–268.

8 Vinholes J *et al.* (1996) Metabolic effects of pamidronate in patients with metastatic bone disease. *European Journal of Cancer.* **5**: 159–175.
9 Vorreuther R (1993) Bisphosphonates as an adjunct to palliative therapy of bone metastases from prostatic carcinoma. A pilot study on clodronate. *British Journal of Urology.* **72**: 792–795.
10 O'Rourke N *et al.* (1995) Double-blind, placebo-controlled, dose response trial of oral clodronate in patients with bone metastases. *Journal of Clinical Oncology.* **13**: 929–934.
11 Mannix K *et al.* (2000) Using bisphosphonates to control the pain of bone metastases: evidence-based guidelines for palliative care. *Palliative Medicine.* **14**: 455–461.
12 DesHarnais-Castel L *et al.* (2001) A microcosting analysis of zoledronic acid and pamidronate therapy in patients with metastatic bone disease. *Supportive Care in Cancer.* **9**: 545–551.
13 Johnson M and Fallon M (1998) Symptomatic hypocalcaemia with oral clodronate. *Journal of Pain and Symptom Management.* **15**: 140–142.
14 Ralston S (1994) Pathogenesis and management of cancer associated hypercalcaemia. In: G Hanks (ed) *Cancer Surveys: Palliative Medicine: problem areas in pain and symptom management.* Cold Spring Harbor Laboratory Press, pp.179–196.
15 Purohit O *et al.* (1995) A randomised, double-blind comparison of intravenous pamidronate and clodronate in hypercalcaemia of malignancy. *British Journal of Cancer.* **72**: 1289–1293.
16 Major P *et al.* (2001) Zoledronic acid is superior to pamidronate in the treatment of hypercalcaemia of malignancy. a pooled analysis of two randomized, controlled clinical trials. *Journal of Clinical Oncology.* **19**: 558–567.

ZOLEDRONIC ACID — BNF 6.6.2

Class: Bisphosphonate.

Indications: Tumour-induced hypercalcaemia; †bone pain.

Pharmacology

Zoledronic acid is a third-generation bisphosphonate and the most potent currently available.[1,2] In patients with hypercalcaemia, zoledronic acid 4mg compared to **pamidronate** 90mg is more effective in achieving normocalcaemia (90% vs 70%) and provides a longer median duration of response, approximately 5 weeks vs 3 weeks (see Table 7.1, p.216).[3] In patients who do not respond or relapse following zoledronic acid 4mg or **pamidronate**, 8mg can be given, with normocalcaemia achieved in 50% of patients. However, the median duration of response in this group is only 2 weeks.[3] The use of zoledronic acid to impede the development of bone metastases is being explored.[4] *In vitro*, zoledronic acid is a more potent inhibitor of prostate cancer cell growth than **pamidronate**.[5] *In vivo*, it is as effective as **pamidronate** in reducing skeletal complications in patients with osteolytic bone lesions due to breast cancer or multiple myeloma.[6] Zoledronic acid is tolerated as well as **pamidronate** but, because of concerns about raised creatinine concentrations in a few patients, the 8mg dose is no longer being encouraged in non-cancer studies.[4] Routine monitoring of renal function is advised. Zoledronic acid is administered IV over 5–15min.[3,6] It has a long terminal elimination halflife on account of its slow release from bone back into the systemic circulation. It is excreted unchanged by the kidney. No data are available for patients with severe renal impairment, but no dosage adjustment is necessary for patients with mild-to-moderate renal impairment.
Onset of action normocalacemia achieved by a median of 4 days (ranging up to 10).
Plasma half-life 1.75h; terminal elimination halflife 1 week.
Duration of action 30–40 days.

Cautions

Severe renal impairment (serum creatinine >400micromol/L).

Undesirable effects

For full list, see manufacturer's SPC.
Very common: transient fever maximal within 1–2 days in about 1/3 of patients.[7]
Common: confusion, bradycardia, nausea, creatinine elevation, fatigue, arthralgia, taste change, thirst, hypocalcaemia, hypophosphataemia.
Rare (<0.1%): pancytopenia.

Dose and use

Tumour-induced hypercalcaemia (corrected serum calcium >3mmol/L)
Patients should be well hydrated. Give 4–8mg IV in 100ml 0.9% sodium chloride or 5% glucose over 15min. The higher dose is reserved for refractory hypercalcaemia.

Supply

Zometa® (Novartis 01276 692255)
Injection 4mg vial = £195.00.

1 Green J *et al.* (1994) Preclinical pharmacology of CGP 42′446 a new, potent, heterocyclic bisphosphonate compound. *Journal of Bone and Mineral Research.* **9**: 745–751.
2 Body J (1997) Clinical research update: zoledronate. *Cancer.* **80**: 1699–1701.
3 Major P *et al.* (2001) Zoledronic acid is superior to pamidronate in the treatment of hypercalcaemia of malignancy. a pooled analysis of two randomized, controlled clinical trials. *Journal of Clinical Oncology.* **19**: 558–567.
4 Cheer S and Noble S (2001) Zoledronic acid. *Drugs.* **61**: 799–805.
5 Lee M *et al.* (2001) Bisphosphonate treatment inhibits the growth of prostate cancer cells. *Cancer Research.* **61**: 2602–2608.
6 Berenson J *et al.* (2001) Zoledronic acid reduces skeletal-related events in patients with osteolytic metastases. *Cancer.* **91**: 1191–1200.
7 Fleisch H (1998) Bisphosphonates: mechanisms of action. *Endocrine Reviews.* **19**: 80–100.

CORTICOSTEROIDS — BNF 6.3.2

Indications: Suppression of inflammatory and allergic disorders, cerebral oedema, nausea and vomiting with chemotherapy, †see Box 7.B.

Box 7.B Unlicensed indications for corticosteroids in advanced cancer[1,2]

Inclusion does not mean that a corticosteroid is necessarily the treatment of choice.

Specific
Spinal cord compression[3]
Nerve compression
Dyspnoea
  pneumonitis (after radiotherapy)
  lymphangitis carcinomatosa
  tracheal compression/stridor
Superior vena caval obstruction
Obstruction of hollow viscus
  bronchus
  ureter
  bowel[6,7]
Radiation-induced inflammation
Rectal discharge (give PR)

Pain relief
Nerve compression
Spinal cord compression[3]
Bone pain

Anticancer hormone therapy
Breast cancer[4]
Prostate cancer[5]
Haematological malignancies
Lymphoproliferative disorders

General
To improve appetite
To enhance sense of wellbeing

Pharmacology

The adrenal cortex secretes **hydrocortisone** (cortisol) which has glucocorticoid activity and weak mineralocorticoid activity. It also secretes aldosterone which has mineralocorticoid activity. Thus, in deficiency states, physiological replacement is best achieved with a combination of **hydrocortisone** and **fludrocortisone**, a mineralocorticoid. When comparing the relative anti-inflammatory (glucocorticoid) potencies of corticosteroids, their water-retaining properties (mineralocorticoid effect) should also be borne in mind (Table 7.3). Hydrocortisone is not used

Table 7.3 Selected pharmacokinetic details of commonly used corticosteroids[8,9]

Drug	*Anti-inflammatory potency*	*Approximate equivalent dose (mg)*	*Sodium-retaining potency*	*Oral bio-availability (%)*	*Onset of action*	*Peak plasma concentration*	*Plasma halflife (h)*	*Duration of action (h)*	*Relative affinity for lung tissue*	*Daily dose (mg) above which adrenal suppression possible*	
										Males	*Females*
Hydrocortisone	1	20	1	96	No data	No data	1.5	8–12	1	20–30	15–25
Prednisolone	4	5	0.25	75–85	No data	1h PO	3.5	12–36	1.6	7.5–10	7.5
Dexamethasone	25–50[a]	0.5–1	<0.01	78	8–24h IM[b]	1–2h PO	4.5	36–54	1	1–1.15	1
Betamethasone				98	No data	10–36min IV	6.5	24–48			

a. thymic involution assay
b. acute allergic reactions.

for long-term disease suppression because large doses would be required and these would cause troublesome fluid retention. On the other hand, the moderate anti-inflammatory effect of hydrocortisone makes it the first-choice corticosteroid for topical use in inflammatory skin conditions; undesirable effects are minimal, both topical and systemic. **Prednisolone** is the most frequently used corticosteroid for disease suppression but **dexamethasone,** with high glucocorticoid activity but insignificant mineralocorticoid effect, is particularly suitable for high-dose therapy. It is 6–12 times more potent than prednisolone, i.e. 2mg of dexamethasone is approximately equivalent to 15–25mg of prednisolone (Box 7.C); it has a long duration of action (Table 7.3). Some esters of **betamethasone** and of **beclometasone** exert a marked topical effect; use is made of this property with skin applications and bronchial inhalations.

For pharmacokinetic details, see Table 7.3.

Box 7.C Approximate equivalent anti-inflammatory doses of corticosteroids[a]

Hydrocortisone	20mg
Prednisolone	5mg
Methylprednisolone	4mg
Triamcinolone	4mg
Betamethasone	750microgram
Dexamethasone	750microgram

a. this list takes no account of either mineralocorticoid effects or variations in duration of action.[10]

Cautions

Diabetes mellitus, psychotic illness. Fourfold increased risk of peptic ulcer if co-administered with a NSAID (but no increased risk if used alone).[11] Corticosteroids antagonise oral hypoglycaemics and insulin (glucocorticoid effect), antihypertensives and diuretics (mineralocorticoid effect). Increased risk of hypokalaemia if high doses of corticosteroids are prescribed with β_2-sympathomimetics (e.g. **salbutamol**, **terbutaline**) or **carbenoxolone**. The metabolism of corticosteroids is accelerated by **aminoglutethimide** (**dexamethasone** only), anti-epileptics (**carbamazepine**, **phenobarbital**, **phenytoin**, **primidone**) and **rifampicin**. This effect is more pronounced with long-acting glucocorticoids; **phenytoin** may reduce the bio-availability of **dexamethasone** to 25–50%, and larger doses (double or more) will be needed when prescribed concurrently.[12] **Dexamethasone** itself can affect plasma **phenytoin** concentrations (may either rise or fall); the effect of concurrent use should be monitored.

Undesirable effects

For full list, see manufacturer's SPC.
See Boxes 7.D–7F.

Dose and use

Patients expected to take corticosteroids for 3 weeks or more, should be supplied with a *Steroid Treatment Card* (Box 7.G). Apart from **hydrocortisone**, corticosteroids can be given in a single daily dose o.m.; this eases compliance and reduces the likelihood of corticosteroid-induced insomnia. Even so, **temazepam** or **diazepam** o.n. is sometimes needed to counter insomnia or agitation. The initial daily dose varies according to indication and fashion.

Replacement therapy: **hydrocortisone** 20mg o.m., 10mg each evening with **fludrocortisone** 100–300microgram.
Anorexia: **dexamethasone** 2–4mg or **prednisolone** 15–30mg.[18,19]
Anti-emetic: e.g. **dexamethasone** 8–20mg o.m.[20–22]
Raised intracranial pressure: **dexamethasone** 8-16mg o.m.[23,24]
Spinal cord compression: **dexamethasone** 16mg o.m.[16]

Box 7.D Undesirable effects of corticosteroids

Glucocorticoid effects
Diabetes mellitus
Osteoporosis
Avascular bone necrosis
Mental disturbances
- insomnia
- paranoid psychosis
- depression
- euphoria

Muscle wasting and weakness (see Box 7.E)
Peptic ulceration (if given with an NSAID)[11]
Infection (increased susceptibility)
- candidiasis
- septicaemia (may delay recognition)
- tuberculosis (may delay recognition)
- chickenpox and measles (increased severity)[a]

Suppression of growth (in child)

Mineralocorticoid effects
Sodium and water retention
→ oedema
Potassium loss
Hypertension

Cushing's syndrome
Moonface
Striae
Acne

Steroid cataract
If prednisolone 15mg or equivalent taken daily for several years = 75% risk

a. if exposed to infection, should be given immunoglobulin either varicella-zoster or normal.

Box 7.E Corticosteroid myopathy[13,14]

Onset generally in the third month of treatment with dexamethasone ⩾4mg daily or prednisolone ⩾40mg daily. Can occur earlier and with lower doses.

If the chronological sequence fits with corticosteroid myopathy, a presumptive diagnosis should be made and the following steps taken:

- explanation to patient and family
- discuss need to compromise between maximising therapeutic benefit and minimising undesirable effects
- halve corticosteroid dose (generally possible as a single step)
- consider changing from dexamethasone to prednisolone (non-fluorinated corticosteroids cause less myopathy)
- attempt further reductions in dose at intervals of 1–2 weeks
- arrange for physiotherapy (disuse exacerbates myopathy)
- emphasise that weakness should improve after 3–4 weeks (provided cancer-induced weakness does not supervene).

Box 7.F Steroid pseudorheumatism

Patients receiving corticosteroids for rheumatoid arthritis occasionally develop diffuse pains, malaise and pyrexia, so-called steroid pseudorheumatism.[15]

It is sometimes also seen in cancer patients receiving large doses of corticosteroids or when a very high dose is reduced rapidly to a lower dose. Most likely to be affected are those:

- receiving 100mg of prednisolone daily for several days in association with chemotherapy
- with spinal cord compression given dexamethasone 96mg IV daily for 3 days[3] (followed by a rapidly reducing oral dose)[a]
- on high doses of dexamethasone to reduce raised intracranial pressure associated with brain metastases
- reducing to an ordinary maintenance dose after a prolonged course.

a. such a high dose is unnecessary; 10mg IV is as effective as 96mg.[16,17]

Box 7.G Patient information about corticosteroids

Following concern about severe chickenpox associated with systemic corticosteroids, the CSM has issued a notice that *every* patient prescribed a systemic corticosteroid should receive the **patient information leaflet** supplied by the relevant manufacturer.

Steroid treatment cards (see below) should also be issued where appropriate. Doctors and pharmacists can obtain supplies of the card from:

England and Wales
Department of Health, PO Box 777, London, SE1 6XH (Tel 0541 555455)

Scotland
Banner Business Supplies, 20 South Gyle Crescent, Edinburgh EH12 9EB (Tel 0131 479 3279)

STEROID TREATMENT CARD

I am a patient on STEROID treatment which must not be stopped suddenly

- If you have been taking this medicine for more than three weeks, the dose should be reduced gradually when you stop taking steroids unless your doctor says otherwise.
- Read the patient information leaflet given with the medicine.
- Always carry this card with you and show it to anyone who treats you (for example a doctor, nurse, pharmacist or dentist). For one year after you stop the treatment, you must mention that you have taken steroids.
- If you become ill, or if you come into contact with anyone who has an infectious disease, consult your doctor promptly. If you have never had chickenpox, you should avoid close contact with people who have chickenpox or shingles. If you do come into contact with chickenpox, see your doctor urgently.
- Make sure that the information on the card is kept up to date.

Stopping corticosteroids

If after 7–10 days the corticosteroid fails to achieve the desired effect, it should be stopped. It is often possible to stop corticosteroids abruptly (Box 7.H).[25] However, if there is uncertainty about disease or symptom resolution, withdrawal should be guided by monitoring disease activity or the symptom.

After whole-brain radiation, **dexamethasone** 4mg should be maintained for at least 1 week and the dose then reduced at the rate of 1mg/week.[26] In dying patients who are no longer able to swallow medication, it is generally acceptable to discontinue corticosteroids abruptly.

Occasionally the patient requests that the **dexamethasone** is stopped because of deterioration, despite the continued use of **dexamethasone**, and an unacceptable quality of life. It is probably best to reduce the **dexamethasone** step by step on a daily basis, because this gives the patient time to reconsider. At the same time prescribe extra analgesics in case headache recurs:

- if on **paracetamol**, prescribe **co-proxamol** p.r.n. (or an alternative weak opioid)
- if on a weak opioid, prescribe **morphine** 10–20mg PO or **diamorphine/morphine** 5–10mg SC p.r.n.
- if >2 p.r.n. doses have been given in the previous 24h, increase the regular analgesic dose

Box 7.H Recommendations for withdrawing systemic corticosteroids[25]

Abrupt withdrawal
Systemic corticosteroids may be stopped abruptly in those whose disease is unlikely to relapse *and* have received treatment for <3 weeks *and* are not in the groups below.

Gradual withdrawal
Gradual withdrawal of systemic corticosteroids is advisable in patients who:
- have received more than 3 weeks' treatment.
- have received prednisolone >40mg daily or equivalent, e.g. dexamethasone 4–6mg
- have had a second dose in the evening
- are taking a short course within 1 year of stopping long-term therapy
- have other possible causes of adrenal suppression.

During corticosteroid withdrawal the dose may initially be reduced rapidly (e.g. halving the dose daily) to physiological doses (prednisolone 7.5mg daily or equivalent) and then more slowly (e.g. 1–2mg per week) to allow the adrenals to recover and to prevent a hypo-adrenal crisis (malaise, profound weakness, hypotension, etc.). The patient should be monitored during withdrawal in case of deterioration.

- if the patient becomes drowsy or swallowing becomes difficult, consider changing PO anti-epileptics to SC **midazolam** and possibly give both **diamorphine** and **midazolam** by CSCI.

If headache is suspected because of grimacing or general restlessness, p.r.n. medication should be given and the dose of the regular opioid increased until the patient appears comfortable. It is important first to exclude the more common reasons for agitation in moribund patients, e.g. full bladder or rectum, pain and stiffness related to immobility.

Supply

Prednisolone (non-proprietary)
Tablets 1mg, 5mg, 28 days @ 15mg o.d. = £2.01.
Tablets e/c 2.5mg, 5mg, 28 days @ 15mg o.d. = £1.20.
Tablets soluble 5mg, 28 days @ 15mg o.d. = £6.16.

Precortisyl Forte® (Aventis Pharma 01732 584000)
Tablets 25mg, 28 days @ 25mg o.d. = £2.35.

Dexamethasone (non-proprietary)
Tablets 500microgram, 2mg, 28 days @ 2mg o.d. = £2.42.
Oral solution 2mg/5ml, 28 days @ 2mg o.d. = £42.00.
***Injection* dexamethasone sodium phosphate** 4mg/ml, 1ml amp = £1.00; 2ml amp = £1.98; 24mg/ml, 5ml vial = £16.66.
***Injection* dexamethasone sodium phosphate** 5mg/ml, 1ml amp = £0.83; 2ml vial = £1.27.

Decadron® (MSD 01992 467272)
Tablets 500microgram, 28 days @ 2mg o.d. = £3.58.

1 Hanks GW *et al.* (1983) Corticosteroids in terminal cancer – a prospective analysis of current practice. *Postgraduate Medical Journal.* **59**: 702–706.

2 Hardy J *et al.* (2001) A prospective survey of the use of dexamethasone on a palliative care unit. *Palliative Medicine.* **15**: 3–8.

3 Greenberg H *et al.* (1979) Epidural spinal cord compression from metastatic tumour: results with a new treatment protocol. *Annals of Neurology.* **8**: 361–366.

4 Minton MJ *et al.* (1981) Corticosteroids for elderly patients with breast cancer. *Cancer.* **48**: 883–887.

5 Tannock I *et al.* (1989) Treatment of metastatic prostatic cancer with low-dose prednisolone: evaluation of pain and quality of life as pragmatic indices of response. *Journal of Clinical Oncology.* **17**: 590–597.

6 Feuer D and Broadley K (1999) Systematic review and meta-analysis of corticosteroids for the resolution of malignant bowel obstruction in advanced gynaecological and gastrointestinal cancers. *Annals of Oncology.* **10**: 1035–1041.

7 Laval G *et al.* (2000) The use of steroids in the management of inoperable intestinal obstruction in terminal cancer patients: do they remove the obstruction? *Palliative Medicine.* **14**: 3–10.

8 Swartz S and Dluhy R (1978) Corticosteroids: clinical pharmacology and therapeutic use. *Drugs.* **16**: 238–255.

9 Demoly P and Chung K (1998) Pharmacology of corticosteroids. *Respiratory Medicine.* **97**: 385–394.

10 British National Formulary (2001) Corticosteroids. In: *British National Formulary* (No. 41). British Medical Association and Royal Pharmaceutical Society of Great Britain, London, pp.336.

11 Piper JM *et al.* (1991) Corticosteroid use and peptic ulcer disease: role of nonsteroidal anti-inflammatory drugs. *Annals of Internal Medicine.* **114**: 735–740.

12 Chalk J *et al.* (1984) Phenytoin impairs the bioavailability of dexamethasone in neurological and neurosurgical patients. *Journal of Neurology, Neurosurgery and Psychiatry.* **47**: 1087–1090.

13 Dropcho EJ and Soong S-J (1991) Steroid induced weakness in patients with primary brain tumours. *Neurology.* **41**: 1235–1239.

14 Eidelberg D (1991) Steroid myopathy. In: DA Rottenberg (ed) *Neurological Complications of Cancer Treatment.* Butterworth-Heineman, Boston, pp.185–191.

15 Rotstein J and Good R (1957) Steroid pseudorheumatism. *AMA Archives of Internal Medicine.* **99**: 545–555.

16 Vecht C *et al.* (1989) Initial bolus of conventional versus high-dose dexamethasone in metastatic spinal cord compression. *Neurology.* **39**: 1255–1257.

17 Delattre J-Y *et al.* (1988) High dose versus low dose dexamethasone in experimental epidural spinal cord compression. *Neurosurgery.* **22**: 1005–1007.

18 Moertel C *et al.* (1974) Corticosteroid therapy for preterminal gastrointestinal cancer. *Cancer.* **33**: 1607–1609.

19 Twycross RG and Guppy D (1985) Prednisolone in terminal breast and bronchogenic cancer. *Practitioner.* **229**: 57–59.

20 Gralla RJ (1989) An outline of anti-emetic treatment. *European Journal of Cancer and Clinical Oncology.* **25 (suppl 1)**: 7–11.

21 Editorial (1991) Ondansetron versus dexamethasone for chemotherapy-induced emesis. *Lancet.* **338**: 478.

22 Sridhar K *et al.* (1992) Five-drug antiemetic combination for cisplatin chemotherapy. *Cancer Investigation.* **10**: 191–199.

23 Galicich JH and French LA (1961) The use of dexamethasone in the treatment of cerebral oedema resulting from brain tumours and brain surgery. *American Practitioner.* **12**: 169.

24 Kirkham S (1988) The palliation of cerebral tumours with high-dose dexamethasone: a review. *Palliative Medicine.* **2**: 27–33.

25 Committee on Safety of Medicines and Medicines Control Agency (1998) Withdrawal of systemic corticosteroids. *Current Problems in Pharmacovigilance.* **24**: 5–7.

26 Vecht C *et al.* (1994) Dose-effect relationship of dexamethasone on Karnofsky performance in metastatic brain tumors. A randomized study of doses of 4, 8 and 16 mg per day. *Neurology.* **44**: 675–680.

DEMECLOCYCLINE — BNF 5.1 & 6.5.2

Class: Tetracycline antibiotic.

Indications: Symptomatic hyponatraemia caused by the syndrome of inappropriate ADH secretion (SIADH).

Pharmacology

Demeclocycline counteracts the effect of antidiuretic hormone (ADH) and causes a nephrogenic diabetes insipidus.[1–3] In SIADH, the manufacturer's literature states that demeclocycline, should be used only if fluid restriction is ineffective. However, in palliative care, fluid restriction to 700–1000ml/24h (or a daily urine output of <500ml) is burdensome and primary treatment of SIADH is preferable. Treatment is only necessary if the hyponatraemia is symptomatic (Box 7.I).

Box 7.I Clinical features of SIADH

Plasma sodium 110–120 mmol/L	**Plasma sodium <110 mmol/L**
Anorexia	Multifocal myoclonus
Nausea and vomiting	Drowsiness
Lassitude	Seizures
Confusion	Coma
Oedema	

SIADH may be caused by many different medical conditions.[4] It has been observed in conjunction with various drugs, notably tricyclic antidepressants, SSRIs, **carbamazepine**, phenothiazines, **lorazepam**, barbiturates. SIADH should be considered in all patients who develop hyponatraemia, drowsiness, confusion or convulsions while taking a tricyclic antidepressant or SSRI. Most cases associated with SSRIs involve elderly people, particularly women.[5,6]

The diagnosis of SIADH is based on the following criteria:[7]

- hyponatraemia (<130mmol/L)
- low plasma osmolality (<270mosmol/L)
- raised urine osmolality (>100mosmol/L)
- urine sodium concentration
  - always >20mmol/L
  - often >50mmol/L
- normal plasma volume.

In practice, a plasma sodium concentration of ≤120mmol/L is sufficient to make a clinical diagnosis of SIADH in the absence of:

- severe vomiting
- diuretic therapy
- hypo-adrenalism
- hypothyroidism
- several renal failure.

Cautions

The absorption of demeclocycline is reduced by the concurrent administration of **iron**, **calcium**, **zinc**, **magnesium**, **aluminium** and **zinc**. Demeclocycline depresses plasma prothrombin activity and, if used concurrently, the dose of **warfarin** may need to be reduced. Warn the patient not to expose skin to direct sunlight or sunlamps because of the risk of photosensitivity.

Undesirable effects

For full list, see manufacturer's SPC.

Nausea, vomiting, diarrhoea, renal impairment (more likely with daily dose of 1200mg),[8] photosensitivity.

Dose and use

Treat the patient and not the biochemical results.

If symptomatic:

- starting dose 300mg b.d. on an empty stomach, e.g. 1h a.c., avoiding milk, antacids and **iron** preparations
- increase if necessary to 300mg q.d.s. after 1 week.

In patients unable to take demeclocycline PO, it can be given PR dispersed in 5ml of a methylcellulose carrier.[9]

Supply

Ledermycin® (Wyeth 01628 604377)
Capsules 150mg, 28 days @ 300mg b.d.= £23.12.

1 deTroyer A (1977) Demeclocycline. Treatment for syndrome of inappropriate antidiuretic hormone secretion. *Journal of the American Medical Association.* **237**: 2723–2726.

2 Forrest J *et al.* (1978) Superiority of demeclocycline over lithium in the treatment of chronic syndrome of inappropriate secretion of antidiuretic hormone. *New England Journal of Medicine.* **298**: 173–177.

3 Miyagawa C (1986) The pharmacologic management of the syndrome of inappropriate secretion of antidiuretic hormone. *Drug Intelligence and Clinical Pharmacy.* **20**: 527–531.

4 Twycross R and Wilcock A (2001) *Symptom Management in Advanced Cancer* (3e). Radcliffe Medical Press, Oxford.

5 ADRAC (Adverse Drug Reactions Advisory Committee) (1996) Selective serotonin reuptake inhibitors and SIADH. *Medical Journal of Australia.* **164**: 562.

6 Liu B *et al.* (1996) Hyponatremia and the syndrome of inappropriate secretion of antidiuretic hormone associated with the use of selective serotonin reuptake inhibitors: a review of spontaneous reports. *Canadian Medical Association Journal.* **155**: 519–527.

7 Saito T (1996) SIADH and other hyponatremic disorders: diagnosis and therapeutic problems. *Nippon Jinzo Gakkai Shi.* **38**: 429–434.

8 Trump D (1981) Serious hyponatremia in patients with cancer: management with demeclocycline. *Cancer.* **47**: 2908–2912.

9 Hussain I *et al.* (1998) Rectal administration of demeclocycline in a patient with syndrome of inappropriate ADH secretion. *International Journal of Clinical Practice.* **52**: 59.

DESMOPRESSIN — BNF 6.5.2

Class of drug: Vasopressin analogue.

Indications: Pituitary diabetes insipidus, refractory nocturia.

Contra-indications: Renal impairment, cardiovascular disease, hypertension.

Pharmacology

Desmopressin is an analogue of the pituitary antidiuretic hormone, vasopression. It increases water resorption by the renal tubules, thereby reducing urine volume. Desmopressin has a longer duration of action than **vasopressin** and **lypressin**, an alternative analogue.
Bio-availability 3–4% intranasal; 0.1–5% PO.
Onset of action 1h intranasal; 2h PO.
Plasma halflife 0.4–4h intranasal; 1.5–2.5h PO.
Duration of action 5–24h intranasal; 6–8h PO.

Serious drug interactions: the concurrent use of drugs which increase the endogenous secretion of vasopressin increases the risk of symptomatic hyponatraemia, e.g. antidepressants.

Undesirable effects

For full list, see manufacturer's SPC.

Water retention and hyponatraemia; in the most serious cases this may result in hyponatraemic convulsions. Patients should be warned to restrict fluids in the evenings; also to stop taking desmopressin if they develop persistent vomiting or diarrhoea. The effect of desmopressin is potentiated by **indometacin** (and possibly other NSAIDs).

Dose and use

Keep to the recommended starting doses to minimise the risk of hyponatraemic seizures:

- starting doses 200–400microgram PO o.n.; 10–20microgram intranasally o.n.
- increase to higher dose only if lower one ineffective.

Supply

Desmopressin (non-proprietary)
Nasal spray 10microgram/metered spray, 28 days @ 20microgram o.n. = £26.13.

Desmotabs® (Ferring 01753 214800)
Tablets 200microgram, 28 days @ 200microgram o.n.= £29.00.

Desmospray® (Ferring 01753 214800)
Nasal spray 10microgram/metered spray, 28 days @ 20microgram o.n.= £31.36.

Nocutil® (Norgine 01895 826600)
Nasal spray 10microgram/metered spray, 28 days @ 20microgram o.n. = £19.60.

DDAVP® (Ferring 01753 214800)
Tablets 100microgram, 200microgram, 28 days @ 200microgram o.n.= £28.59.
Intranasal solution 100microgram/ml in 2.5ml dropper bottle and catheter, 28 days @ 20microgram o.n.= £21.28.

DRUGS FOR DIABETES MELLITUS — BNF 6.1

Indications: Diabetes mellitus not controlled by diet only.

Contra-indications: Chlorpropamide and **glibenclamide** should not be used in the elderly and those with renal or hepatic impairment. **Metformin** should not be used in patients with renal failure because of the risk of lactic acidosis; best avoided in all elderly debilitated patients, particularly those with associated hepatic or cardiac dysfunction.

Pharmacology

Glucose intolerance is one of the first metabolic consequences of cancer and is found in nearly 40% of non-diabetic cancer patients given an oral or IV glucose tolerance test.[1] Corticosteroids are the most common precipitant of diabetes in advanced cancer.[2] Thiazide diuretics and **furosemide** (frusemide) may also produce hyperglycaemia. In the non-cancer population, patients newly presenting with diabetes are symptomatic (e.g. thirst) with a fasting blood glucose of ≥12mmol/L. However, the renal threshold increases considerably with age and it is common for older patients to be asymptomatic with a fasting blood glucose of 15–18mmol/L, occasionally more. In newly diagnosed symptomatic patients, a short-acting sulphonylurea such as **gliclazide** or **tolbutamide** should be prescribed with a realistic safe target, e.g. fasting blood glucose 8–12mmol/L. The dose should be reduced if the fasting blood glucose is consistently <8mmol/L. For pharmacokinetic details, see Table 7.4.

Table 7.4 Pharmacokinetic details of oral hypoglycaemics

	Gliclazide	*Tolbutamide*
Bio-availability	78%	>95%
Onset of action	3–4h	1–3h
Time to peak plasma concentration	2–4h	3–5h
Plasma halflife	10–12h	4.5–6.5h
Duration of action	12–24h	≤12h

Insulin is often needed in newly diagnosed diabetics with advanced cancer. Patients with pre-existing non-insulin dependent diabetes and on maximal doses of **gliclazide** or **tolbutamide**, sometimes require **insulin** in addition if prescribed a corticosteroid, e.g. **soluble insulin**

10units o.d. at 1800h. Less may be needed in an emaciated patient and more if obese. The dose is monitored to achieve a fasting blood glucose of 8–12mmol/L. With the appropriate dose of **isophane insulin**, an inability to eat does not matter as it provides only a basal insulin supply. A sliding scale of **soluble insulin** is only occasionally necessary. Note:

- it is unnecessary to maintain theoretically ideal blood glucose levels to avoid long-term complications
- rigid dietary control is not indicated when life expectancy is short
- when stable, monitoring is generally adequate with a *fasting blood glucose* fingerprick test twice a week.

Urine tests for glucose may well be adequate. For most patients, glycosuria 1+ and 2+ reflect satisfactory (asymptomatic) control; no glycosuria would trigger a decrease in hypoglycaemic therapy and 3+ an increase.[3] Initial comparison of the urine glucose with the blood glucose will detect patients with an increased renal threshold for glucose (associated with renal impairment) and those with a low threshold (renal glycosuria).

Cautions

After discontinuation, **chlorpropamide** and **glibenclamide** can produce hypoglycaemia for 48–72h, and up to 96h if there is renal or hepatic impairment. 1/3 of diabetics lose their adrenergic warning symptoms of hypoglycaemia within 20 years of developing diabetes; autonomic neuropathy may remove both the warning symptoms and the counter-regulatory mechanism of an adrenaline (epinephrine)-induced increase in blood glucose (Box 7.J). Malnourished patients with reduced hepatic glycogen stores will also have a reduced capacity to counteract hypoglycaemia.[4]

Box 7.J Treatment of hypoglycaemia

Hypoglycaemia should be treated with glucose 10–20g PO; this is contained in 3 sugar lumps, Lucozade 60ml or milk 200ml. If drowsy and swallowing unsafe, precede oral glucose with glucagon 1mg IM or IV. Give 25–50ml of glucose 50% IV if no improvement within 10min.

Dose and use

Gliclazide: starting dose 40–80mg o.m. (with breakfast); increase if necessary every 3 days to a maximum of 160mg b.d. (maximum single dose 160mg).

Tolbutamide: starting dose 500mg b.d.; increase if necessary every 3 days to a maximum of 1g b.d.

Insulin: if the fasting blood glucose is >12mmol/L, the patient is symptomatic and already taking the maximal dose of an oral hypoglycaemic, prescribe **isophane insulin** 10units o.d. at 1800h and adjust the dose according to response. A *preprandial* sliding scale of short-acting **soluble insulin** is occasionally necessary (Table 7.5).

Table 7.5 Preprandial sliding scale of insulin[a]

Preprandial blood glucose (mmol/L)	*Soluble insulin dose (units)*
10–15	6
>15–18	8
>18–22	10
>22[b]	12

a. responses to insulin vary widely and sliding scales need to be individualised
b. patients with marked hyperglycaemia should have monitoring 2h after meals as well until the blood glucose is better controlled.

Supply

Gliclazide (non-proprietary)
Tablets 80mg, 28 days @ 80mg o.m.= £2.96.

Diamicron® (Servier 01753 662744)
Tablets 80mg, 28 days @ 80mg o.m.= £3.27.

Tolbutamide (non-proprietary)
Tablets 500mg, 28 days @ 500mg b.d.= £3.08.

1 Glicksman A and Rawson R (1956) Diabetes and altered carbohydrate metabolism in patients with cancer. *Cancer.* **9**: 1127–1134.
2 Poulson J (1997) The management of diabetes in patients with advanced cancer. *Journal of Pain and Symptom Management.* **13**: 339–346.
3 Kovner V (1998) Management of diabetes in advanced cancer: urine sugar tests. *Journal of Pain and Symptom Management.* **15**: 147–148.
4 Holroyde C *et al.* (1975) Altered glucose metabolism in metastatic carcinoma. *Cancer Research.* **35**: 3710–3714.

*OCTREOTIDE — BNF 8.3.4.3

Class: Synthetic hormone.

Indications: Symptoms associated with unresectable hormone-secreting tumours, e.g. carcinoid, VIPomas, glucagonomas, gastrinomas, insulinomas, acromegaly and thyrotrophinomas; bleeding oesophageal varicies;[1] †pancreatic and enterocutaneous fistulas;[2] †prevention of complications after elective pancreatic surgery;[3] †intractable diarrhoea related to high output ileostomies, AIDS, radiation, chemotherapy or bone marrow transplant;[2,4] †inoperable bowel obstruction in patients with cancer;[5,6] †hypertrophic pulmonary osteoarthopathy,[7] †ascites,[8,9] †buccal fistula,[10] †death rattle, †reduction of tumour-related secretions.[8]

Pharmacology

Octreotide is a synthetic analogue of somatostatin with a longer duration of action. Somatostatin is an inhibitory hormone found throughout the body. In the hypothalamus it inhibits the release of growth hormone, TSH, prolactin and ACTH. It inhibits the secretion of insulin, glucagon, gastrin and other peptides of the gastro-enteropancreatic system (i.e. peptide YY, neurotensin, VIP and substance P), reducing splanchnic blood flow, portal blood flow, gastro-intestinal motility, gastric, pancreatic and small bowel secretion, and increases water and electrolyte absorption.[11] In Type 1 diabetes mellitus, octreotide decreases insulin requirements. However, in Type 2 diabetes, octreotide suppresses both insulin and glucagon release, leaving plasma glucose concentrations either unchanged or slightly elevated.[12,13] Octreotide has a direct anticancer effect on solid tumours of the gastro-intestinal tract and prolongs survival.[14–16] In hormone-secreting tumours, octreotide improves symptoms by inhibiting hormone secretion, e.g.:

- 5HT in carcinoid (improving flushing and diarrhoea)
- VIP in VIPomas (improving diarrhoea)
- glucagon in glucagonomas (improving rash and diarrhoea).

In patients with cancer and inoperable bowel obstruction octreotide rapidly improves symptoms in ≥75% of patients.[5,6,17] Doses of ≤1200microgram daily were used but a beneficial effect is generally apparent with ≤600microgram daily. Octreotide 300microgram daily appears to reduce NG tube output more effectively and rapidly than **hyoscine *butylbromide*** 60mg daily, although both allowed NG tube removal after about 5 days.[17] However, at Sir Michael Sobell House octreotide is rarely used because of its expense and a low success rate (≈20%) when used after standard UK palliative care regimens for bowel obstruction.[10]

Octreotide is reported to improve mucous discharge from rectal carcinomas[8] and to reduce the rate of formation of malignant ascites.[8,9] Octreotide may interfere with ascitic fluid formation through a reduction in splanchnic blood flow, reduced plasma levels of aldosterone and antidiuretic hormone, improving diuresis[18] or as a result of a direct tumour antisecretory effect. Octreotide could be considered in patients with rapidly accumulating ascites requiring frequent paracentesis despite diuretic therapy (see **spironolactone**, p.31). Octreotide may also help resolve chylous ascites[19,20] and pleural effusion secondary to cirrhosis.[21,22] Octreotide has also provided rapid pain relief in a patient with hypertrophic pulmonary osteo-arthropathy that had not improved with more traditional analgesia.[7] Octreotide reduces salivary production and may be of use in buccal fistulas[10] and death rattle that has failed to respond to antimuscarinic drugs[23] (see **hyoscine *hydrobromide*** p.118, **hyoscine *butylbromide*** p.5, **glycopyrronium** p.287).

At doses far below those necessary for an antisecretory effect (e.g. 1microgram SC t.d.s.), octreotide protects the stomach from NSAID-related injury, probably via its ability to reduce NSAID-induced neutrophil adhesion to the microvasculature.[24] Somatostatin receptors have been identified on leucoytes and, in rats, octreotide has been shown to suppress inflammation.[25] Octreotide is also of value in chronic non-malignant pancreatic pain caused by hypertension in the scarred pancreatic ducts.[26,27] Suppressing exocrine function by administering **pancreatin** supplements also reduces pain in 50–75% of patients with chronic pancreatitis.[28] The benefit reported with octreotide could therefore be secondary to its antisecretory action.[29] Octreotide is generally given as a bolus SC or by CSCI.[30] It can be given IV when a rapid effect is required. Octreotide has also been administered IT.[31] Long-acting depot preparations are also available for octreotide and **lanreotide**.[32] Their use has been evaluated only in hormone-secreting tumours.
Onset of action 30min.
Time to peak plasma concentration 30min SC.
Plasma halflife 1.5h SC.
Duration of action 8h.

Cautions

Insulinoma (may potentiate hypoglycaemia). In diabetes mellitus, insulin and oral hypoglycaemic requirements may be reduced.

Undesirable effects

For full list, see manufacturer's SPC.
Bolus injection SC is painful (but less if the vial is warmed to room temperature), dry mouth, flatulence (lowers oesophageal sphincter tone).

Dose and use

Dose varies according to indication (Table 7.6). Some of the recommendations are based on experience with only a small number of patients, so the dose should always be titrated according to effect. Once improvement in the symptom is achieved, reduction to the lowest dose that maintains symptom control can be tried.

Table 7.6 Dose recommendations for SC octreotide

Indication	*Starting dose*	*Usual maximum*
Hormone-secreting tumours		
acromegaly	100–200microgram t.d.s.	600microgram daily[11]
carcinoid, VIPomas, glucagonomas	50–100microgram t.d.s; increased to 200microgram t.d.s.	1500microgram daily, rarely 6000microgram daily[33]
Intractable diarrhoea	50–500microgram daily	1500microgram daily,[34] occasionally higher[35]
Intestinal obstruction	250–500microgram daily	750microgram daily, occasionally higher
Tumour-antisecretory effect	50–100microgram b.d.	600microgram daily[8]
Ascites	200–600microgram daily	600microgram daily[9]
Hypertrophic pulmonary osteo-arthropathy	100microgram b.d.[7]	

When given by CSCI, using 0.9% saline as diluent, octreotide is miscible with **dexamethasone**, **diamorphine**, **haloperidol**, **hyoscine butylbromide** and **midazolam**; precipitation may occur with **cyclizine**.
Depot preparations
Depot preparations of octreotide 10–30mg, given every 4 weeks, are available. Alternatively, **lanreotide** (Somatuline® LA) 30mg, given every 2 weeks (sometimes every 7–10 days), and **lanreotide** (Somatuline® Autogel) 30–90mg, given every 4 weeks, can be used. In palliative care,

these long-acting preparations are most likely to be used in patients with a chronic intestinal fistula or intractable diarrhoea. Generally, they will be used only when symptoms have first been controlled with SC octreotide. The octreotide preparation requires *deep IM injection* into the gluteal muscle. In acromegaly, stop the SC dose of octreotide when the first depot injection is given; for other neuro-endocrine tumours continue the SC dose for a further 2 weeks.

Supply

Octreotide

Sandostatin® (Novartis 01276 692255)
Injection 50microgram/ml, 1ml amp = £3.47; 100microgram/ml, 1ml amp = £6.53; 200microgram/ml, 5ml vial = £5.10 (14 day expiry once started); 500microgram/ml, 1ml amp = £31.65.

Sandostatin LAR® (Novartis 01276 692255)
Depot injection (microsphere powder for aqueous suspension) 10mg vial = £637.50; 20mg vial = £850.00; 30mg vial = £1062.50 (all supplied with diluent and syringe), for IM injection every 28 days.

Lanreotide

Somatuline® LA (Ipsen 01753 627777)
Depot injection (copolymer microparticles for aqueous suspension) 30mg vial = £334.25, for IM injection every 14 days (sometimes every 7–10 days).

Somatuline® Autogel (Ipsen 01753 627777)
Depot injection (pre-filled syringe) 60mg = £542; 90mg = £722; 120mg = £932, for deep SC injection every 28 days.

1 Sung J (1993) Octreotide infusion or emergency sclerotherapy for variceal haemorrhage. *Lancet.* **342**: 637–641.
2 Harris A (1992) Octreotide in the treatment of disorders of the gastrointestinal tract. *Drug Investigation.* **4**: 1–54.
3 Bassi C *et al.* (1994) Prophylaxis of complications after pancreatic surgery: results of a multicenter trial in Italy. Italian Study Group. *Digestion.* **55**: 41–47.
4 Crouch M *et al.* (1996) Octreotide acetate in refractory bone marrow transplant-associated diarrhea. *Annals of Pharmacotherapy.* **30**: 331–336.
5 Mercadante S *et al.* (1993) Octreotide in relieving gastrointestinal symptoms due to bowel obstruction. *Palliative Medicine.* **7**: 295–299.
6 Riley J and Fallon M (1994) Octreotide in terminal malignant obstruction of the gastro-intestinal tract. *European Journal of Palliative Care.* **1**: 23–25.
7 Johnson S *et al.* (1997) Treatment of resistant pain in hypertrophic pulmonary arthropathy with subcutaneous octreotide. *Thorax.* **52**: 298–299.
8 Harvey M and Dunlop R (1996) Octreotide and the secretory effects of advanced cancer. *Palliative Medicine.* **10**: 346–347.
9 Caims W and Malone R (1999) Octreotide as an agent for the relief of malignant ascites in palliative care patients. *Palliative Medicine.* **13**: 429–430.
10 Lam CM and Wong SY (1996) Use of somatostatin analog in the management of traumatic parotid fistula. *Surgery.* **119**: 481.
11 Gyr KE and Meier R (1993) Pharmacodynamic effects of Sandostatin® in the gastrointestinal tract. *Digestion.* **54**: 14–19.
12 Davies RR *et al.* (1989) Somatostatin analogues in diabetes mellitus. *Diabetic Medicine.* **6**: 103–111.
13 Lunetta M *et al.* (1997) Effects of octreotide on glycaemic control, glucose disposal, hepatic glucose production and counterregulatory hormone secretion in type 1 and type 2 insulin treated diabetic patients. *Diabetes Research and Clinical Practice.* **38**: 81–89.
14 Cascinu S *et al.* (1995) A randomised trial of octreotide vs best supportive care only in advanced gastrointestinal cancer patients refractory to chemotherapy. *British Journal of Cancer.* **71**: 97–101.
15 Pandha H and Waxman J (1996) Octreotide in malignant intestinal obstruction. *Anti-cancer Drugs.* **7**: 5–10.

16 Kouroumalis E *et al.* (1998) Treatment of hepatocellular carcinoma with octreotide: a randomised controlled study. *Gut.* **42**: 442–447.
17 Ripamonti C *et al.* (2000) Role of octreotide, scopolamine butylbromide, and hydration in symptom control of patients with inoperable bowel obstruction and nasogastric tubes: a prospective randomized trial. *Journal of Pain and Symptom Management.* **19**: 23–34.
18 Oezbakir O *et al.* (1997) Effects of somatostatin and octreotide on renal functions in the patients with ascites due to postnecrotic cirrhosis. *Journal of Hepatology.* **26 (suppl 1)**: 248.
19 Widjaja A *et al.* (1999) Octreotide for therapy of chylous ascites in yellow nail syndrome. *Gastroenterology.* **116**: 1017–1018.
20 Ferrandiere M *et al.* (2000) Chylous ascites following radical nephrectomy: efficacy of octreotide as treatment of ruptured thoracic duct. *Intensive Care and Medicine.* **26**: 484–485.
21 Dumortier J *et al.* (2000) Successful treatment of hepatic hydrothorax with octreotide. *European Journal of Gastroenterology and Hepatology.* **12**: 817–820.
22 Pfammatter R *et al.* (2001) Treatment of hepatic hydrothorax and reduction of chest tube output with octreotide. *European Journal of Gastroenterology and Hepatology.* **13**: 977–980.
23 Corcoran R (2001) Personal communication.
24 Scheiman J *et al.* (1997) Reduction of NSAID induced gastric injury and leucocyte endothelial adhesion by octreotide. *Gut.* **40**: 720–725.
25 Karalis K *et al.* (1994) Somatostatin analogues suppress the inflammatory reaction in vivo. *Journal of Clinical Investigations.* **93**: 2000–2006.
26 Donnelly PK *et al.* (1991) Somatostatin for chronic pancreatic pain. *Journal of Pain and Symptom Management.* **6**: 349–350.
27 Okazaki K *et al.* (1988) Pressure of papillary zone and pancreatic main duct in patients with chronic pancreatitis in the early state. *Scandinavian Journal of Gastroenterology.* **23**: 501–506.
28 Mossner J *et al.* (1989) Influence of treatment with pancreatic extracts on pancreatic enzyme secretion. *Gut.* **3**: 1143–1149.
29 Lembcke B *et al.* (1987) Effect of the somatostatin analogue sandostatin on gastrointestinal, pancreatic and biliary function and hormone release in man. *Digestion.* **36**: 108–124.
30 Mercadante S (1995) Tolerability of continuous subcutaneous octreotide used in combination with other drugs. *Journal of Palliative Care.* **11**: 14–16.
31 Chrubasik J (1985) *Spinal infusion of opiates and somatostatin.* Hygieneplan, Germany.
32 Scherubl H *et al.* (1994) Treatment of the carcinoid syndrome with a depot formulation of the somatostatin analogue lanreotide. *European Journal of Cancer.* **30A**: 1590–1591.
33 Harris A and Redfern J (1995) Octreotide treatment of carcinoid syndrome: analysis of published dose-titration data. *Alimentary Pharmacology and Therapeutics.* **9**: 387–394.
34 Cello J *et al.* (1991) Effect of octreotide on refractory AIDS-associated diarrhea. A prospective, multicenter clinical trial. *Annals of Internal Medicine.* **115**: 705–710.
35 Petrelli N *et al.* (1993) Bowel rest, intravenous hydration, and continous high-dose infusion of octreotide acetate for the treatment of chemotherapy-induced diarrhea in patients with colorectal carcinoma. *Cancer.* **72**: 1543–1546.

PROGESTOGENS — BNF 6.4.1.2 & 8.3.2

Class: Sex hormones.

Indications: †Postcastration hot flushes (women and men), anticancer hormonal therapy. The licensed indications for **megestrol** are limited to breast and endometrial cancers whereas the licence for **medroxyprogesterone** also includes renal cell cancer (Farlutal®, Provera®) and prostate cancer (Farlutal® only).

Contra-indications: Hepatic impairment.

Pharmacology

There are two main groups of progestogens, **progesterone** and its analogues (**dydrogesterone**, **hydroxyprogesterone**, and **medroxyprogesterone**) and **testosterone** and its analogues (**norethisterone** and **norgestrel**). Progesterone analogues are less androgenic than the **testosterone** analogues; neither **progesterone** nor **dydrogesterone** causes virilisation. Other synthetic derivatives are variably metabolised into **testosterone** and **oestrogen**; undesirable effects vary with the preparation and the dose.

Hormonal manipulation has an important role in the treatment of metastatic cancers of the breast, prostate and endometrium. Treatment is not curative but may induce remission in 15–30% of patients, occasionally for years. Tumour response and treatment toxicity need to be monitored and treatment changed if progression occurs or undesirable effects exceed benefit.

Progestogens have been shown to stimulate appetite and weight gain in patients with AIDS or cancer, particularly those with breast cancer.[1,2] The impact is more long-lasting than with corticosteroids. Progestogens are relatively expensive and should be used selectively. Doses of **megestrol** of up to 1600mg/day have been used and there is evidence of a dose-response effect;[3] elderly patients may respond to 80mg/day. For pharmacokinetic details see Table 7.7.

Table 7.7 Selected pharmacokinetic data

	Medroxyprogesterone	*Megestrol*
Bio-availability	1–10%	No data
Time to peak plasma concentration	2–7h	1–3h
Plasma halflife	38–46h	13–105h (mean about 30h)

Undesirable effects

For full list, see manufacturer's SPC.

Urticaria, acne, weight gain, fluid retention, hypertension, nausea, constipation, fatigue, depression, insomnia. Alopecia, hirsutism, jaundice (all rare).

Dose and use

Appetite stimulation and weight gain

- **medroxyprogesterone acetate** 400mg o.m. *or* **megestrol acetate** 80–160mg o.m.
- consider doubling the dose if initial poor response.[4,5]

The effect of progestogens may be enhanced by the concurrent use of an NSAID, e.g. **ibuprofen** 400mg t.d.s.[6]

Hot flushes after surgical or chemical castration

Medroxyprogesterone acetate 5–20mg b.d.–q.d.s. *or* **megestrol acetate** 40mg o.m.[7] The effect manifests after 2–4 weeks. **Diethylstilbestrol** and **cyproterone** (has weak progestogen activity) are also of benefit.[8]

Supply

Medroxyprogesterone acetate

Farlutal® (Pharmacia 01908 661101)
Tablets 100mg, 250mg, 500mg, 28 days @ 500mg o.m. = £54.26.

Provera® (Pharmacia 01908 661101)
Tablets 100mg, 200mg, 400mg, 28 days @ 400mg o.m. = £43.58.

Provera® (Pharmacia 01908 661101)
Tablets 2.5mg, 5mg, 28 days @ 5mg b.d. = £6.89.

Megestrol acetate

Megace® (Bristol-Myers Squibb 020 8572 7422)
Tablets 40mg, 160mg, 28 days @ 160mg o.m. = £27.35.

1 Aisner J *et al.* (1990) Appetite stimulation and weight gain with megestrol acetate. *Seminars in Oncology.* **17**: 2–7.

2 Strang P (1997) The effect of megestrol acetate on anorexia, weight loss and cachexia in cancer and AIDS patients (review). *Anticancer Research.* **17**: 657–662.

3 Downer S *et al.* (1993) A double blind placebo controlled trial of medroxyprogesterone acetate (MPA) in cancer cachexia. *British Journal of Cancer.* **67**: 1102–1105.

4 Donnelly S and Walsh TD (1995) Low-dose megestrol acetate for appetite stimulation in advanced cancer. *Journal of Pain and Symptom Management.* **10**: 182–183.

5 Vadell C *et al.* (1998) Anticachectic efficacy of megestrol acetate at different doses and versus placebo in patients with neoplastic cachexia. *American Journal of Clinical Oncology.* **21**: 347–351.
6 McMillan D *et al.* (1997) A pilot study of megestrol acetate and ibuprofen in the treatment of cachexia in gastrointestinal cancer patients. *British Journal of Cancer.* **76**: 788–790.
7 Loprinzi CL *et al.* (1996) Megestrol acetate for the prevention of hot flushes. *New England Journal of Medicine.* **331**: 347–352.
8 Miller J and Ahmann F (1992) Treatment of castration-induced menopausal symptoms with low dose diethylstilbestrol in men with advanced cancer. *Urology.* **40**: 499–502.

STANOZOLOL

Class: Anabolic steroid (17α-alkyl androgen).

Indications: †Itch associated with obstructive jaundice when stenting of the common bile duct is contra-indicated and skin care alone is inadequate, †muscle wasting and weakness in AIDS.

Pharmacology

Cholestatic itch is central in origin and is associated with enhanced opioidergic tone.[1,2] In intrahepatic cholestasis, an opioid antagonist is the treatment of choice (Figure 7.1).[3] However, when opioids are needed for concurrent cancer pain, a 17α-alkyl androgen should be used instead (Figure 7.2).[4] The mechanism of action is unknown.

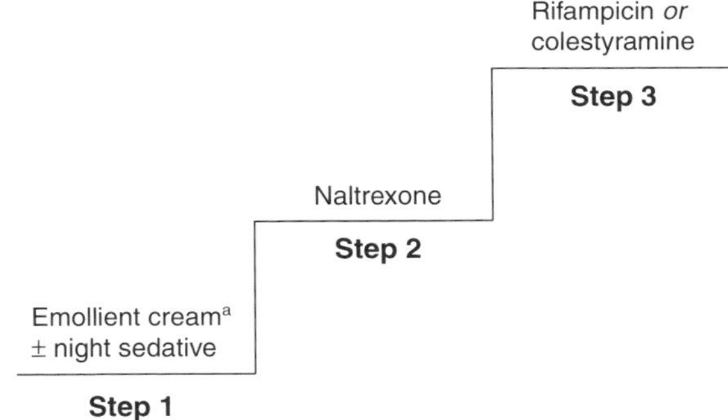

Figure 7.1 A treatment ladder for itch in intrahepatic cholestasis.

a. many patients have a dry skin and the first step is always to correct this.

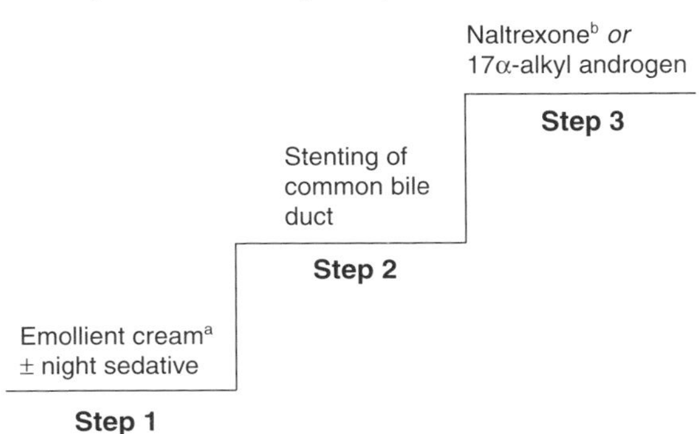

Figure 7.2 A treatment ladder for itch in obstructive jaundice caused by extrahepatic cancer.

a. many patients have a dry skin and the first step is always to correct this
b. contra-indicated in patients needing opioids for pain relief.

17α-alkyl androgens are directly toxic to hepatocytes.[5] It is possible that the effect of stanozolol is mediated via focal cell damage, thereby limiting the ability of the cholestatic liver to produce enkephalins. Certainly, androgens themselves can cause cholestatic jaundice and have occasionally caused serious liver impairment.[6] The beneficial effect of 17 α-alkyl androgens was discovered serendipitously some 50 years ago when the co-incidental use of **methyltestosterone** in a patient with primary biliary cirrhosis resulted in the amelioration of the associated itch.[7] 17α-alkyl androgens are more potent in this respect than other androgens, e.g. **methyltestosterone** is more potent than **testosterone** itself.[8] This is probably because of a marked reduction in first-pass hepatic metabolism in androgens with a 17α-alkyl radical. Stanozolol also has additional effects on the liver which are not shared by **testosterone**.[9] Benefit is maintained even if the cholestasis is exacerbated by the androgen itself.[8] Androgens and oestrogens sometimes also relieve non-specific pruritus in the elderly.[10] An anecdotal report suggests that some patients with AIDS may benefit from stanozolol 2mg t.d.s. in terms of weight gain (1.6–4kg in 2 months) and increased strength.[11] However, confirmation in placebo-controlled studies is required.
Bio-availability no data.
Onset of action <7 days.
Time to peak plasma concentration no data.
Plasma halflife 8h; slow metaboliser 39h.
Duration of action 24–36h.

Undesirable effects

Acne, oedema, cramp. Can enhance the effects of **insulin** and **warfarin**. In women with a normal or long life expectancy, masculinisation (amenorrhoea, hirsutes and deep voice) is a problem but may be contained by reducing the dose from o.d. to 3 times weekly or even less.[8] Occasional severe hepatotoxicity.

Dose and use

Itch

Moisturising the skin with an emollient is a prerequisite for success.
- 5–10mg o.d.; benefit noticed after about 1 week.[12,13]

Alternative regimens (not UK) include:
- **norethandrolone** 10mg b.d.–t.d.s.
- **methyltestosterone** 25mg o.d. SL.

The production of stanozolol was discontinued world-wide in March 2002. It is possible that **danazol** (also a 17α-alkyl androgen) 200mg o.d.–t.d.s. can be used instead, but as yet there are no clinical reports to support such 'beyond licence' use.

Supply

Tablets manufacture discontinued world-wide; in UK use **danazol** instead.

1 Jones E and Bergasa N (1990) The pruritus of cholestasis. From bile acids to opiate agonists. *Hepatology.* **11**: 884–887.
2 Jones E and Dekker R (2000) Florid opioid withdrawal-like reaction precipitated by naltrexone in a patient with chronic cholestasis. *Gastroenterology.* **118**: 431–432.
3 Jones E and Bergasa N (1999) The pruritus of cholestasis. *Hepatology.* **29**: 1003–1006.
4 Twycross R *et al.* Itch: scratching more than the surface. Submitted for publication.
5 Welder A *et al.* (1995) Toxic effects of anabolic-androgen steroids in primary rat hepatic cell cultures. *Journal of Pharmacological and Toxicological Methods.* **33**: 187–195.
6 Gurakar A *et al.* (1994) Androgenic/anabolic steroid-induced intrahepatic cholestasis: a review with four additional case reports. *Journal of Oklahoma State Medical Association.* **87**: 399–404.
7 Ahrens E (1950) Primary biliary cirrhosis. *Medicine.* **29**: 299–364.
8 Lloyd-Thomas H and Sherlock S (1952) Testosterone therapy for the pruritus of obstructive jaundice. *British Medical Journal.* **2**: 1289–1291.
9 Fernandez L *et al.* (1994) Stanozolol and danazol, unlike natural androgens, interact with the low affinity glucocorticoid-binding sites from male rat liver microsomes. *Endocrinology.* **134**: 1401–1408.

10 Feldman S *et al.* (1942) Treatment of senile pruritus with androgens and estrogens. *Archives of Dermatology and Syphilology Chicago.* **46**: 112–127.
11 Berger J *et al.* (1993) Effect of anabolic steroids on HIV-related wasting myopathy. *Southern Medical Journal.* **86**: 865–866.
12 Sherlock S (1981) *Diseases of the Liver and Biliary System* (6e). Blackwell Scientific, Oxford.
13 Sherlock S and Dooley J (1993) *Diseases of the Liver and Biliary System* (9e). Blackwell Scientific, Oxford.

THALIDOMIDE — BNF 5.1.10

Class: Immunomodulator.

Indications: †Lepromatous leprosy (erythema nodosum leprosum), †graft versus host disease (GVHD), †recurrent aphthous stomatitis in HIV infection and connective tissue disease (Behcet's syndrome), †paraneoplastic sweating, †paraneoplastic itch, †cachexia in HIV and cancer, †intractable irinotecan-induced diarrhoea, †discord lupus erythematosus, †rheumatoid arthritis, †prevention of graft rejection.[1,2]

Contra-indications: Thalidomide should *never* be used in women who are pregnant or may become so.[3]

Pharmacology

Thalidomide is an immunomodulator with anti-angiogenic, anti-cytokine and anti-integrin properties.[4] It was withdrawn from use as a non-barbiturate hypnotic with anti-emetic properties in the early 1960s after it became apparent that it caused severe congenital abnormalities (absent or shortened limbs) when given to women in the first trimester of pregnancy.[5] Subsequently, it has been found to have immunomodulatory properties with potential for the treatment of various conditions.[6] Thalidomide inhibits the synthesis of the pro-inflammatory cytokine, tumour necrosis factor α (TNF-α) by monocytes.[7] It also inhibits chemotaxis of neutrophils and monocytes. Thalidomide antagonises PGE_2, PGF_2, histamine, serotonin and acetylcholine.[8] It also effects several other mechanisms associated with inflammation and immunomodulation.[9] These properties probably account for the prevention of irinotecan-induced diarrhoea,[10] and for the amelioration of paraneoplastic sweating[11] and paraneoplastic itch.[12] Thalidomide inhibits angiogenesis, a property which is the basis for investigational studies in oncology.[13,14] Whereas thalidomide itself inhibits TNFα production, metabolites may be responsible for its anti-angiogenic properties.

Apart from teratogenicity in pregnant women, the most serious undesirable effect is peripheral neuropathy.[9] This is caused by axonal degeneration without demyelination, with sensory nerves affected predominantly.[15] Neuropathy occurs in up to 30% of cases. The likelihood of developing neuropathy increases with cumulative dosage but has been reported after only 2.8g.[16] It is not related to age. Symptoms include numbness, paraesthesia, hyperaethesia for pain and temperature of the hands and feet, and leg cramps. The lower limbs are more commonly involved than the upper limbs. Findings include diminished ankle jerks and decreased sensation to vibration and position.[17] Although thalidomide is sometimes continued despite electrophysiological abnormalities, if a patient develops symptomatic neuropathy thalidomide should be stopped to decrease the likelihood of chronic painful neuropathy.[16,17] Thalidomide appears to undergo non-enzymatic hydrolysis in plasma; hepatic metabolism is minor. Studies in patients with hepatic and renal insufficiency have not been peformed. Thalidomide causes an increase in plasma **paracetamol** concentration but this is not clinically important.[8]

Bio-availability 67–93% PO in *animals*, no data in humans.
Onset of action varies from 2 days for lepromatous leprosy and paraneoplastic sweating to 1–2 months for GVHD and 2–3 months for rheumatoid arthritis.
Time to peak plasma concentration 2–6h, delayed by food.
Plasma halflife 6h (200mg/24h)–18h (800mg/24h).[9]
Duration of action $>$24h.

Cautions

Treat as a 'cytotoxic' when handling. Pregnant women or women planning to become pregnant should *not* handle thalidomide. Because it is not known if thalidomide is present in semen, men taking thalidomide should use latex condoms when having sex.

Thalidomide potentiates the sedative properties of barbiturates and alcohol, and increases the likelihood of extrapyramidal effects with **chlorpromazine** and **reserpine**.[8] Thalidomide should be used cautiously with drugs that cause drowsiness, neuropathy or reduce the effectiveness of oral contraception (HIV protease inhibitors, **rifampicin**, **rifabutin**, **phenytoin** and **carbamazepine**).[8,18]

Undesirable effects

Teratogenicity if given to pregnant women in the first trimester and peripheral neuropathy in up to 30% of patients. In clinical trials, 10–20% of patients stopped taking thalidomide, mostly because of drowsiness, skin rashes and peripheral neuropathy.[19–22] Rash may occur even when thalidomide is given with dexamethasone. Drowsiness and sedation are dose-dependent. Myelosuppression is rare. Thalidomide can increase HIV viral load.[23]

A dose-dependent decrease in supine systolic and diastolic pressures is seen up to 2h after dosing.[24] Headache, dizziness, and delirium occur more often at higher doses.[18,24] Other undesirable effects include dry mouth, constipation, bradycardia, altered temperature sensitivity, irregular menstrual cycles, hypothyroidism and oedema.[13,18,25,26] Cancer patients may have an increased susceptibility to thalidomide-associated undesirable effects, including thrombo-embolism.[25]

Dose and use

Aphthous ulcers in HIV+ disease: 100–200mg o.n. for 10 days.[27]
Paraneoplastic sweating: 100–200mg o.n.[11,28]
Cachexia in HIV+ disease and cancer: 100–200mg o.n.[29,30]
Intractable irinotecan-induced diarrhoea: 400mg o.n.[10,31]
Female patients prescribed thalidomide must be counselled about the need for contraception and male patients must undertake to use a condom. Written consent should be obtained.[32]

Supply

In the UK it is unlicensed and available only via Hospital Supply as a named patient supply (see Special orders and named patient supplies, p.349); the prescriber's name and department and the clinical indication must be supplied when ordering.

Thalidomide (IDIS 020 8410 0700)
Tablets 100mg, 28days @ 200mg o.n. = £72.80.

Sauramide (Penn 01495 711222)
Capsules 100mg, 28 days @ 200mg o.n. = £143.26.

1 Calabrese L and Fleischer A (2000) Thalidomide: current and potential clinical applications. *American Journal of Medicine.* **108**: 487–495.
2 Jacobson J (2000) Thalidomide: a remarkable comeback. *Expert Opinion in Pharmacotherapy.* **1**: 849–863.
3 Committee on Safety of Medicines (1994) CSM guidance on prescribing. *Current Problems in Pharmacovigilance.* **20**: 8.
4 Davis M and Dickerson E (2001) Thalidomide: dual benefits in palliative medicine and oncology. *American Journal of Hospice and Palliative Care.* **18**: 347–351.
5 Marriott J *et al.* (1999) Thalidomide as an emerging immunotherapeutic agent. *Trends in Immunology Today.* **20**: 538–540.
6 Peuckmann V *et al.* (2000) Potential novel uses of thalidomide: focus on palliative care. *Drugs.* **60**: 273–292.
7 Sampaio E *et al.* (1991) Thalidomide selectively inhibits tumour necrosis factor alpha production by stimulated human monocytes. *Journal of Experimental Medicine.* **173**: 699–703.
8 Radomsky C and Levine N (2001) Thalidomide. *Dermatologic Clinics.* **19**: 87–103.
9 Bousvaros A and Mueller B (2001) Thalidomide in gastrointestinal disorders. *Drugs.* **61**: 777–787.
10 Govindarajan R *et al.* (2000) Effect of thalidomide on gastrointestinal toxic effects of irinotecan. *Lancet.* **356**: 566–567.
11 Deaner P (1998) Thalidomide for distressing night sweats in advanced malignant disease. *Palliative Medicine.* **12**: 208–209.
12 Smith J *et al.* (2002) Use of thalidomide in the treatment of intractable itch. Poster abstract 21, Palliative Care Congress, Sheffield, UK.
13 Adlard J (2000) Thalidomide in the treatment of cancer. *Anticancer Drugs.* **11**: 787–791.

14 Eisen T (2000) Thalidomide in solid tumors: the London experience. *Oncology (Huntingt).* **14**: 17–20.
15 Fullerton P and O'Sullivan D (1968) Thalidomide neuropathy: a clinical, electrophysiological, and histological follow up study. *Journal of Neurology, Neurosurgery and Psychiatry.* **31**: 543–551.
16 Gardner-Medwin J *et al.* (1994) Clinical experience with thalidomide in the management of severe oral and genital ulceration in conditions such as Behcet's disease. *Annals of Rheumatic Diseases.* **128**: 443–450.
17 Ochonisky S *et al.* (1994) Thalidomide neuropathy incidence and clinico-electrophysiologic findings in 42 patients. *Archives of Dermatology.* **130**: 66–69.
18 Thomas D and Kantarjian H (2000) Current role of thalidomide in cancer treatment. *Current Opinion in Oncology.* **12**: 564–573.
19 Vogelsang G *et al.* (1992) Thalidomide for the treatment of chronic graft-versus-host disease. *New England Journal of Medicine.* **326**: 1055–1058.
20 Hamuryudan V *et al.* (1998) Thalidomide in the treatment of the mucocutaneous lesions of the Behcet syndrome. A randomized, double-blind, placebo-controlled trial. *Annals of Internal Medicine.* **128**: 443–450.
21 Ehrenpreis E *et al.* (1999) Thalidomide therapy for patients with refractory Crohn's disease: an open label trial. *Gastroenterology.* **117**: 1271–1277.
22 Vasilauskas E *et al.* (1999) An open label study of low-dose thalidomide in chronically active, steroid-dependent Crohn's disease. *Gastroenterology.* **117**: 1278–1287.
23 Marriott J *et al.* (1997) A double-blind placebo-controlled phase II trial of thalidomide in asymptomatic HIV-positive patients: clinical tolerance and effect on activation markers and cytokines. *AIDS Research and Human Retroviruses.* **13**: 1625–1631.
24 Noormohamed F *et al.* (1999) Pharmacokinetics and hemodynamic effects of single oral doses of thalidomide in asymptomatic human immunodeficiency virus-infected subjects. *AIDS Research and Human Retroviruses.* **15**: 1047–1052.
25 Clark T *et al.* (2001) Thalidomid (Thalidomide) capsules: A review of the first 18 months of spontaneous postmarketing adverse event surveillance, including off-label prescribing. *Drug Safety.* **24**: 87–117.
26 Galani E *et al.* (2000) Thalidomide and dexamethasone combination for refractory multiple myeloma. *Annals of Oncology.* **4**: 97.
27 Jacobson J *et al.* (1997) Thalidomide for the treatment of oral aphthous ulcers in patients with human immunodeficiency virus infection. *New England Journal of Medicine.* **336**: 1487–1493.
28 Calder K and Bruera E (2000) Thalidomide for night sweats in patients with advanced cancer. *Palliative Medicine.* **14**: 77–78.
29 Boasberg P *et al.* (2000) Thalidomide induced cessation of weight loss and improved sleep in advanced cancer patients with cachexia. *ASCO Online.* **Visited 21**: Abstract 2396.
30 Mantovani G *et al.* (2001) Managing cancer-related anorexia/cachexia. *Drugs.* **61**: 499–514.
31 Govindarajan R (2000) Irinotecan and thalidomide in metastatic colorectal cancer. *Oncology (Huntingt).* **14 (12 suppl 13)**: 29–32.
32 Powell R and Gardner-Medwin J (1994) Guidelines for the clinical use and dispensing of thalidomide. *Postgraduate Medical Journal.* **70**: 901–904.

8: URINARY TRACT DISORDERS

INDORAMIN BNF 7.4

Class: Selective α_1-adrenoceptor antagonist.

Indications: Hesitancy of micturition, hypertension.

Contra-indications: Symptomatic postural hypotension, cardiac failure, concurrent use of MAOI.

Pharmacology

Indoramin is a α-adrenoceptor antagonist which acts selectively and competitively on post-synaptic α_1-adrenoceptors, causing a decrease in peripheral vascular resistance, relaxation of the bladder neck and contraction of the detrusor.[1–3] In palliative care, indoramin is used for hesitancy of micturition associated with benign prostatic hypertrophy.[4,5] Other selective α_1-antagonists are available, namely **prazosin**, **tamsulosin** and **terazosin**.[6] All may cause severe hypotension, particularly with the first dose and in patients receiving diuretics or other antihypertensive medication.[7] Low cost is the only advantage in using **prazosin**; this has to be balanced against ease of compliance with **tamsulosin** and **terazosin** (o.d. compared to b.d.). Indoramin is probably the safest in debilitated patients.[6] Muscarinic drugs and anticholinesterases are sometimes preferable to an α-adrenoceptor antagonist, e.g. **bethanechol** 10–25mg t.d.s., **distigmine** 5mg o.d. If necessary, one of these may be used concurrently with indoramin. Indoramin is also licensed for use in the management of hypertension.[8–11]

Bio-availability 30% PO.

Onset of action 30–60min; maximum benefit 4–8 weeks.

Time to peak plasma concentration 1–4h.

Plasma halflife 4–5h.

Duration of action 12–24h.

Cautions

Alcohol increases the rate and extent of absorption of indoramin and should be avoided during initial dose titration. If the patient is taking antihypertensives, the dose should be reduced and the blood pressure monitored. **Baclofen** enhances the hypotensive effect. Epilepsy (seizures reported in animal studies).

Undesirable effects

For full list, see manufacturer's SPC.

Drowsiness, dizziness, postural hypotension.

Dose and use

Hesitancy of micturition

- starting dose 20mg b.d. (the first dose taken in bed at night); 20mg o.n. in elderly
- increase dose if necessary by 20mg every 2 weeks to a maximum of 100mg/day.

Hypertension
Doses tend to be higher, e.g. 25mg b.d., and increasing if necessary by 25–50mg every 2 weeks to a maximum of 200mg/day.

Supply
Doralese® (GSK 0800 221441)
Tablets 20mg, 28 days @ 20mg b.d.= £11.48.

Baratol® (Shire 01256 894000)
Tablets 25mg, 50mg, 28 days @ 25mg b.d.= £6.00.

Although the 20mg tablets are marketed for hesitancy of micturition and the 25mg and 50mg tablets for hypertension, use of the 25mg tablets for hesitancy would reduce drug costs.

---

1 Shanks R (1986) The clinical pharmacology of indoramin. *Journal of Cardiovascular Pharmacology.* **8 (suppl 2)**: S8–15.
2 Kenny B *et al.* (1996) Evaluation of the pharmacological selectivity profile of alpha 1 adrenoceptor antagonists at prostatic alpha 1 adrenoceptors: binding, functional and in vivo studies. *British Journal of Pharmacology.* **118**: 871–878.
3 Pupo A *et al.* (1999) Effects of indoramin in rat vas deferens and aorta: concomitant alpha 1-adrenoceptor and neuronal uptake blockade. *British Journal of Pharmacology.* **127**: 1832–1836.
4 Iacovou J and Dunn M (1987) Indoramin – an effective new drug in the management of bladder outflow obstruction. *British Journal of Urology.* **60**: 526–528.
5 Stott M and Abrams P (1991) Indoramin in the treatment of prostatic bladder outflow obstruction. *British Journal of Urology.* **67**: 499–501.
6 Clifford G and Farmer R (2000) Medical therapy for benign prostatic hyperplasia: a review of the literature. *European Urology.* **38**: 2–19.
7 Hieble J and Ruffolo R (1996) The use of alpha-adrenoceptor antagonists in the pharmacological management of benign prostatic hypertrophy: an overview. *Pharmacological Research.* **33**: 145–160.
8 Archibald J and Turner P (1983) Indoramin in the treatment of hypertension. A mini-review update. *South African Medical Journal.* **63**: 307–309.
9 Holmes B and Sorkin E (1986) Indoramin. A review of its pharmacodynamic and pharmacokinetic properties, and therapeutic efficacy in hypertension and related vascular, cardiovascular and airway diseases. *Drugs.* **31**: 467–499.
10 Cubeddu L (1988) New alpha 1-adrenergic receptor antagonists for the treatment of hypertension: role of vascular alpha receptors in the control of peripheral resistance. *American Heart Journal.* **116**: 133–162.
11 Studer J and Piepho R (1993) Antihypertensive therapy in the geriatric patient: II. A review of alpha 1-adrenergic blocking agents. *Journal of Clinical Pharmacology.* **33**: 2–13.

OXYBUTYNIN — BNF 7.4.2

Class: Antimuscarinic.

Indications: Frequency of micturition not caused by infective cystitis, bladder spasms.

Contra-indications: Bladder outflow obstruction, intestinal atony, glaucoma, myasthenia gravis.

Pharmacology
Oxybutynin has an antispasmodic action on the detrusor muscle of the bladder and an antimuscarinic (anticholinergic) effect on bladder innervation.[1] This helps to prevent bladder spasm and increase bladder capacity. The plasma halflife of oxybutynin increases in the elderly, generally allowing smaller doses to be given less frequently. An alternative drug may be more appropriate for some patients (Box 8.A).

Bio-availability 100% PO.
Onset of action 30–60min.
Time to peak plasma concentration 30–60min.
Plasma halflife first phase 40min; second phase 2–3h (4–5h in the elderly).
Duration of action 6–10h.

Box 8.A Drugs for urinary frequency and bladder spasms

Antimuscarinics are the drugs of choice even though treatment may be limited by other antimuscarinic effects:
- oxybutynin 2.5–5mg b.d.–q.d.s.; also has a topical anaesthetic effect on the bladder mucosa[2]
- tolterodine 2mg b.d. is as effective as oxybutynin 5mg t.d.s. but fewer antimuscarinic effects;[3] it is more expensive
- amitriptyline 25–50mg o.n.
- propantheline 15–30mg b.d.–t.d.s.

Sympathomimetics, e.g. terbutaline 5mg t.d.s.

Musculotropic drugs, flavoxate 200–400mg t.d.s.

NSAIDs, e.g.:
- flurbiprofen 50–100mg b.d.
- naproxen 250–500mg b.d.

Topical analgesics, e.g. phenazopyridine 100–200mg t.d.s. (not UK).

Vasopressin analogues, e.g. desmopressin, are of value in refractory nocturia; hyponatraemia is a possible complication.

Undesirable effects

For full list, see manufacturer's SPC.
Dry mouth, other antimuscarinic effects (see p.4), cognitive impairment and delirium in the elderly,[4] nausea, abdominal discomfort.

Dose and use

- starting dose 2.5–5mg b.d.
- increase if necessary to 5mg q.d.s.

Supply

Oxybutynin (non-proprietary)
Tablets 2.5mg, 3mg, 5mg, 28 days @ 5mg b.d.= £9.67.

Cystrin® (Sanofi-Synthelabo 01483 505515)
Tablets 3mg, 5mg, 28 days @ 5mg b.d.= £15.25.

Ditropan® (Sanofi-Synthelabo 01483 505515)
Tablets 2.5mg, 5mg, 28 days @ 5mg b.d.= £15.25.
Oral solution 2.5mg/5ml, 28 days @ 5mg b.d.= £17.84.

Ditropan® XL (Sanofi-Synthelabo 01483 505515)
Tablets m/r 5mg, 10mg, 28 days @ 10mg o.d.= £17.71.

1 Andersson K (1988) Current concepts in the treatment of disorders of micturition. *Drugs*. **35**: 477–494.
2 Robinson T and Castleden C (1994) Drugs in focus: 11. Oxybutynin hydrochloride. *Prescribers' Journal*. **34**: 27–30.
3 Hills C *et al.* (1998) Tolterodine. *Drugs*. **55**: 813–820.
4 Donnellan C *et al.* (1997) Oxybutynin and cognitive dysfunction. *British Medical Journal*. **315**: 1363–1364.

METHENAMINE HIPPURATE AND NITROFURANTOIN BNF 5.1.13

Class: Urinary antiseptics.

Indications: Prophylaxis against cystitis.

Contra-indications: Methenamine hippurate should not be used in severe renal failure (creatinine clearance <10ml/min) or metabolic acidosis. Nitrofurantoin should not be given with a creatinine clearance of <60ml/min or elevated plasma creatinine.

Pharmacology

In an acid environment (pH <5), methenamine (hexamine) hippurate dissociates into methenamine and hippuric acid. Methenamine is then converted to formaldehyde which is responsible for the bactericidal effect.[1] Urea-splitting bacteria tend to raise the pH of urine and could thereby inhibit the formation of formaldehyde; however, hippuric acid maintains an acidic environment. Nearly all bacteria are sensitive to formaldehyde at concentrations of ≥20microgram/ml. In catheterised patients, methenamine hippurate reduces sediment and catheter blockage, and doubles the interval between catheter changes.[2]

Nitrofurantoin is an alternative urinary antiseptic. Because of its rapid excretion from the blood, nitrofurantoin reaches significant concentrations only in the bladder.[3] Nitrofurantoin is reduced by flavoproteins to reactive intermediates which inactivate or alter bacterial ribosomal proteins and other macromolecules. As a result, protein synthesis, aerobic metabolism, DNA synthesis, RNA synthesis and cell wall synthesis are inhibited. This broad mode of action is probably the reason why acquired bacterial resistance to nitrofurantoin is rare.

For pharmacokinetic details, see Table 8.1.

Table 8.1 Pharmacokinetics of urinary antiseptics PO

	Methenamine hippurate	*Nitrofurantoin*
Bio-availability	No data	90%
Onset of action	3h	2.5–4.5h
Plasma halflife	4h	60min
Duration of action	No data	5–8h

Cautions

Methenamine hippurate should not be administered concurrently with **sulphonamides** because of the possibility of crystalluria. Concurrent administration with **magnesium salts** reduces the absorption of nitrofurantoin. Neither drugs should be given concurrently with alkalising agents such as **potassium citrate** because of the need for an acid urinary environment.

Undesirable effects

For full list, see manufacturer's SPC.

Both methenamine hippurate and nitrofurantoin may cause gastro-intestinal symptoms, e.g. dyspepsia, nausea, vomiting.

Dose and use

Neither methenamine hippurate nor nitrofurantoin should be used to treat acute infection of the upper urinary tract.

- methenamine hippurate 1g b.d.[4]
- nitrofurantoin 50–100mg o.n.[5]

Supply

Methenamine hippurate
Hiprex® (3M 01509 611611)
Tablets 1g, 28 days @ 1g b.d. = £6.60.

Nitrofurantoin
Macrodantin® (Goldshield 020 8649 8500)
Capsules 100mg, 28 days @ 100mg o.n. = £5.38.
Furadantin® (Goldshield 020 8649 8500)
Tablets 100mg, 28 days @ 100mg o.n. = £5.07.

1 Strom JJ and Jun H (1993) Effect of urine pH and ascorbic acid on the rate of conversion of methenamine to formaldehyde. *Biopharmaceutics and Drug Disposition.* **14**: 61–69.
2 Norberg A *et al.* (1980) Randomized double-blind study of prophylactic methenamine hippurate treatment of patients with indwelling catheters. *European Journal of Clinical Pharmacology.* **18**: 497–500.
3 Hooper D (1995) Urinary tract agents: nitrofurantoin and methenamine. In: G Mandell *et al.* (eds) *Mandell, Douglas and Bennett's Principles and Practice of Infectious Diseases.* Churchill Livingstone, New York, pp.376–381.
4 Cronberg S *et al.* (1987) Prevention of recurrent acute cystitis by methenamine hippurate: double blind controlled crossover longterm study. *British Medical Journal.* **294**: 1507–1508.
5 Brumfitt W *et al.* (1981) Prevention of recurrent urinary infections in women: a comparative trial between nitrofurantoin and methenamine hippurate. *Journal of Urology.* **126**: 71–74.

CRANBERRY JUICE

Class: Herbal remedy.

Indications: Prophylaxis against cystitis.

Pharmacology

Cranberry (and blueberry) juice contains a large polymer of unknown structure which inhibits bacterial adherence to the bladder mucosa. It reduces the frequency of symptomatic urinary tract infections with *Escherichia coli.*[1] Although sometimes recommended, the addition of **ascorbic acid** (vitamin C) is not necessary. However, two recent reviews cast doubt on the efficacy of cranberry juice.[2,3]
Pharmacokinetic data not available.

Dose and use

Drink as fruit juice 180ml b.d.

Supply

Available OTC.

1 Avorn J *et al.* (1994) Reduction of bacteriuria and pyuria after ingestion of cranberry juice. *Journal of the American Medical Association.* **271**: 751–754.
2 Harkins K (2000) What's the use of cranberry juice? *Age and Ageing.* **29**: 9–12.
3 Jepson R *et al.* (2000) Cranberries for preventing urinary tract infections. *Cochrane Library.* **2**.

CATHETER PATENCY SOLUTIONS BNF 7.4.4

Deposit which forms on the surface of indwelling urinary catheters is composed chiefly of phosphate crystals. To minimise this a latex catheter should be changed at least every 6 weeks. If the catheter is to be left for longer periods a silicone catheter should be used together with the appropriate use of catheter maintenance solutions. Repeated blockage usually indicates that the catheter needs to be changed. In some patients blockage is caused by blood clots.

Bladder washouts do not cure infection; their main purpose is to reduce the frequency of catheter blockage.[1] There is no evidence that **chlorhexidine** has any advantage over **sodium chloride**; it may cause irritation or lead to the emergence of resistant bacterial strains.[2,3]

Supply and use

A range of prepacked 100ml solutions is available. Administer washouts daily; reduce to alternate days or change to sodium chloride once problem resolved.

Sodium chloride 0.9% recommended for flushing of debris and small blood clots.
Uriflex S® (SSL 01565 624000)
Sachet 100ml = £2.40.
Uro-Tainer Sodium Chloride® (Braun 0114 225 9000)
Sachet 100ml = £2.45.

Chlorhexidine 0.02% antiseptic solution aimed at preventing or reducing bacterial growth, particularly *Escherichia coli* and *Klebsiella*; ineffective against most *Pseudomonas* species.
Uriflex C® (SSL 01565 624000)
Sachet 100ml = £2.40.
Uro-Tainer Chlorhexidine® (Braun 0114 225 9000)
Sachet 100ml = £2.60.

Solution G 3.23% citric acid solution containing magnesium, reduces encrustation.
Uriflex G® (SSL 01565 624000)
Sachet 100ml = £2.40.
Uro-Tainer Suby G® (Braun 0114 225 9000)
Sachet 100ml = £2.60.

BNF also contains **Mandelic acid** 1% and **Solution R**.

1 Getliffe K (1996) Bladder instillations and bladder washouts in the management of catheterized patients. *Journal of Advanced Nursing*. **23**: 548–554.

2 Baillier L (1987) Chlorhexidine resistance among bacteria isolated from urine of catheterized patients. *Journal of Hospital Infection*. **10**: 83–86.

3 Davies AJ *et al.* (1987) Does instillation of chlorhexidine into the bladder of catheterized geriatric patients help reduce bacteria? *Journal of Hospital Infections*. **9**: 72–75.

9: NUTRITION AND BLOOD

Anaemia
Epoetin
Ferrous sulphate

Vitamins
Ascorbic acid (vitamin C)
Multivitamin preparations
Phytomenadione (vitamin K_1)

Potassium

Magnesium

ANAEMIA — BNF 9.1

Anaemia is common in cancer and other forms of chronic disease. The main causes are:

- anaemia of chronic disease
- iron deficiency
- folate deficiency
- malignant infiltration of the marrow
- haemolytic anaemia
- renal failure.

It is important to distinguish between the various types of anaemia because treatment differs. The commonest form in cancer is anaemia of chronic disease (ACD). This is a paraneoplastic phenomenon and relates partly to suppression of endogenous erythropoietin production (Figure 9.1).[1]

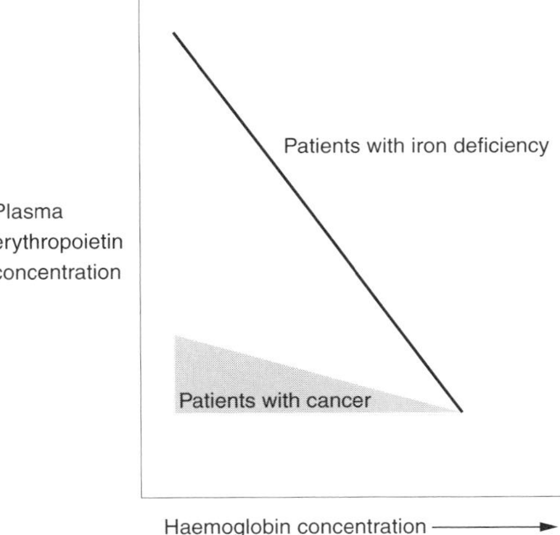

Figure 9.1 Relationship between haemoglobin and erythropoietin concentration in patients with iron deficiency and cancer-associated anaemia.[1]

Diagnostic features are:
- normochromic-normocytic anaemia (hypochromic-microcytic in iron deficiency)
- reticulocytopenia
- low plasma iron
- low/low-normal plasma transferrin concentration (TIBC) (high/high-normal in iron deficiency)
- high/high-normal plasma ferritin concentration (low in iron deficiency)
- hypoplastic bone marrow appearances
- increased marrow iron stores
- reduced iron within maturing erythroblasts.

About 75% of patients with ACD respond to **epoetin** treatment. In patients already transfusion-dependent, about half will become transfusion-independent.[2] **Epoetin** clearly has several advantages when compared with blood transfusion (Table 9.1). A full analysis of the costs suggests that treatment with **epoetin** is probably no more expensive than intermittent blood transfusions, particularly when personal factors are taken into account.[3]

Table 9.1 Comparison of epoetin and blood transfusion

	Epoetin	*Transfusion*
Rise in haemoglobin	Long-lasting	Transient (2–4 weeks)
Speed of effect	4–6 weeks	Immediate
Safety	Undesirable effects rare and generally minor	Risk of transfusion reaction and infection[4]
Inconvenience	SC injection thrice weekly or less	IV infusion every 4 weeks

1 Miller C *et al.* (1990) Decreased erythropoietin response in patients with the anemia of cancer. *New England Journal of Medicine.* **322**: 1689–1692.

2 Seidenfeld J *et al.* (2001) Epoetin treatment of anemia associated with cancer therapy: a systematic review and meta-analysis of controlled clinical trials. *Journal of the National Cancer Institute.* **93**: 1204–1214.

3 Engert A (2000) Recombinant human erythropoietin as an alternative to blood transfusion in cancer-related anaemia. *Disease Management and Health Outcomes.* **8**: 259–272.

4 Williamson L *et al.* (1999) Serious hazards of transfusion (SHOT) initiative: analysis of the first two annual reports. *British Medical Journal.* **319**: 16–19.

EPOETIN — BNF 9.1.3

Class: Erythrostimulant.

Indications: Anaemia associated with chronic renal failure, cancer chemotherapy, †chronic disease.

Contra-indications: Uncontrolled hypertension.

Pharmacology

Epoetin is recombinant human erythropoietin, the hormone responsible for the maintenance of erythropoiesis.[1] The drug binds to and activates receptors on erythroid progenitor cells which then develop into mature erythrocytes.[2] Epoetin increases the reticulocyte count, haemoglobin concentration (Hb) and haematocrit in a dose-proportional manner. Epoetin is available in two forms, alfa and beta; they are both synthesised in Chinese hamster ovary cells by gene technology.[3] They are identical with endogenous human erythropoietin in amino acid and carbohydrate composition. Clinically they are equally effective but epoetin beta is more potent in terms of absolute reticulocyte response.[3,4] Despite reduced bio-availability, the reticulocyte response is more sustained when epoetin is given SC rather than IV, permitting a 30% reduction in dose.[2] Epoetin is probably metabolised by the liver; less than 10% is eliminated unchanged by the kidneys. Response to epoetin in patients receiving anticancer therapy has been shown in controlled trials and confirmed by meta-analysis.[5] Response is greatest with squamous cell cancers (head and neck, oesophagus, lung) and multiple myeloma; it is less with other cancers, particularly Hodgkin's lymphoma. In myelodysplastic syndrome the response is <10%.[6] The likelihood of a positive response can be predicted with a high degree of accuracy from measurements of erythropoietin and Hb at baseline and after 2 weeks. A positive response is 95% likely if:

- there is adequate bone marrow reserve (neutrophils $>1.5 \times 10^9$/L and platelets $>100 \times 10^9$/L) *and*
- the initial serum erythropoietin concentration is <100milli-units/ml *and*
- the Hb increases by >0.5g/dl after 2 weeks.[7]

The converse predicts a lack of response with similar accuracy; and epoetin treatment should be stopped. In some patients, concurrent iron deficiency restricts response.[8] A low serum ferritin concentration is unequivocal evidence of diminished iron stores; it occurs in no other circumstance. (In cancer, the serum ferritin is generally raised because it is an acute phase protein.) When there is definite iron deficiency, elemental iron 200–300mg/day should be given for 4 weeks and the situation then reviewed before a decision is made to use epoetin.

An excessive increase in red cell mass is avoided by:

- reducing the dose by 25–50% if the Hb increases by >2g/dl/month
- aiming to maintain a Hb of 11g/dl in women and 12g/dl in men
- discontinuing treatment if the Hb increases to >14g/dl, restarting with 25–50% of the previous dose once Hb falls below 12g/dl.

In addition to producing a sustained rise in Hb, epoetin also significantly reduces fatigue and increases energy, activity level and quality of life. The improvement in these parameters increases incrementally up to a Hb of about 12g/dl.[9–11] There is some evidence that raising the Hb with epoetin increases survival by a median of some 6 months in cancer patients receiving non-platinum chemotherapy.[12]

Darbepoetin alfa (novel erythropoiesis stimulating protein, NESP) is a new modified epoetin produced by similar gene technology but with 8 more sialic acid side chains than epoetin alfa and beta.[13,14] This results in greater bio-availability, a longer halflife and a longer duration of action.[15] Darbepoetin is licensed for use in anaemia associated with chronic renal failure, and has also been used successfully in anaemia associated with chemotherapy and anaemia of chronic disease in cancer.[16,17] Darbepoetin is as effective as epoetin alfa and beta. However, because it needs to be given only every 1–2 weeks and is no more expensive, darbepoetin is likely to supplant epoetin alfa and beta.

Bio-availability alfa 20%; beta 20–40%; darbepoetin 37% SC.
Onset of action apparent 2–3 weeks after starting treatment.
Time to peak plasma concentration alfa and beta 12–18h SC; darbepoetin 34h (24–72h).
Plasma halflife alfa 4–5h IV, 24h SC; beta 4–12h IV, 13–28h SC; darbepoetin 25h IV, 49h (27–89h) SC.
Duration of action alfa and beta, about 1 week; darbepoetin about 2 weeks.

Cautions

Epilepsy, severe hepatic impairment. Uncontrolled hypertension should be stabilised with anti-hypertensives before commencing treatment with epoetin.

Blood pressure, Hb and platelet counts should be routinely monitored; avoid a rate of rise of Hb of >2g/dl per month or a Hb level of >14g/dl (see Dose and use).

Undesirable effects

For full list, see manufacturer's SPC.

The injections are often painful, epoetin beta less than epoetin alfa.[18,19] Epoetin beta prepared without albumin (Recormon®) is even less likely to cause pain,[18] as is the use of a pen injector.[20] Flu-like symptoms may occur, particularly at the start of treatment. If the anaemia is corrected rapidly, headaches, elevated blood pressure and seizures may occur; these are mostly restricted to patients with renal failure and are largely prevented by adherence to the manufacturers' dose recommendations. Thrombocytosis occurs rarely. Pure red cell aplasia has occurred very rarely following months or years of therapy. Most patients had detectable anti-erythropoietin anti-bodies. Treatment should be stopped and patients not transferred to any other erythropoietin.

Dose and use

Epoetin alfa and beta; anaemia of chronic disease in cancer

The first dose should be given under medical supervision because of rare reports of anaphylaxis. Although the SPC recommends SC injections 3 times weekly, equal benefit is seen in chemotherapy/radiation therapy-induced anaemia with a larger injection once weekly.[21–23]

- starting dose 450units/kg SC weekly
- *after 2 weeks,* if Hb increases by >1.3g/dl → reduce the dose to 300units/kg/week
- *after 4 weeks,* if Hb increases >1g/dl → continue indefinitely
  if Hb increases by >2g/dl → halve the dose to 225units/kg/week
  if Hb increases <1g/dl → double the dose to 900units/kg/week (Table 9.2)
- *at any time,* if Hb increases to >14g/dl → stop treatment and restart with 25% of the previous dose when Hb falls below 12g/dl.

Table 9.2 Calculating the dose of epoetin[a]

Weight	*Initial dose (450units/kg/week)*	*Dose for non-responders (900units/kg/week)*
40–50kg	20 000units/week	40 000units/week
51–60kg	25 000units/week	50 000units/week
61–70kg	30 000units/week	60 000units/week
71–80kg	33 000units/week	66 000units/week
81–90kg	38 000units/week	76 000units/week
91–100kg	42 000units/week	84 000units/week

a. for average weight within each range, rounded up or down for convenience.

Epoetin alfa and beta; anaemia of chronic renal disease

The dosing schedule is very different and includes both SC and IV routes. There are also additional cautions. *For details, see manufacturer's SPC.*

Darbepoetin

The recommended starting dose is 0.45microgram/kg/week IV/SC. In some patients, darbepoetin will need to be given only every 2 weeks. If switching from epoetin alfa or beta to darbepoetin, the initial dose of darbepoetin (microgram/week) can be determined by dividing the total weekly dose of recombinant human epoetin (unit/week) by 200.

Supply

Epoetin alfa

Eprex® (Janssen-Cilag 01494 567567)

The manufacturer operates a guarantee scheme whereby, if there has not been a satisfactory response to treatment after 8 weeks, Ortho Biotech will replace the epoetin used free of charge.

Injection 1000units/0.5ml, 2000units/ml, 4000units/ml, 10 000units/ml, 40 000units/ml vials, 28 days @ 40 000units/week = £1340.80.

Injection prefilled syringe 1000units, 2000units, 3000units, 4000units, 5000units, 6000units, 7000units, 8000units, 9000units, 10 000units (an auto-injector device is available for use with the 10 000units/ml prefilled syringes), 28 days @ 40 000units/week = £1340.80.

Epoetin beta

NeoRecormon® (Roche 01707 366000)

The manufacturer offers a standardised set of blood tests to predict whether or not there is a high probability of a response to epoetin. The tests are carried out by the manufacturer once a week. A free service is also provided whereby a nurse visits patients at home to teach them over 3–4 visits how to self-administer epoetin SC.

Injection (prefilled syringe) 500units, 1000units, 2000units, 3000units, 4000units, 5000units, 6000units, 10 000units, 28 days @ 40 000units/week = £1340.80.
Injection (multidose vial) 50 000units,100 000units, 28 days @ 40 000units/week = £1340.80; stable for one month after reconstitution if stored in a refrigerator.
Injection (Reco-pen®) (double chamber cartridge containing epoetin beta and solvent for SC use); 10 000units, 20 000units, 60 000units, 28 days @ 40 000units/week = £1340.80.

Darbepoetin alfa
Aranesp® (Amgen 01223 420305)
Injection (prefilled syringe) 10microgram/0.4ml, 15microgram/0.375ml, 20microgram/0.5ml, 30microgram/0.3ml, 40microgram/0.4ml, 50microgram/0.5ml, 60microgram/0.3ml, 80microgram/0.4ml, 100microgram/0.5ml, 150microgram/0.3ml, 28 days @ 200microgram/week = £1340.80.

1 Engert A (2000) Recombinant human erythropoietin as an alternative to blood transfusion in cancer-related anaemia. *Disease Management and Health Outcomes.* **8**: 259–272.
2 Dunn C and Markham A (1996) Epoetin beta. A review of its pharmacological properties and clinical use in the management of anaemia associated with chronic renal failure. *Drugs.* **51**: 299–318.
3 Storring P *et al.* (1998) Epoetin alfa and beta differ in their erythropoietin isoform compositions and biological properties. *British Journal of Haematology.* **100**: 79–89.
4 Halstenson C *et al.* (1991) Comparative pharmacokinetics and pharmacodynamics of epoetin alfa and epoetin beta. *Clinical Pharmacology and Therapeutics.* **50**: 702–712.
5 Seidenfeld J *et al.* (2001) Epoetin treatment of anemia associated with cancer therapy: a systematic review and meta-analysis of controlled clinical trials. *Journal of the National Cancer Institute.* **93**: 1204–1214.
6 Ludwig H and Fritz E (1998) Anemia of cancer patients: patient selection and patient stratification for epoetin treatment. *Seminars in Oncology.* **25 (suppl 7)**: 35–38.
7 Ludwig H *et al.* (1994) Prediction of response to erythropoietin treatment in chronic anemia of cancer. *Blood.* **84**: 1056–1063.
8 Beguin Y (1998) Prediction of response to optimize outcome of treatment with erythropoietin. *Seminars in Oncology.* **25 (suppl 7)**: 27–34.
9 Demetri G *et al.* (1998) Quality-of-life benefit in chemotherapy patients treated with epoetin alfa is independent of disease response or tumor type: results from a prospective community oncology study. Procrit Study Group. *Journal of Clinical Oncology.* **16**: 3412–3425.
10 Cleeland C *et al.* (1999) Identifying haemoglobin level for optimal quality of life: results of an incremental analysis. *Proceedings of the American Society of Clinical Oncology.* **18**: Abstract 2215.
11 Littlewood T *et al.* (1999) Efficacy and quality of life outcomes of epoetin alfa in a double blind, placeo-controlled multicentre study of cancer patients receiving non-platinum containing chemotherapy. *Proceedings of the American Society of Clinical Oncology.* **Abstract**: 2217.
12 Littlewood T *et al.* (2000) Possible relationship of haemoglobin levels with survival in anemic cancer patients receiving chemotherapy. *Proceedings of the American Society of Clinical Oncology.* **19**: Abstract 2381.
13 Demetri G (2001) Anaemia and its functional consequences in cancer patients: current challenges in management and prospects for improving therapy. *British Journal of Cancer.* **84**: 31–37.
14 Egrie J and Browne J (2001) Development and characterization of novel erythropoiesis stimulating protein (NESP). *British Journal of Cancer.* **84**: 3–10.
15 Heatherington A *et al.* (2001) Pharmacokinetics of novel erythropoiesis stimulating protein (NESP). *British Journal of Cancer.* **84**: 11–16.
16 Glaspy J *et al.* (2001) A dose-finding and safety study of novel erythropoiesis stimulating protein (NESP) for the treatment of anaemia in patients receiving multicycle chemotherapy. *British Journal of Cancer.* **84**: 17–23.
17 Smith R *et al.* (2001) Novel erythropoiesis stimulating protein (NESP) for the treatment of anaemia of chronic disease associated with cancer. *British Journal of Cancer.* **84**: 24–30.
18 Frenken L *et al.* (1991) Assessment of pain after subcutaneous injection of erythropoietin in patients receiving haemodialysis. *British Medical Journal.* **303**: 288.

19 Lui S *et al.* (1991) Pain after subcutaneous injection of erythropoietin. *British Medical Journal.* **303**: 856.
20 Ruiz P *et al.* (2000) Tolerability of the epoetin-beta multidose formulation (Reco-Pen) in patients with renal anaemia. *Clinical Drug Investigations.* **20**: 151–158.
21 Gabrilove J *et al.* (1999) Once-weekly dosing of epoetin alfa is similar to three-times weekly dosing in increasing haemoglobin and quality of life. *Proceedings of the American Society of Clinical Oncology.* **18**: Abstract 2216.
22 Cheung W *et al.* (2000) The pharmacokinetics and pharmacodynamics of epoetin alfa once weekly versus epoetin alfa 3 times weekly. *Journal of the American Society of Hematology.* **96**: Abstract 1270.
23 Shasha D *et al.* (2000) Once-weekly dosing of epoetin alfa increases hemoglobin and improves quality of life in anemic cancer patients receiving radiation therapy either concomitantly or sequentially with chemotherapy. *Presented at the American Society of Hematology, San Francisco, CA. December 1–5.*

FERROUS SULPHATE — BNF 9.1.1

Class: Elemental salt.

Indications: Iron deficiency anaemia.

Contra-indications: Anaemia of chronic disease.

Pharmacology

Ferrous salts are better absorbed than ferric salts. Because there are only marginal differences in terms of efficiency of iron absorption, the choice of ferrous salt is based mainly on the incidence of undesirable effects and cost. Undesirable effects relate directly to the amount of elemental iron and an apparent improvement in tolerance on changing to another salt may be because of a lower elemental iron content (Table 9.3). M/r preparations are designed to reduce undesirable effects by releasing iron gradually as the capsule or tablet passes along the bowel. However, these preparations are likely to carry most of the iron past the first part of the duodenum into parts of the bowel where iron absorption is poor. Such preparations have no therapeutic advantage and should not be used.

Some oral preparations contain **ascorbic acid** to aid absorption, or the iron is in the form of a chelate. These modifications have shown experimentally to produce a modest increase in absorption of iron. However, the therapeutic advantage is minimal and cost may be increased. There is no clinical justification for the inclusion of other therapeutically active ingredients, such as the B group of vitamins (except **folic acid** for pregnant women). In the treatment of iron deficiency, the haemoglobin concentration should rise by about 1g/dl/week. After the haemoglobin has risen to normal, treatment should be continued for a further 3 months in an attempt to replenish the iron stores. Epithelial tissue changes such as atrophic glossitis and koilonychia also improve but generally more slowly.

Table 9.3 Elemental ferrous iron content of different iron salts

Iron salt	*Amount*	*Ferrous content*
Ferrous fumarate	200mg	65mg
Ferrous sulphate, dried	200mg	65mg
Ferrous sulphate	300mg	60mg
Ferrous gluconate	300mg	35mg
Ferrous succinate	100mg	35mg

Undesirable effects

For full list, see manufacturer's SPC.

Dyspepsia, nausea, epigastric pain, constipation, diarrhoea. Elderly patients are more likely to develop constipation, occasionally leading to faecal impaction; m/r preparations are more likely to cause diarrhoea.

Dose and use

The diagnosis of iron deficiency should be confirmed before iron supplements are prescribed (see Anaemia, p.247):

- prescribe dried ferrous sulphate 200mg b.d. (elemental iron 130mg)
- if undesirable gastro-intestinal effects occur, reduce the dose or change to an alternative iron salt.

Supply

Ferrous sulphate (non-proprietary)
Tablets 200mg (65mg iron), 28 days @ 200mg b.d.= £1.79.

Ferrous fumarate
Fersamal® (Goldshield 020 8649 8500)
Oral syrup 140mg (45mg iron)/5ml, 28 days @ 10ml b.d.= £6.58.

Galfer® (Galen 028 3833 4974)
Oral syrup 140mg (45mg iron)/5ml, 28 days @ 10ml b.d.= £9.07.

ASCORBIC ACID (VITAMIN C) — BNF 9.6.3

Class: Vitamin.

Indications: Scurvy, †decubitus ulcers, †furred tongue (topical), †urinary infection.

Pharmacology

Ascorbic acid (vitamin C) is a powerful reducing agent. It is obtained from fresh fruit and vegetables, particularly blackcurrant and kiwifruit; it cannot be synthesised by the body. It is involved in the hydroxylation of proline to hydroxyproline, which is necessary for the formation of collagen. The failure of this accounts for most of the clinical effects found in deficiency (scurvy), e.g. keratosis of hair follicles with 'corkscrew hair', perifollicular haemorrhages, swollen spongy infected and bleeding gums, loose teeth, spontaneous bruising and haemorrhage, anaemia and failure of wound healing. Repeated infections are also common. In healthy adults, a dietary intake of 30–60mg/day is necessary; in scurvy, a rapid clinical response is seen with 100–200mg/day. Absorption occurs mainly from the proximal small intestine by a saturable process. In health, body stores of ascorbic acid are about 1.5g, although larger stores may occur with intakes higher than 200mg daily. It is excreted as oxalic acid, unchanged ascorbic acid and small amounts of dehydro-ascorbic acid. Ascorbic acid is used to acidify urine in patients with alkaline urine and recurrent urinary infections.

A beneficial effect of megadose ascorbic acid therapy has been claimed for many conditions,[1] including the common cold, asthma, atherosclerosis, cancer, psychiatric disorders, increased susceptibility to infections related to abnormal leucocyte function, infertility, and osteogenesis imperfecta. Ascorbic acid has also been tried in the treatment of wound healing, pain in Paget's disease and opioid withdrawal. There are few controlled studies to substantiate these claims. High-dose vitamin C is not effective against advanced cancer.[2] Vitamin C alone or with β-carotene and vitamin E does not prevent the development of colorectal adenoma.[3] However, ascorbic acid does reduce the severity of a cold but not its incidence.[4] On the other hand, enthusiasm for high-dose ascorbic acid for HIV+ people waned after many died from disease progression.[5] Although it has been postulated that ascorbic acid might help prevent ischaemic heart disease, in contrast to other anti-oxidant vitamins, little benefit is seen in controlled studies.[6,7] Of more concern are data which indicate that a daily dose as small as 500mg has a pro-oxidant effect which could result in genetic mutation.[8]

Undesirable effects

For full list, see manufacturer's SPC.

Excess ascorbic acid (>3g/day) may result in acidosis, diarrhoea, glycosuria, oxaluria and renal stones. Tolerance may be induced with prolonged use of large doses, resulting in symptoms of deficiency when intake is returned to normal.

Dose and use

Furred tongue

- place 1/4 of 1g effervescent tablet on the tongue and allow it to dissolve; repeat up to q.d.s. for <1 week.

Acidification of urine

- 100–200mg b.d.; test urine with litmus paper until constant acid result is obtained.

Enhancement of healing

- 100mg b.d. for 4 weeks.

Scurvy

- 100mg b.d. for 4 weeks.

Supply

Ascorbic acid (non-proprietary)

Tablets 50mg, 100mg, 200mg, 500mg, 28 days @ 100mg b.d.= £0.50.

Tablets effervescent 1g, 28 days @ 1/4 of a tablet q.d.s. = £3.44 (~~NHS~~).

1 Ovesen L (1984) Vitamin therapy in the absence of obvious deficiency. What is the evidence? *Drugs*. **27**: 148–170.

2 Moertel C *et al.* (1985) High-dose vitamin C versus placebo in the treatment of patients with advanced cancer who have had no prior chemotherapy. A randomized double-blind comparison. *New England Journal of Medicine*. **312**: 137–141.

3 Greenberg E *et al.* (1994) A clinical trial of antioxidant vitamins to prevent colorectal adenoma. Polyp Prevention Study Group. *New England Journal of Medicine*. **331**: 141–147.

4 Hemila H (1994) Does vitamin C alleviate the symptoms of the common cold? a review of current evidence. *Scandinavian Journal of Infectious Diseases*. **26**: 1–6.

5 Abrams D (1990) Alternative therapies in HIV infection. *AIDS*. **4**: 1179–1187.

6 Rimm E (1993) Vitamin E consumption and the risk of coronary heart disease in men. *New England Journal of Medicine*. **328**: 1450–1456.

7 Stampfer M (1993) Vitamin E consumption and the risk of coronary disease in women. *New England Journal of Medicine*. **328**: 1444–1449.

8 Podmore I *et al.* (1998) Vitamin C exhibits pro-oxidant properties. *Nature*. **392**: 559.

MULTIVITAMIN PREPARATIONS — BNF 9.6.7

Indications: Vitamin deficiency (e.g. sore red tongue, angular stomatitis, painful neuropathy).

Dose and use

Multivitamin capsules 1 b.d.–t.d.s.

Supply

Vitamins (available OTC)

Capsules (ascorbic acid 15mg, nicotinamide 7.5mg, riboflavin 500microgram, thiamine 1mg, vitamin A 2500 units, vitamin D 300 units), 28 days @ 1 b.d. = £0.59.

PHYTOMENADIONE (VITAMIN K_1) BNF 9.6.6

Class: Vitamin.

Indications: Vitamin K deficiency, reversal of anticoagulant effects of **warfarin**, †bleeding tendency in patients with hepatic impairment in advanced cancer.

Pharmacology

Phytomenadione (vitamin K_1) is the active form of vitamin K. It is necessary for the production of blood clotting factors and proteins involved in bone calcification. Because vitamin K is fat-soluble, patients with fat malabsorption may become deficient, particularly in biliary obstruction or hepatic disease. Oral coumarin anticoagulants (e.g. **warfarin**) act by interfering with vitamin K metabolism in the liver and their effects are antagonised by giving exogenous vitamin K. Vitamin K is not indicated routinely in severe liver failure, nor even in moribund patients with manifestations of a bleeding diathesis (e.g. petechiae, purpura, multiple bruising, nose and gum bleeds) and it should not be used merely to prevent an imminent inevitable death. Its use is limited to conscious patients with a reasonable performance status for whom other supportive measures are deemed appropriate (e.g. blood transfusion).
Plasma halflife 1.5–3h.

Cautions and undesirable effects

For full list, see manufacturer's SPC.
Konakion®, a proprietary preparation of phytomenadione containing polyethoxylated castor oil, has been associated with anaphylaxis.

Dose and use

Partial reversal of warfarin anticoagulation
- the recommendations of the British Society of Haematology should be followed (see BNF 2.8.2).

Correction of a bleeding tendency in liver failure
- give Konakion® MM 10mg by slow IV injection, repeat p.r.n.

Prevention of vitamin K deficiency in malabsorption
- use an oral water-soluble preparation, i.e. menadiol sodium phosphate 10mg o.d.

Supply

Menadiol phosphate (non-proprietary)
Tablets (as 10mg **menadiol sodium phosphate**), 100 = £32.33.

Phytomenadione
Konakion® (Roche 01707 366000)
Tablets 10 = £1.77. *To be chewed/dissolved in mouth.*
Injection 2mg/ml, 0.5ml amp = £0.23. For IM and slow IV use; *must not be diluted.*

Konakion® MM (Roche 01707 366000)
Colloidal injection 10mg/ml, 1ml amp = £0.43. Konakion® MM may be administered by slow IV injection or by IV infusion in 5% glucose; *not for IM injection.*

POTASSIUM BNF 9.2.1.1

Class: Elemental salt.

Indications: Hypokalaemia (<3.5mmol/L).

Pharmacology

In palliative care, hypokalaemia is most common in patients receiving diuretics, particularly if also taking a corticosteroid and/or a NSAID. Hypokalaemia is also associated with chronic diarrhoea and persistent vomiting. Correction of hypokalaemia is important in patients taking digoxin or other anti-arrhythmic drugs because of the risk of an arrhythmia. Potassium supplements are seldom required with small doses of diuretics given to treat hypertension. When larger doses of thiazide or loop diuretics are given to eliminate oedema, potassium-sparing diuretics (e.g. **amiloride**) rather than potassium supplements are recommended for the prevention of hypokalaemia. Dietary supplements can help maintain plasma potassium; 10mmol of potassium is contained in a large banana and in 250ml of orange juice.

Cautions
Smaller doses must be used if there is renal insufficiency (common in the elderly) so as to avoid switching from hypokalaemia to hyperkalaemia.

Undesirable effects
For full list, see manufacturer's SPC.
Nausea and vomiting, often resulting in poor compliance. Liquid or effervescent preparations are distasteful.

Dose and use
Whenever possible orange juice and bananas should be used as a palatable source of potassium. To minimise nausea and vomiting, potassium supplements are best taken during or after a meal.
Prevention of hypokalaemia
- amiloride 5–10mg o.d. (see BNF 2.2.3)
- potassium chloride 2–4g daily (24–48mmol) = Slow K® 3–6 tablets or Sando-K® 2–4 tablets.

Treatment of hypokalaemia
The aim is to give 60–80mmol daily:
- Sando-K® 2 tablets t.d.s.

Supply
Sando-K® (HK Pharma 01462 433993)
***Tablets effervescent* potassium bicarbonate** and **chloride** = potassium 470mg (12mmol K^+) and chloride 285mg (8mmol Cl^-), 28 days @ 2 t.d.s. = £12.85.

Slow-K® (Alliance 01249 466966)
***Tablets m/r* potassium chloride** 600mg (8mmol K^+ and 8mmol Cl^-), 28 days @ 2 t.d.s. = £4.62.

MAGNESIUM — BNF 9.5.1.3

Class: Metal element.

Indications: hypomagnesaemia, constipation, †arrhythmia, †asthma, †eclampsia, †myocardial infarction.

Pharmacology
Magnesium is the second most abundant intracellular ion and is an essential component of numerous biochemical and physiological functions, particularly in muscle and nerve tissue. This includes all functions involving adenosine triphosphate. It also acts as an NMDA-receptor-channel blocker (see **ketamine**, p.289) which probably accounts for its analgesic effect.[1–3] Magnesium competes with calcium for absorption in the small intestine, probably by active transport. Magnesium salts are generally poorly absorbed PO and have a laxative effect. The normal serum magnesium is 0.7–1.1mmol/L. Magnesium is excreted by the kidneys, 3–12mmol/24h. Magnesium and calcium share the same transport system in the renal tubules and there is a reciprocal relationship between the amounts excreted. The minimum daily dietary requirement of magnesium is 10–20mmol.

Magnesium deficiency can result from an inadequate dietary intake, alcoholism, reduced absorption (e.g. small bowel resection, cholestasis, pancreatic insufficiency), excessive loss from the bowel (e.g. diarrhoea, stoma, fistula) or kidney (e.g. due to interstitial nephritis, acute tubular necrosis, aminoglycosides, **amphotericin**, **cisplatin**, **cyclosporin** or loop diuretic). When magnesium deficiency develops acutely, the symptoms may be obvious and severe, particularly muscle cramps, which aids diagnosis (Box 9.A). In chronic deficiency, symptoms may be insidious in onset, less severe and non-specific.

Box 9.A Symptoms and signs of magnesium deficiency and excess

Magnesium deficiency	**Magnesium excess**
Muscle	Muscle
weakness	weakness
tremor	hypotonia
twitching	loss of reflexes
cramps	Sensation of warmth (IV)
tetany (positive Chvostek's sign)	Flushing (IV)
Paraesthesia	Drowsiness
Apathy	Slurred speech
Depression	Double vision
Delirium	Delirium
Choreiform movements	Hypotension
Epileptic seizures	Cardiac arrhythmia
Prolonged QT interval	Respiratory depression
Cardiac arrhythmia	Nausea and vomiting
Increased pain(?)	Thirst
Hypomagnesaemia[a]	Hypermagnesaemia
Hypokalaemia	
Hypocalcaemia	
Hypophosphataemia	

a. not always present.

Hypermagnesaemia is rare and is seen most often in patients with renal impairment who take OTC medicines containing magnesium. Serum concentrations >4mmol/L produce drowsiness, vasodilation, slowing of atrio-ventricular conduction and hypotension. Over 6mmol/L there is profound CNS depression and muscle weakness (Box 9.A). **Calcium gluconate** IV is used to help reverse the effects of hypermagnesaemia.

When drugs such as **cisplatin** cause severe renal wasting of magnesium, hypomagnesaemia is generally present and aids diagnosis. If necessary, this can be confirmed by the high urinary excretion of magnesium. In deficiency states which develop more insidiously the serum magnesium is an insensitive guide to total body stores and hypomagnesaemia is not always present.[4] In this situation, the finding of a low urinary excretion of magnesium helps diagnosis. *Hypokalaemia not responding to supplementation (± hypocalcaemia) should also raise the possibility of magnesium deficiency.* The best method for detecting magnesium deficiency is the magnesium loading test (Box 9.B).[4–7]

Cautions

Renal failure.

Undesirable effects

For full list, see manufacturer's SPC.

Flushing, sweating and sensation of warmth IV; diarrhoea PO. Also see Box 9.A.

Dose and use

Magnesium supplements can be given IV or PO. If the cause of the magnesium deficiency persists, maintenance therapy will be required.

Box 9.B The magnesium loading test[5]

Collect pre-infusion urine sample for urinary magnesium (Mg)/creatinine (Cr) ratio mmol/L.

By IVI over 4h, give 0.1mmol/kg of magnesium, using magnesium sulphate 500mg (2mmol)/ml diluted to 50ml with 5% glucose.

Simultaneously start a 24h urine collection for magnesium and creatinine.

Calculate % magnesium retention:

$$1-\left[\frac{\text{24h urinary Mg (mmol)} - (\text{pre-infusion urinary Mg/Cr ratio (mmol/L)} \times \text{24h urinary Cr (mmol)})}{\text{dose of magnesium infused (mmol)}}\right]\times 100$$

$>$20% retention implies probable deficiency
$>$50% retention implies definite deficiency.

Prevention

- magnesium-rich foods, e.g. meat, seafood, green leafy vegetables, cereals and nuts
- potassium-sparing diuretics also preserve magnesium, e.g. **amiloride**.

Replacement

Because the degree of deficiency is difficult to determine from the serum magnesium, replacement is empirical, guided by symptoms, serum magnesium and renal function. In renal impairment, reduce doses by 50% and monitor serum magnesium daily. When there is need to replace $>$1mmol/kg of magnesium, the route of choice is IV, generally given in divided doses over 3–5 days:[8, 9]

- typically 50mmol is given on the first day, followed by 25mmol/day until the deficiency is corrected; give as 12.5–25ml of magnesium sulphate 500mg (2mmol)/ml added to 250ml 0.9% saline or 5% dextrose (equivalent to a concentration of 0.1–0.2mmol/ml) over at least 90min
- to avoid venous irritation the maximum recommended concentration for IVI is 200mg (0.8mmol)/ml
- to avoid saturating renal tubular resorption of magnesium, with resultant urinary loss, the rate of IVI should not exceed 0.6mmol/min.

Maintenance

PO is used unless poorly tolerated or ineffective, e.g. malabsorption. The main limiting factor is diarrhoea, generally seen at doses $\geqslant$40mmol/day. It may be reduced by taking magnesium with food. Suitable preparations include:

- magnesium hydroxide (Milk of Magnesia®), contains magnesium 7.1mmol/5ml
- magnesium sulphate powder (Epsom Salts) dissolved in water, contains 4mmol/1g powder
- magnesium glycerophosphate, contains magnesium 4mmol/1g tablet (unlicensed).

Supply

Magnesium glycerophosphate (4mmol elemental magnesium/1g magnesium glycerophosphate)
Tablets 1g (4mmol), 100 = £32.50. (Unlicensed, available as a named patient supply from IDIS (020 8410 0700); see Special orders and named patient supplies, p.349.)

Magnesium hydroxide (17mmol elemental magnesium/1g magnesium hydroxide)
Oral suspension magnesium hydroxide mixture BP (Cream of Magnesia) contains hydrated magnesium oxide 415mg (7.1mmol)/5ml, *do not store in a cold place*; available OTC as Milk of Magnesia®.

Magnesium sulphate (4mmol elemental magnesium/1g magnesium sulphate)
Oral powder available OTC as Epsom Salts; *an oral preparation can be prepared extemporaneously*.
Injection 500mg (2mmol)/ml, 2ml, 5ml and 10ml amp = £2.69, £2.28 and £3.05 respectively.

1 Mauskop A *et al.* (1995) Intravenous magnesium sulphate relieves migraine attacks in patients with low serum ionised magnesium levels: a pilot study. *Clinical Science*. **89**: 633–636.
2 Tramer M *et al.* (1996) Role of magnesium sulphate in postoperative analgesia. *Anesthesiology*. **84**: 340–347.

3 Crosby V *et al.* (2000) The safety and efficacy of a single dose (500mg or 1g) of intravenous magnesium sulfate in neuropathic pain poorly responsive to strong opioid analgesics in patients with cancer. *Journal of Pain and Symptom Management.* **19**: 35–39.
4 Dyckner T and Wester P (1982) Magnesium deficiency – guidelines for diagnosis and substitution therapy. *Acta Medica Scandinavica.* **661**: 37–41.
5 Ryzen E *et al.* (1985) Parenteral magnesium testing in the evaluation of magnesium deficiency. *Magnesium.* **4**: 137–147.
6 Crosby V *et al.* (2000) The importance of low magnesium in palliative care. *Palliative Medicine.* **14**: 544.
7 Crosby V (2001) Personal communication.
8 Flink E (1969) Therapy of magnesium deficiency. *Annals of the New York Academy of Science.* **162**: 901–905.
9 Miller S (1995) Drug-induced hypomagnesaemia. *Hospital Pharmacy.* **30**: 248–250.

10: MUSCULOSKELETAL AND JOINT DISEASES

Depot corticosteroid injections

Hyaluronidase

Rubifacients and other topical preparations

Skeletal muscle relaxants
Baclofen
Dantrolene sodium
Tizanidine
Quinine

DEPOT CORTICOSTEROID INJECTIONS BNF 10.1.2.2

Indications: Inflammation of joints and soft tissues, †pain in superficial bones (e.g. rib, scapula, iliac crest), †pain caused by spinal metastases.

Contra-indications: Untreated local or systemic infection.

Pharmacology

Corticosteroids have an anti-inflammatory effect, i.e. they reduce the concentration of algesic substances present in inflammation which sensitise nerve endings.[1] When injected locally, they also have a direct inhibitory effect on spontaneous activity in excitable damaged nerves.[2]

Cautions

May mask or alter presentation of infection in immunocompromised patients; such patients should not receive live vaccines and may need to take precautions if exposed to chickenpox. Depot preparations may result in symptomatic hyperglycaemia for several days in patients with diabetes mellitus and suppression of the hypothalamic-pituitary-adrenal axis for up to 4 weeks. Pneumothorax may follow injection of a rib.

Undesirable effects

For full list, see manufacturer's SPC.

Occasionally, a patient develops lipodystrophy (local fat necrosis), resulting in indentation of the overlying skin. Antagonism of antihypertensive, antidiabetic and diuretic drugs. Enhanced effect of potassium-losing drugs. Also see Corticosteroids, p.219.

Dose and use

Intralesional injection[3]

- infiltrate the skin and SC tissues overlying the point of maximal bone tenderness with local anaesthetic
- with the tip of the needle pressing against the tender bone, inject depot **methylprednisolone** 80mg in 2ml.

In addition for rib lesions, reposition the needle under the rib and inject 5ml of **bupivacaine** 0.5% to anaesthetise the intercostal nerve. Complete or good relief occurs in more than 2/3 of patients. If of benefit, injections can be repeated if the pain returns but not more than every 2 weeks.

Epidural injection[3,4]
Depot **methylprednisolone** 80mg in 2ml. A single ED injection is given, or daily for 3 days, via an indwelling cathether. The effect of ED corticosteroids is unpredictable and may not peak until 1 week after injection; some patients obtain weeks of benefit from one injection. Further injections can be given at monthly or longer intervals. Depot corticosteroids cannot be injected through an epidural bacterial filter.

Supply

Methylprednisolone acetate
Depo-Medrone® (Pharmacia 01908 661101)
Depot injection (aqueous suspension) 40mg/ml, 1ml vial = £2.87; 2ml vial = £5.15; 3ml vial = £7.47.

1 Pybus P (1984) Osteoarthritis: a new neurological method of pain control. *Medical Hypothesis*. **14**: 413–422.
2 Twycross R (1994) *Pain Relief in Advanced Cancer* (2e). Churchill Livingstone, Edinburgh.
3 Rowell NP (1988) Intralesional methylprednisolone for rib metastases: an alternative to radiotherapy? *Palliative Medicine*. **2**: 153–155.
4 Devor M *et al.* (1985) Corticosteroids reduce neuroma hyperexcitability. In: HL Fields *et al.* (eds) *Advances in Pain Research and Therapy*. Raven Press, New York, pp.451–455.

HYALURONIDASE BNF 10.3

Class: Enzyme.

Indications: To enhance diffusion of SC injections and infusions (hypodermoclysis), †inflammatory reactions caused by CSCI.

Contra-indications: Local infection or local malignancy.

Pharmacology

Hyaluronidase has a rapid temporary depolymerising action on hyaluronic acid, a mucopolysaccharide component of the intracellular matrix, thereby rendering the tissues more permeable to injected or excess fluids.[1] The natural process of repair to the intercellular matrix takes about 24h; repeat injections are therefore time-contingent (o.d. at most) and *not* related to the volume of fluid infused. *Hyaluronidase is not generally necessary when the daily SC infusion is ≤2L/24h.*[2–4]
Onset of action within minutes.
Duration of action about 24h.

Undesirable effects

For full list, see manufacturer's SPC.
Occasional allergy.

Dose and use

Hyaluronidase is not used at Hayward House or Sir Michael Sobell House.
Hypodermoclysis
1500units dissolved in 1ml WFI or 0.9% sodium chloride and administered SC *before* starting a slow infusion of 500–1000ml over 4–8h:[2]
- prime the tubing attached to the butterfly needle with hyaluronidase 0.5ml
- position the butterfly needle SC
- inject remainder of hyaluronidase (0.5ml)
- commence infusion.

Some centres inject *150*units SC before a *1h* infusion of 500ml SC (2 parts 5% dextrose and 1 part 0.9% saline).[5–7]

CSCI skin reaction

Start with hyaluronidase 1500units *as for hypodermoclysis* and repeat every 24h p.r.n.

Supply

Guidelines for the use of hyaluronidase in hypodermoclysis are available from the manufacturers.

Hyalase® (CP 01978 661261)

Injection (ovine) 1500unit amp = £7.60.

1 Menzel E and Farr C (1998) Hyaluronidase and its substrate hyaluronan: biochemistry, biological activities and therapeutic uses. *Cancer Letter.* **131**: 3–11.

2 Constans T *et al.* (1991) hypodermoclysis in dehydrated elderly patients: local effects with and without hyaluronidase. *Journal of Palliative Care.* **7**: 10–12.

3 Rochon P *et al.* (1997) A systematic review of the evidence for hypodermoclysis to treat dehydration in older people. *Journals of Gerontology. Series A, Biological sciences and medical sciences.* **52**: 169–176.

4 Bruera E *et al.* (1999) A randomized controlled trial of local injections of hyaluronidase versus placebo in cancer patients receiving subcutaneous hydration. *Annals of Oncology.* **10**: 1255–1258.

5 Bruera E *et al.* (1995) Comparison of two different concentrations of hyaluronidase in patients receiving one-hour infusions of hypodermoclysis. *Journal of Pain and Symptom Management.* **10**: 505–509.

6 Regnard C (1996) Comparison of concentrations of hyaluronidase. *Journal of Pain and Symptom Management.* **12**: 147.

7 Viola R and Scott J (1996) Comparison of concentrations of hyaluronidase. *Journal of Pain and Symptom Management.* **12**: 147–148.

RUBIFACIENTS AND OTHER TOPICAL PREPARATIONS BNF 10.3.2

Indications: Muscle, tendon and joint pains (rubifacients, topical NSAIDs), severe skin reaction to an indwelling SC cannula and/or phlebitis (kaolin poultices).

Contra-indications: Inflamed or broken skin.

Pharmacology

Rubifacients act by counter-stimulation of the skin, thereby closing the pain 'gate' in the dorsal horn of the spinal cord.[1,2] Algipan Rub® contains capsicin, glycol salicylate and methyl nicotinate. **Kaolin** poultices applied warm also act by counter-stimulation, substituting the pleasure of warmth for the stinging/burning of the skin reaction.

Topically applied **salicylates** and certain other NSAIDs can achieve high local SC concentrations and therapeutically effective concentrations within synovial fluid and peri-articular tissues similar to those seen after oral administration.[3–5] The benefit of topical **ibuprofen** has been demonstrated in a randomised controlled trial; a trial with **piroxicam** failed to show benefit.[6,7]

Onset of action immediate.

Duration of action 3–6h.

Cautions

Large quantities of topical NSAIDs have been associated with systemic effects, e.g. hypersensitivity, rash, asthma and renal impairment.[8]

Dose and use

Algipan Rub® applied b.d.–q.d.s. according to results and patient preference.
Topical NSAIDs applied b.d.–q.d.s.
Kaolin poultices generally applied b.d.
The patient should be advised to wash hands after application.

Supply

Algipan Rub® (Whitehall Laboratories 01628 669011)
***Cream* capsicin, glycol salicylate, methyl nicotinate** 40g, available OTC.

Benzydamine
Difflam® (3M 01509 611611)
Cream 3%, 100g = £6.69.

Ibuprofen
Ibugel® (Dermal 01462 458866)
Gel 5%, 100g, available OTC.
Forte gel 10%, 100g = £6.50.
Also see **ibuprofen**, p.152).

Kaolin
Kaolin Poultice K/L Pack® (K/L 01294 215951)
Poultice 4 × 100g pouches = £5.72.

1 Melzack R (1971) Phantom limb pain: implications for treatment of pathologic pain. *Anesthesiology.* **35**: 409–419.
2 Anonymous (1976) The pain paradox. *Lancet.* **i**: 945–946.
3 Mondino A *et al.* (1983) Kinetic studies of ibuprofen on humans. Comparative study for the determination of blood concentrations and metabolites following local and oral administration. *Med Welt.* **34**: 1052–1054.
4 Chlud K and Wagener H (1987) Percutaneous nonsteroidal anti-inflammatory drug (NSAID) therapy with particular reference to pharmacokinetic factors. *EULAR Bulletin.* **2**: 40–43.
5 Peters H *et al.* (1987) Percutaneous kinetics of ibuprofen (German). *Aktuelle Rheumatologie.* **12**: 208–211.
6 Kageyama T (1987) A double blind placebo controlled multicenter study of piroxicam 0.5% gel in osteoarthritis of the knee. *European Journal of Rheumatology and Inflammation.* **8**: 114–115.
7 Anonymous (1990) More topical NSAIDs: worth the rub? *Drugs and Therapeutics Bulletin.* **28**: 27–28.
8 O'Callaghan C *et al.* (1994) Renal disease and use of topical NSAIDs. *British Medical Journal.* **308**: 110–111.

SKELETAL MUSCLE RELAXANTS — BNF 10.2.2

Skeletal muscle relaxants are used to relieve painful chronic muscle spasm and CNS spasticity, e.g. in paraplegia, post-stroke, multiple sclerosis and sometimes in motor neurone disease. †**Baclofen** is also used to relieve hiccup.

Baclofen, **diazepam** and **tizanidine** act principally on spinal and supraspinal sites within the CNS; **dantrolene** and **quinine** act on muscle (Table 10.1). The use of **diazepam** as a muscle relaxant is discussed elsewhere (see pp.67 & 70).

Table 10.1 Oral drugs used to treat spasticity

Agent	*Starting dose*	*Maximum dose*	*Adverse effects*	*Monitoring*	*Precautions*
Diazepam	2mg b.d. or 5mg o.n.	60mg/day	Weakness, sedation, cognitive impairment, depression	Cumulation, prolongation of plasma halflife with cimetidine	Withdrawal syndrome
Baclofen	5mg o.d.–t.d.s.	20mg q.d.s.	Weakness, sedation, fatigue, dizziness, nausea, hepatotoxicity	Periodic LFT	Abrupt cessation is associated with seizures
Tizanidine	2–4mg o.n.	12mg t.d.s.	Drowsiness, dry mouth, dizziness, hepatotoxicity	Periodic LFT	Do not use with antihypertensives or clonidine
Dantrolene	25mg o.d.	100mg q.d.s.	Weakness, sedation, diarrhoea, hepatotoxicity	Periodic LFT	

BACLOFEN BNF 10.2.2

Class: Skeletal muscle relaxant.

Indications: Painful muscle spasm, CNS spasticity, †hiccup.

Contra-indications: Peptic ulcer.

Pharmacology

Baclofen is a chemical congener of the naturally occurring neurotransmitter, GABA (gamma-aminobutyric acid). It acts upon the GABA-receptor, inhibiting the release of excitatory amino acids glutamate and aspartate, principally at the spinal level.[1]
Bio-availability >90% PO.
Onset of action 3–4 days.
Time to peak plasma concentration 0.5–3h.
Plasma halflife 3.5h; 4.5h in the elderly.
Duration of action 6–8h.

Cautions

Withdrawal: serious adverse psychiatric reactions can occur with abrupt withdrawal (agitation, delirium, delusions, hallucinations, paranoia and psychosis). Discontinue by gradual dose reduction over 1–2 weeks, or longer if symptoms occur.[2]

History of peptic ulceration, severe psychiatric disorders, epilepsy, liver disease (monitor LFT), renal impairment (reduce dose), respiratory impairment, diabetes mellitus, hesitancy of micturition (may precipitate urinary retention), patients who use spasticity to maintain posture or to aid function. Drowsiness may affect skilled tasks/driving; effects of alcohol enhanced.

Undesirable effects

For full list, see manufacturer's SPC.
Hypotonia and sedation (increase dose slowly particularly in the elderly), euphoria, insomnia, depression, tremor, nystagmus, paraesthesias, convulsions, muscular pain and weakness, respiratory or cardiovascular depression, hypotension, dry mouth, gastro-intestinal and urinary disturbances. Rarely visual disorders, taste alterations, sweating, rash, blood glucose changes, altered liver function tests, and a paradoxical increase in spasticity.

Dose and use

Starting doses are the same for muscle spasm, spasticity and hiccup:

- start with 5mg b.d.–t.d.s., preferably p.c, and increase if necessary by 5mg b.d.–t.d.s. every 3 days
- effective doses for hiccup are often relatively low e.g. 5–10mg t.d.s. although higher doses may be necessary
- for spasticity, the effective dose is generally ≤20mg t.d.s. (maximum 100mg daily)
- effective doses for muscle spasm fall somewhere in the middle.

With spasticity, if no improvement with maximum tolerated dose after 6 weeks, withdraw gradually.

Supply

Baclofen (non-proprietary)
Tablets 10mg, 28 days @ 5mg t.d.s.= £1.53.

Lioresal® (Cephalon 0800 783 4869)
Tablets 10mg, 28 days @ 5mg t.d.s.= £5.42.
Oral solution 5mg/5ml, 28 days @ 5mg t.d.s.= £12.53.

Baclofen is also available for use in neurorehabilitation units as an intrathecal injection.

1 Kochak GM *et al.* (1985) The pharmacokinetics of baclofen derived from intestinal infusion. *Clinical Pharmacology and Therapeutics*. **38**: 251–257.
2 Anonymous (1997) Reminder: severe withdrawal reactions with baclofen. *Current Problems in Pharmacovigilance*. **23**: 3.

DANTROLENE SODIUM — BNF 10.2.2

Class: Skeletal muscle relaxant.

Indications: CNS spasticity.

Contra-indications: Hepatic impairment (may cause severe liver damage).

Pharmacology

Dantrolene acts directly on skeletal muscle reducing the amount of intracellular calcium available for contraction. It produces fewer central undesirable effects than **baclofen** and **diazepam** and, if necessary, it can be used in conjunction with them.
Bio-availability 35% PO.
Onset of action up to 1 week.
Time to peak plasma concentration up to 3h.
Plasma halflife 5–9h.
Duration of action no data.

Cautions

The dose of dantrolene must be built up slowly, not more than 25mg per week.

Undesirable effects

For full list, see manufacturer's SPC.
Transient drowsiness, dizziness, muscle weakness, diarrhoea. Rarely severe hepatotoxicity develops after 1–6 months in people over 30 years of age; fatalities have occured only with doses over 200mg/24h.[1,2]

Dose and use

- starting dose 25mg o.d.
- increased by 25mg *weekly*
- usual effective dose 75mg t.d.s.; maximum dose 100mg q.d.s.

Some centres increase the dose more rapidly because of the patient's limited prognosis.

Supply

Dantrium® (Procter & Gamble 01932 896000)
Capsules 25mg, 100mg, 28 days @ 75mg t.d.s.= £31.88.

1 Utili R *et al.* (1977) Dantrolene-associated hepatic injury. Incidence and character. *Gastroenterology*. **72**: 610–616.
2 Wilkinson S *et al.* (1979) Hepatitis from dantrolene sodium. *Gut*. **20**: 33–36.

TIZANIDINE — BNF 10.2.2

Class: Skeletal muscle relaxant.

Indications: CNS spasticity.

Contra-indications: Severe hepatic impairment.

Pharmacology

Tizanidine, like **clonidine**, is a central α_2-receptor agonist within the CNS at supraspinal and spinal levels. This results in inhibition of spinal polysynaptic reflex activity. This reduces the sympathetic outflow which in turn reduces muscle tone. Tizanidine has no direct effect on skeletal muscle, the neuromuscular junction or on monosynaptic spinal reflexes. Tizanidine reduces pathologically increased muscle tone, including resistance to passive movements, and alleviates painful spasms and clonus.[1] In spasticity, tizanidine is comparable in efficacy to **diazepam** and **baclofen**.[2] Tizanidine is well absorbed but undergoes extensive first-pass metabolism in the liver to inactive metabolites which are mostly excreted by the kidneys. Wide interpatient variability in the effective plasma concentrations means that the optimal dose must be titrated over 2–4 weeks for each patient. Maximum effects occur within 2h of administration.[3]
Bio-availability 40% PO.
Onset of action 1–2h; peak response = 8 weeks.
Time to peak plasma concentration 1.5h.
Plasma halflife 2.5h; up to 14h ± 10 in renal failure.[4]
Duration of action no data.

Cautions

Renal impairment; elderly; concurrent administration with drugs which prolong QT interval; concurrent administration with hypotensive agents or digoxin which may potentiate hypotension or bradycardia. Liver function tests should be monitored monthly for the first 4 months.

Undesirable effects

For full list, see manufacturer's SPC.
Drowsiness, weakness and dry mouth in more than 2/3 of those taking it,[5] although drowsiness and weakness may be less than with **diazepam** and **baclofen**.[6] Also reduction in blood pressure and dizziness. Less frequently insomnia, bradycardia, hallucinations and hepatotoxicity.

Dose and use

- starting dose 2mg o.d.
- increase by 2mg every 3–4 days according to response
- above 2mg, the doses should be divided and given b.d.–q.d.s.
- usual dose up to 24mg in 3–4 divided doses; maximum 36mg daily.

A slow titration helps minimise undesirable effects. Elderly patients and those with renal impairment (creatinine clearance <25ml/min) should undergo an even slower titration. Because of the prolonged plasma halflife, slow titration with a *single* daily dose is recommended by the manufacturers.

Supply

Zanaflex® (Elan 01438 765100)
Tablets 2mg, 4mg, 28 days @ 8mg t.d.s = £125.58.

1 Wallace J (1994) Summary of combined clinical analysis of controlled clinical trials with tizanidine. *Neurology*. **44**: S60–S69.
2 Lataste X *et al.* (1994) Comparative profile of tizanidine in the management of spasticity. *Neurology*. **44**: S53–S59.
3 Wagstaff A and Bryson H (1997) Tizanidine. A review of its pharmacology, clinical efficacy and tolerability in the management of spasticity associated with cerebral and spinal disorders. *Drugs*. **53**: 435–452.
4 Ohnhaus E (1986) Pharmacokinetic study with Sirdalud (tizanidine, DS 103-282) in patients with renal insufficiency.
5 Nance P *et al.* (1997) Relationship of the antispasticity effect of tizanidine to plasma concentration in patients with multiple sclerosis. *Archives of Neurology*. **54**: 731–736.

6 Smith H and Barton A (2000) Tizanidine in the management of spasticity and musculoskeletal complaints in the palliative care population. *American Journal of Hospice and Palliative Care.* **17 (1)**: 50–58.

QUININE **BNF 10.2.2**

Class: Antimalarial.

Indications: Nocturnal calf and foot cramps.

Pharmacology

Quinine reduces the amount of intracellular calcium available for muscle contraction. Controlled trials show that quinine reduces the frequency of cramps by about 25% in ambulatory patients and improves sleep,[1] but does not always reduce cramp severity.[2] However, benefit was generally less in 3 unpublished trials then in 4 published ones.[3] Maximum benefit takes up to 4 weeks. Smoking can block the effect of quinine.[4]
Bio-availability 76–88% PO.
Onset of action <1h.
Time to peak plasma concentration 1–3h PO.
Plasma halflife 8–12h.
Duration of action 4–8h.

Cautions

Quinine is very toxic in overdosage and fatalities have occurred in children.

Undesirable effects

For full list, see manufacturer's SPC.
Tinnitus, other symptoms of cinchonism (i.e. headache, hot flushed skin, nausea, abdominal pain, rashes, visual disturbances/temporary blindness, confusion), hypersensitivity reactions including angioedema, blood disorders including thrombocytopenia and DIC, acute renal failure, hypoglycaemia (unlikely with oral administration).

Dose and use

- quinine *sulphate* 200–300mg o.n.[5–7] *or* 200mg with evening meal and 100mg o.n.[5]
- quinine *bisulphate* 300mg o.n.

Stop if no benefit after 4 weeks; interrupt treatment every few months to see if quinine is still needed.

Supply

Quinine base 100mg = quinine *sulphate* 121mg or quinine *bisulphate* 169mg. Thus, quinine bisulphate 300mg contains 177mg of quinine base, and quinine sulphate 300mg contains 248mg, whereas quinine sulphate 200mg contains 165mg; *i.e. quinine bisulphate 300mg is approximately equivalent to quinine sulphate 200mg.*

Quinine sulphate (non-proprietary)
Tablets 200mg, 300mg, 28 days @ 200mg o.n. = £1.46.

Quinine bisulphate (non-proprietary)
Tablets 300mg, 28 days @ 300mg o.n. = £1.06.

1 Man-Son-Hing M and Wells G (1998) Quinine for nocturnal leg cramps. A meta-analysis including unpublished data. *Journal of General Internal Medicine.* **13**: 600–606.
2 Connolly PS *et al.* (1992) The treatment of nocturnal leg cramps: a crossover trial of quinine versus vitamin E. *Archives of Internal Medicine.* **152**: 1877–1880.
3 Anonymous (2001) Quinine for nocturnal leg cramps. *Bandolier.* **8 (6)**: 4–5.
4 Kasdon D (1986) Controversies in the surgical management of spasticity. *Clinical Neurosurgery.* **35**: 523–529.

5 Jansen P *et al.* (1997) Randomised controlled trial of hydroquinine in muscle cramps. *Lancet.* **349**: 528–532.
6 Warburton A *et al.* (1987) A quinine a day keeps the leg cramps away? *British Journal of Clinical Pharmacology.* **23**: 459–465.
7 Man-Son-Hing M and Wells G (1995) Meta-analysis of efficacy of quinine for treatment of nocturnal leg cramps in elderly people. *British Medical Journal.* **310**: 13–17.

11: EAR, NOSE AND OROPHARYNX

MOUTHWASHES — BNF 12.3.4

Mouthwashes cleanse and freshen the mouth. **Compound Sodium Chloride Mouthwash** BP is probably as beneficial as any. Mouthwashes or mouth swabs containing glycerin should *not* be used because glycerin tends to have a rebound drying effect. Mouthwashes containing an oxidising agent, such as **hydrogen peroxide** and **sodium perborate**, froth when in contact with oral debris and help to debride a heavily furred tongue. **Sodium bicarbonate mouthwash** is probably equally effective, as is gentle brushing with a child's soft toothbrush. **Ascorbic acid** (**vitamin C**) effervescent tablets can also be used for debriding the tongue (see p.253); they taste nice but are expensive. **Chlorhexidine** inhibits the formation of plaque on teeth and may be a useful adjunct to other measures for oral infection or when toothbrushing is not possible. However, **chlorhexidine** mouthwash contains alcohol and may cause rebound dryness. **Povidone-iodine** is useful for mucosal infections but does not inhibit plaque. It should not be used for more than 2 weeks because a significant amount of iodine is absorbed.

Supply and use

Teledont® (Available OTC)
Mouthwash solution-tablets (**sodium benzoate** BP, **oil of mentha** BP, **thymol** BP, **menthol** BP, **oil of cinnamon** BP, **saccharin** BP), 10 = £1.95. Dissolve in 50–60ml water and rinse mouth p.r.n.

Ascorbic acid (non-proprietary)
Tablets effervescent 1g, 10 = £1.23 (~~NHS~~). Place 1/4 of 1g tablet on the tongue and allow it to dissolve q.d.s. p.r.n.

Sodium Chloride Mouthwash, Compound BP
Mouthwash **sodium bicarbonate** 1%, **sodium chloride** 1.5% (peppermint) can be prepared extemporaneously. Dilute 15ml with equal volume of warm water.

Chlorhexidine gluconate (non-proprietary)
Mouthwash 0.2%, 300ml (original, aniseed or mint) = £1.93. Rinse the mouth with 10ml for 1min b.d.

Corsodyl® (GSK Consumer Health 020 8560 5151)
Mouthwash 0.2%, 300ml (original or mint) = £1.93; 600ml (mint) = £3.85. Rinse the mouth with 10ml for 1min b.d.
Oral spray 0.2%, 60ml (mint) = £4.10. Apply b.d. to tooth and gingival surfaces (maximum of 12 actuations b.d.).
Dental gel 1%, 50g = £1.21. Brush on teeth b.d.

Hexetidine
Oraldene® (Parke Davis 023 8062 0500)
Mouthwash or gargle 0.1%, 100ml = £1.31; 200ml = £2.02. Use 15ml undiluted b.d.–t.d.s.

ARTIFICIAL SALIVA BNF 12.3.5

Artificial salivas help to provide relief of dry mouth. They should be used only in conjunction with standard oral hygiene and mouth care. Patients should be encouraged to adopt helpful strategies such as sucking boiled sweets and sipping ice-cooled drinks.[1] The proportion of patients prescribed an artificial saliva varies widely between palliative care services.

Ideally artificial saliva should be of a neutral pH and contain electrolytes (including fluoride) to correspond approximately to the composition of saliva. Proprietary artificial salivas available in the UK include:

- pastilles containing acacia, malic acid etc. (Salivix®)
- porcine gastric mucin spray and lozenges (AS Saliva Orthana®)
- carmellose-based sprays (Glandosane®, Luborant®, Salivace®, Saliveze®)
- hydroxyethylcellulose-based gel (Oralbalance®); contains salivary peroxidase which enhances the production of hypothiocyanite, an antibacterial ion.

Luborant is licensed for any condition giving rise to a dry mouth; AS Saliva Orthana®, Salivace®, Saliveze®, Glandosane®, Oralbalance® and Salivix® pastilles have approval for dry mouth associated with radiotherapy or sicca syndrome. AS Saliva Orthana® has a sorbitol base which is cooling to taste. Artificial salivas are generally used frequently, including before and during meals. Studies suggest that mucin-based preparations are less sticky but, paradoxically, remain in the mouth for longer and need to be taken less often.[2,3] Many patients find no additional benefit with carmellose-based preparations compared with frequent tea, coffee, milk or fruit juice.

Supply and use

Salivix® (Provalis 01244 288888)
Pastilles (sugar-free) **acacia, malic acid**, etc. 50 = £2.86. Use p.r.n.

AS Saliva Orthana® (AS Pharma 01908 371025)
Lozenges **mucin** 65mg, **xylitol** 59mg in **sorbitol**, 45 = £3.03. Use p.r.n.
Oral spray gastric **mucin** 3.5%, **xylitol** 2%, **sodium fluoride** 4.2mg/ml, 50ml = £3.95; 450ml refill = £23.47. Apply 2–3 sprays p.r.n.

Luborant® (Antigen 01704 562777)
Oral spray **sorbitol** 1.8g and **carmellose sodium** 390mg in 60ml, 60ml unit = £3.96. Apply 2–3 sprays q.d.s. p.r.n. (*NB: may be difficult to obtain.*)

Oralbalance® (Anglian 01438 743070)
Saliva replacement gel **lactoperoxidase, glucose oxidase** and **xylitol** in gel, 50g tube = £3.69. Apply p.r.n.

Biotene® (Anglian 01438 743070)
Mouthwash and ***toothpaste*** (Unlicensed, available as named patient items from Anglian; see Special orders and named patient supplies, p.349.) Also available with the saliva replacement gel as a total package for dry mouth (Oralbalance® system).

1 Twycross R and Wilcock A (2001) *Symptom Management in Advanced Cancer* (3e). Radcliffe Medical Press, Oxford.
2 S'Gravenmade E *et al.* (1974) The effect of mucin-containing artificial saliva on severe xerostomia. *International Journal of Oral Surgery*. **3**: 435–439.
3 Vissink A *et al.* (1983) A clinical comparison between commercially available mucin- and CMC-containing saliva substitutes. *International Journal of Oral Surgery*. **12**: 232–238.

PILOCARPINE BNF 12.3.5

Class: Parasympathomimetic.

Indications: Xerostomia (dry mouth) after radiation for head and neck cancer, dry mouth (and dry eyes) in Sjogren's syndrome and †drug-induced dry mouth.

Contra-indications: Intestinal obstruction, uncontrolled asthma and COPD, narrow-angle glaucoma.

Pharmacology

Pilocarpine is a parasympathomimetic (predominantly muscarinic) with mild β-adrenergic activity which stimulates secretion from exocrine glands, including salivary glands.[1] Most patients with drug-induced dry mouth respond to pilocarpine immediately if they are going to respond, whereas after head and neck radiation the response may be delayed for 4–12 weeks. The response rate is about 90% for drug-induced dry mouth but only about 50% after radiation.[2] In a controlled study, 1/2 of the patients preferred pilocarpine and 1/2 preferred **artificial saliva** (mainly because it was a spray and not a tablet).[2] Undesirable effects were much more common in patients receiving pilocarpine (84% vs 22%), which resulted in 1/4 of the patients withdrawing from the study. **Bethanechol** is used instead of pilocarpine at some centres.[3,4]
Bio-availability 96% PO.
Onset of action 20min (drug-induced dry mouth); up to 3 months (after radiation).
Time to peak plasma concentration no data.
Plasma halflife 1h.
Duration of action 3–5h.

Undesirable effects

For full list, see manufacturer's SPC.
Sweating, dizziness, rhinitis, urinary frequency, diarrhoea, nausea, vomiting, intestinal colic, blurred vision, excess salivation, increased bronchial secretions and increased airway resistance.[2]

Dose and use

In drug-induced dry mouth the effective dose is generally 5mg t.d.s. or less, whereas after radiation the effective dose is generally 5–10mg t.d.s.:

- start with 5mg t.d.s with meals
- if tolerated but response not sufficient, increase the dose after 2 days (if drug-induced) and after 1 week (if radiation-induced)
- maximum dose 10mg t.d.s.
- if no improvement, stop after 2 days (drug-induced) and after 2 weeks (radiation-induced).

It is much cheaper to give pilocarpine eyedrops PO than to prescribe tablets, e.g. pilocarpine 4% 2–3 drops t.d.s. in raspberry syrup or peppermint water = 4–6mg. Maximum cost/month = £5, whereas tablets would cost over £50.

If **bethanechol** is used instead for drug-induced dry mouth:

- start with 10mg t.d.s. with meals
- increase after 2 days to 25mg t.d.s. if initial response poor.

Undesirable effects are comparable to pilocarpine but generally less, either because the equivalent dose is less or the muscarinic receptor binding pattern of **bethanechol** is different.

Supply

Salagen® (Novartis Opthalmics 01276 692255)
Tablets 5mg, 28 days @ 5mg t.d.s.= £51.43.

Oral solution can be prepared extemporaneously by diluting pilocarpine eyedrops (Anon).
Eyedrops 4% (40mg/1ml), 10ml = £1.57.

1 Anonymous (1994) Oral pilocarpine for xerostomia. *Medical Letter on Drugs and Therapeutics*. **36**: 76.

2 Davies A *et al.* (1998) A comparison of artificial saliva and pilocarpine in the management of xerostomia in patients with advanced cancer. *Palliative Medicine*. **12**: 105–111.

3 Epstein J *et al.* (1994) A clinical trial of bethanechol in patients with xerostomia after radiation therapy. A pilot study. *Oral Surgery, Oral Medicine and Oral Pathology*. **77**: 610–614.

4 Everett H (1975) The use of bethanechol chloride with tricyclic antidepressants. *American Journal of Psychiatry*. **132**: 1202–1204.

DRUGS FOR ORAL INFLAMMATION AND ULCERATION BNF 12.3.1

'Stomatitis' is a general term applied to diffuse inflammatory, erosive and ulcerative conditions affecting the mucous membranes of the mouth. Use of the term 'mucositis' tends to be restricted to stomatitis caused by chemotherapy or local radiotherapy. The causes of ulceration of the oral mucosa include trauma, recurrent aphthous ulcers, infection, cancer, and nutritional deficiencies. It is important to determine the cause so that, if appropriate, specific as well as symptomatic treatment is given. For example, teeth and dentures should be checked, and ill-fitting dentures relined. Oral mucositis associated with radiation therapy or chemotherapy is the commonest severe cause of oral inflammation and ulceration in patients with malignant disease.[1] Mouth care before, during and after treatment reduces the severity of mucositis.[2]

Management strategy

In addition to prophylactic measures and disease-specific treatment, a range of options are available.[3] Aphthous ulcers are caused by auto-immunity and opportunistic infection and often respond to topical corticosteroids and/or topical antibiotics (Box 11.A).

Box 11.A Treatment of aphthous ulcers[4]

Antiseptic and antibiotic mouthwashes

Useful when ulcers affect a wide range of oral sites not accessible to covering pastes:

- chlorhexidine gluconate 0.2% mouthwash (Corsodyl®); rinse the mouth with 10ml tetracycline suspension 250mg t.d.s. for 3 days; prepared by mixing the contents of a capsule with a small quantity of water; hold in the mouth for 3min and then spit out.

Corticosteroids

Corticosteroids are useful for recurrent attacks:

- hydrocortisone lozenges 2.5mg 1 q.d.s. for up to 5 days; lozenges are placed at the site of the ulcers and left to dissolve
- triamcinolone 0.1% dental paste (Adcortyl in Orabase®) b.d.–q.d.s. for up to 5 days; smear a thin layer onto the ulcers
- nasal aerosols sprayed into the mouth, when a more potent corticosteroid is needed for sites such as the soft palate and oropharynx, e.g. budesonide (100microgram/metered spray), triamcinolone acetonide (Nasacort®, 55microgram/metered spray)
- hydrocortisone and lidocaine (lignocaine) mouthwash when ulcers are widespread.

Cytoprotective agents

These act either by increasing mucin production (**carbenoxolone**) or by adhering to and coating the raw surface (**carmellose, sucralfate**). The latter can be difficult to apply effectively:

- **carbenoxolone sodium** (Bioral gel®, Bioplex® granules), dissolve granules 2g in 30–50ml of warm water and use q.d.s. as a mouthwash
- **carmellose sodium** (Orabase® protective paste, Orahesive® powder), apply the paste to or sprinkle the powder on the sore area p.c.
- although **sucralfate** is *not* of benefit in chemotherapy or radiation-induced mucositis,[5,6] it may be of benefit in less severe stomatitis; it can be given as a suspension 1g/5ml q.d.s.

Topical analgesics

Topical analgesics have a definite but limited role in the management of painful oral ulceration, including radiation and chemotherapy mucositis. When applied topically their action is of relatively short duration; pain relief cannot be maintained continuously throughout the day.

Benzydamine mouthwash or spray eases the discomfort associated with various causes of sore mouth, including radiation. **Choline salicylate** dental gel provides similar relief, but excessive application or confinement under a denture irritates the mucosa and can cause ulceration.

- **choline salicylate** 8.7% oral gel (Bonjela®), 1–2cm q3h p.r.n.

- **benzydamine** 0.15% oral rinse (Difflam®), a NSAID and a mild local anaesthetic, 15ml q1h p.r.n.; dilute if causes stinging.[7]

Other options include:

- **flurbiprofen** lozenge, 8.75mg q4h p.r.n.
- **diclofenac** dispersible tablets, 50mg t.d.s.; swish around the mouth for 5min before swallowing
- **diphenhydramine** mouthwash (Box 11.B).

Box 11.B The use of diphenhydramine hydrochloride for oral mucositis[8]

Diphenhydramine is an antihistamine with a topical analgesic effect (*not* readily available in the UK). It is generally given as a locally-prepared compound mouthwash.

Proprietary solutions of diphenhydramine (USA) contain alcohol 5–14%; *use solutions with a low alcohol content* to avoid causing additional discomfort.

Formulations include:

- diphenhydramine hydrochloride (25mg/5ml) and magnesium hydroxide in equal parts
- diphenhydramine in kaopectate (equal parts of diphenhydramine elixir 12.5mg/5ml and kaopectate); the pectin in the kaopectate helps the diphenhydramine adhere to inflamed/ulcerated mucosa
- stomatitis cocktail, National Cancer Institute, USA (equal parts of lidocaine (lignocaine) viscous 2%, diphenhydramine elixir 12.5mg/5ml and Maalox®, a proprietary antacid).

Use up to 30ml q2h. Spread around the mouth with the tongue and then swallow or spit out after 2–3min.

Local anaesthetics

With all topical local anaesthetic preparations care must be taken not to produce anaesthesia of the pharynx before meals as this might lead to aspiration and choking:

- **lidocaine** gel 2% (Instillagel®), applied a.c. & p.r.n.
- **cocaine hydrochloride** 2% solution prepared extemporaneously 10ml (200mg) q4h p.r.n.; swish around the mouth for several minutes and then spit out (swallowing 200mg of **cocaine** could lead to agitation and hallucinations)
  *Warning: if **cocaine** is combined with **sodium bicarbonate**, the systemic absorption of cocaine is increased 10-fold*

Topical morphine sulphate

- extemporaneous **morphine** gel (1mg/ml), initially 3ml q8h–q4h; hold in mouth for 10min and then swallow
- **morphine** solutions, Sevredol® is preferable to Oramorph® because it is alcohol-free, take 10mg (5ml) q4h, use as a mouthwash and then swallow.

Systemic analgesics

Non-opioids and opioids should be given as for other pains, balancing benefit against undesirable effects. For severe mucositis (patient unable to eat ± unable to drink) inadequately relieved by topical measures, a parenteral opioid should be administered, e.g. **morphine**. Chemotherapy patients often have a permanent IV access, e.g. Hickman line, and this can be used for patient-controlled analgesia (PCA).[9] In other patients, and in palliative care generally, CSCI is likely to be more convenient. Some patients have benefited from short-term ('burst') treatment with **ketamine** (see Box 13.A, p.291).

Immunomodulation

*†**Thalidomide** (an immunomodulator) 100mg o.d. or b.d. for 10 days is sometimes used in resistant cases of mouth ulceration in patients with AIDS. It is unlicensed because it causes severe congenital abnormalities (absent or shortened limbs) and irreversible peripheral neuropathy. *The use of thalidomide is best limited to centres with the necessary expertise.*

Supply

Orabase® (ConvaTec 01895 628400)
Oral paste **carmellose sodium** 16.7%, **pectin** 16.7% and **gelatin** 16.7%, 30g = £1.84; 100g = £4.10. Apply a thin layer after meals p.r.n.

Orahesive® (ConvaTec 01895 628400)
Powder **carmellose**, **pectin** and **gelatin**, equal parts, 25g = £2.09. Sprinkle on the affected area.

Carbenoxolone
Bioral Gel® (Seven Seas 01482 375234)
Gel 2% in adhesive base, 5g = £2.30. Apply p.c. and o.n.

Bioplex® (Provalis 01244 288888)
Mouthwash granules 1% 20mg/sachet, 24 = £7.23. Dissolve contents of sachet in 30–50ml of warm water and rinse mouth p.c. and o.n.

Triamcinolone acetonide
Adcortyl in Orabase® (Squibb 020 8572 7422)
Oral paste 0.1% in adhesive base, 10g = £1.27. Apply a thin layer to the ulcers b.d.–q.d.s.

Hydrocortisone
Corlan® (Celltech 01753 534655)
Pellets (lozenges) 2.5mg, 20 = £2.10. Dissolve 1 lozenge q.d.s. slowly in the mouth in contact with an ulcer for up to 5 days; if necessary, continue treatment b.d. for 2–3 weeks.

Benzydamine
Difflam® (3M 01509 611611)
Oral rinse 0.15%, 300ml = £3.92. Rinse or gargle 15ml every 1.5–3h p.r.n. for up to 7 days. If the full strength mouthwash stings, dilute with an equal volume of water.
Spray 0.15%, 30ml unit = £3.41. 4–8 sprays to affected area every 1.5–3h.

Choline salicylate
Bonjela® (Reckitt Benckiser 01482 326151)
Oral gel (sugar-free) 8.7%, 15g = £1.70. Apply 1cm of gel with gentle massage q3h p.r.n. (maximum 6 applications daily).

Dinnefords Teejel® (SSL 01565 624000)
Oral gel 8.7%, 10g = £1.36. Apply 1cm of gel with gentle massage q3h p.r.n. (maximum 6 applications daily).

Flurbiprofen
Strefen® (Crookes 0115 968 8922)
Lozenges 8.75mg, 16 = £2.00. Allow 1 lozenge to dissolve in the mouth q3–6h, maximum of 5 lozenges/24h, for maximum of 3 days.

Cocaine hydrochloride
Oral solution 2% can be prepared extemporaneously.

Morphine
Oral gel 0.1% (1mg/ml) can be prepared extemporaneously.

---

1 Wilkes J (1998) Prevention and treatment of oral mucositis following cancer chemotherapy. *Seminars in Oncology.* **25**: 535–551.
2 Larson P *et al.* (1998) The PRO-SELF mouth aware program: an effective approach for reducing chemotherapy-induced mucositis. *Cancer Nursing.* **21**: 263–268.
3 Turhal N *et al.* (2000) Efficacy of treatment to relieve mucositis-induced discomfort. *Supportive Care in Cancer.* **8**: 55–58.
4 Odell E *et al.* (2000) Comprehensive review of treatment for recurrent aphthous stomatitis. URL http://www.umds.ac.uk/dental/opath/daphtrt1.htm and daphtrt2.htm: 1-10
5 Loprinzi C *et al.* (1997) Phase III controlled evaluation of sucralfate to alleviate stomatitis in patients receiving fluorouracil-based chemotherapy. *Journal of Clinical Oncology.* **15**: 1235–1238.
6 Meredith R *et al.* (1997) Sucralfate for radiation mucositis: results of a double-blind randomized trial. *International Journal of Radiation, Oncology, Biology and Physics.* **37**: 275–279.

7 Kim J *et al.* (1985) A clinical study of benzydamine for the treatment of radiotherapy induced mucositis of the orpharynx. *International Journal of Tissue Reaction.* **7**: 215–218.
8 NIH Consensus Development Conference Statement (1989) Oral complications of cancer therapies, prevention and treatment. *NIH Consensus Statement.* **7**: 1–11.
9 Coda B *et al.* (1997) Comparative efficacy of patient-controlled administration of morphine, hydromorphone, or sufentanil for the treatment of oral mucositis pain following marrow transplantation. *Pain.* **72**: 333–346.

CERUMENOLYTICS BNF 12.1.3

Indications: Impacted ear wax (cerumen).

Pharmacology

Ear wax is secreted to provide a protective film on the skin of the external auditory meatus. Keratin is a major constituent of ear wax. Disintegration is facilitated by keratin cell hydration and lysis. Keratolysis is optimal in aqueous solutions. In one study, water and **docusate** 0.5% (Waxsol®) were more effective than **sodium bicarbonate** 5% BP[1] whereas, in a second study, **sodium bicarbonate** 5% and 10% acted more quickly than both water alone and **hydrogen peroxide** (1.5h compared with 3h and 18h at 37°C).[2] In contrast, organic-based OTC preparations had no effect or took ⩾1 week to bring about disintegration and should therefore not be used. Cerumol® (**chlorobutanol** 5%, **paradichlorobenzene** 2%, **arachis oil** 57%) causes meatal irritation, as does **docusate** in high concentrations, i.e. 5%,[1] and are not recommended.

Dose and use

Ear wax should be removed only if it causes deafness or prevents examination of the ear drum. Wax may be removed by syringing with warm water. If necessary soften first with water or **sodium bicarbonate** 5% BP; tap water is more convenient and costs nothing. Aqueous preparations are truly cerumenolytic and 'liquefy' ear wax. Use over several days might obviate the need for syringing. However, syringing is likely to be necessary to remove a firmly impacted plug of ear wax:

- lie the patient down with the affected ear uppermost
- instil a few drops of tap water 15–30min before syringing
- if syringing is unsuccessful, instil water or **docusate** 0.5% or **sodium bicarbonate** ear drops BP b.d. for 3 days, and then repeat syringing.

Some centres use Otex® (**urea-hydrogen peroxide** 5% in **glycerol**) once weekly to prevent recurrent wax impaction, and to obviate the need for further syringing.[3,4]

Supply

Tap water
Ear drops 1ml = £0.00.

Sodium bicarbonate (non-proprietary)
Ear drops 5% 10ml = £1.18.

Docusate sodium
Waxsol® (Norgine 01895 826600)
Ear drops 0.5% 10ml = £1.24.

Urea-hydrogen peroxide
Otex® (DDD 01923 229251)
Ear drops 5% 8ml = £2.64.

1 Bellini M *et al.* (1989) An evaluation of common cerumenolytic agents: an in-vitro study. *Clinical Otolaryngology.* **14**: 23–25.
2 Robinson A and Hawke M (1989) The efficacy of cerumenolytics: everything old is new again. *Journal of Otolaryngology.* **18**: 263–267.

3 Fahmy S and Whitefield M (1982) Multicentre clinical trial of exterol as a cerumenolytic. *British Journal of Clinical Practice*. **36**: 197–204.
4 Freeland A (2001) Personal communication.

12: SKIN

Emollients

Topical antipruritics

Barrier preparations

Topical cleansing agents and disinfectants

EMOLLIENTS — BNF 13.2

Indications: Dry or rough skin.

Pharmacology

Emollients soothe, smooth and hydrate the skin and are indicated for all causes of dry flaky skin (Box 12.A). The essential component is oil (Table 12.1) Some ingredients occasionally cause sensitisation and this should be suspected if the treated area becomes inflamed (allergic dermatitis). Benefit is relatively short-lasting and, depending on the condition of the skin, application may be necessary several times daily. Soap should not be used because it dries the skin. **Aqueous Cream** BP can be used as a soap substitute, and an emollient bath additive can be used when bathing. Topical creams and ointments can cause folliculitis if massaged into the hair follicles; the likelihood of this is reduced by massaging in the direction of hair growth.

Box 12.A Topical applications

Ointments	**Creams**	**Lotions**
Grease-based	Oil-in-water (aqueous) or water-in-oil (oily) emulsions	Solutions, suspensions or emulsions where water evaporates to leave a thin coating of powder
Most hydrating	Less hydrating	Least hydrating; cools as it evaporates
Messy to apply; difficult if skin very hairy	Massage well into skin; cosmetically more acceptable	Shake well before use; apply to the skin without friction

Dose and use

General

A simple preparation such as **Aqueous Cream** BP (containing emulsifying ointment 30%) is generally as effective as more complex proprietary formulations. Diprobase® cream and Oilatum® cream are paraffin-based; they are more convenient to use but more expensive. Apply up to q.d.s.; long-term treatment o.d.–b.d. often advisable (Table 12.2).

Lymphoedema

The choice of emollient depends mainly on the state of the skin (Figure 12.1).

For areas resistant to treatment, consider applying LP/WSP 50/50 and covering with a hydrocolloid dressing (Comfeel®, Granuflex®) for 2 days and then soak, etc. (see footnote c above). Avoid emollients which:

- contain lanolin/wool fat or are strongly scented (can cause allergic dermatitis)
- are expensive, e.g. E45® cream (contains hypo-allergenic lanolin; 500g = £5.61, compared with aqueous cream = £1.10).

Table 12.1 Composition of selected emollients: least oily to most oily

	Preservative	*Perfume*	*Lanolin (wool fat)*
Lotion			
Keri® lotion	+	+	+
Light creams			
Aveeno®	–	–	–
Aqueous BP	+	–	–
Diprobase®	+	–	–
Hydromol®	+	–	–
E45®	+	–	+
Ultrabase®	+	+	–
Oilatum®	+	+	+
Rich creams (more oily)			
Aquadrate®	–	–	–
Unguentum M®	+	–	–
Lipobase®	+	–	–
Hydrous Ointment BP	+	–	+
Ointments (most oily)			
White Soft Paraffin BP	–	–	–
Liquid and White Soft Paraffin BP	–	–	–
Coconut Oil BP	–	–	–
Diprobase®	–	–	–

Table 12.2 Quantities required for b.d. application for 1 week

	Creams and ointments	*Lotions*
Face Groins and genitalia	15–30g	100ml
Both hands	25–50g	200ml
Scalp	50–100g	200ml
Both arms or both legs	100–200g	200ml
Trunk	400g	500ml

For other measures for hyperkeratotic skin, see *Symptom Management in Advanced Cancer.*[1]

Antipruritic emollients

If pruritus is caused by the dry skin, rehydration of the skin will correct it. Thus, all emollients are antipruritic in this sense. Preparations which have more specific antipruritic properties include:

- **aqueous cream + menthol** 1–2%
- **colloidal oatmeal cream** (Aveeno®); popular with children.

Crotamiton 10% (Eurax®) lotion or cream is not antipruritic,[2] and should be used only as a mild topical antiscabetic agent.

Supply

Aqueous Cream BP (non-proprietary)

Cream 100g = 21p. (**Menthol** 1–2% can be added to aqueous cream extemporaneously to enhance its antipruritic effect.)

Colloidal oatmeal

Aveeno® (Bioglan 01462 438444)

Cream 100ml = £3.78.

Lotion 400ml = £6.02.

Both are classified in the UK as a borderline substance.

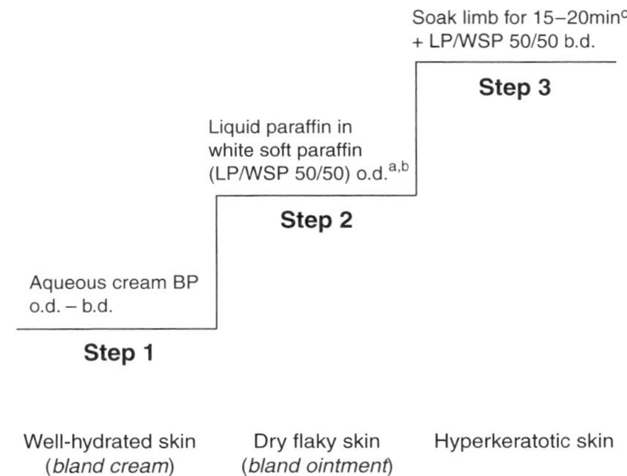

Figure 12.1 Emollients in lymphoedema.

a. ointments are generally not necessary for more than a few days
b. some people prefer Coconut Oil BP because it has a skin-cooling effect. Use the plain variety; added fragrance can cause allergic dermatitis
c. after soaking in a bucket of warm water (to which 15–20ml of LP/WSP 50/50 has been added) and after drying the limb, apply LP/WSP 50/50 using a circular motion; this tends to lift off hyperkeratotic skin.

Paraffin, White Soft BP (non-proprietary)
Ointment white petroleum jelly, 100g = 32p.

Liquid and White Soft Paraffin Ointment (Bell 0151 424 8352)
Ointment liquid paraffin 50%, white soft paraffin 50%, 250g = £0.88; 500g = £1.75.

Bath additives
Balneum® (Crookes 0115 968 8922)
Contains **soya**, 200ml = £2.79; 500ml = £6.06; 1000ml = £11.70.

Oilatum® (Stiefel 01628 524966)
Contains **liquid paraffin** and **wool alcohols**; 250ml = £2.75; 500ml = £4.57.

1 Twycross R and Wilcock A (2001) *Symptom Management in Advanced Cancer* (3e). Radcliffe Medical Press, Oxford.
2 Smith E *et al.* (1984) Crotamiton lotion in pruritus. *International Journal of Dermatology*. **23**: 684–685.

TOPICAL ANTIPRURITICS — BNF 13.3

Indications: Pruritus.

Management strategy

Because pruritus is often associated with dry skin, an emollient (moisturiser) should be tried first. Many proprietary emollients are available but **Aqueous Cream** BP is usually adequate when applied o.d.–b.d. **Menthol** or **phenol** 1–2% can be added extemporaneously on a trial basis if aqueous cream alone is inadequate; both agents are known to have topical antipruritic properties.

In the USA, a veterinary agent, Bag Balm Antiseptic Salve is sometimes used; it is relatively cheap and comprises hydroxyquinoline 0.3% in a petroleum-lanolin base (www.bagbalm.com).

Crotamiton

This is marketed in a 10% cream as Eurax®. It has a mild antiscabetic effect and it is probably this that is responsible for its reputation as an antipruritic. However, in a controlled trial, crotamiton was no more effective than plain aqueous cream,[1] and therefore is not recommended.

Antihistamines

Several topical H_1-antihistamines are available, e.g. **mepyramine** and **diphenhydramine**. The former can cause contact dermatitis and its use is best limited to a few days. Generally available OTC.

Calamine

Calamine lotion (cutaneous suspension) contains **phenol** 0.5%. Its antipruritic effect can be enhanced by the extemporaneous addition of a further 0.5%. However, as the water evaporates, a lotion has a drying effect which is counterproductive.

Alternative calamine preparations are an oily lotion and an aqueous cream. The former contains **arachis** (peanut) **oil** and **lanolin** (wool fat) and the latter **liquid paraffin**; these additives circumvent the problem of drying. However, the pink colour of calamine is cosmetically unacceptable to most people.

Local anaesthetics

Several preparations contain a local anaesthetic. **Benzocaine** and **lidocaine** (lignocaine) are the commonest but some preparations contain **tetracaine** (amethocaine). Apart from **lidocaine**, local anaesthetics can cause contact dermatitis. They are absorbed to a variable extent. Use is best restricted to a few days. All of these products are available OTC.

In pruritus in uraemia, the regular use of Balneum Plus®, a bath oil containing **polidocanol** (mixed lauromacrogols), a non-ionic surfactant with local anaesthetic properties, improves dry skin, reducing pruritus and sleep disturbance.[2] A cream containing **urea** 5% and **polidocanol** 3% (E45® Itch Relief Cream) has been used in dermatitis (atopic and non-atopic) and psoriasis with 90% of patients reporting improvement in the condition of their skin and 50% becoming pruritus-free.[3–5]

Capsaicin

Capsaicin, isolated from pepper plants of the genus *Capsicum,* depletes substance P from C-fibres when applied repeatedly and reduces both pain and pruritus. **Capsaicin** cream 0.025–0.075% is applied 3–5 times daily. Patients should avoid taking a hot shower/bath before application, and should apply the cream using gentle massage, avoiding contact with mucous membranes, eyes and broken/inflamed skin. For the first few days **capsaicin** cream causes a local burning sensation which is poorly tolerated. It has been shown to be effective in itch caused by notalgia paraesthetica and localised pruritus in uraemia.[6]

Strontium nitrate

Topical **strontium nitrate** 10–20% possesses potent antipruritic properties and is effective in reducing pruritus associated with facial peels.[7–9] It acts possibly by selectively blocking neuronal transmission in C-fibres. Commercial preparations are not available.

Supply

Calamine (non-proprietary)
Aqueous cream 4%, 100ml = £0.65.
Lotion (cutaneous suspension) 15%, 200ml = £0.64 (contains **phenol** 0.5%).
Oily lotion 5%, 200ml = £1.06 (contains **arachis** (peanut) **oil**).

E45® Itch Relief Cream (Crookes 0115 968 8922)
Cream **urea** 5%, **polidocanol** 3%, 50g = £2.10.

Capsaicin
Axsain® (Elan 01438 765100)
Cream 0.075%, 45g = £15.04.

Zacin® (Elan 01438 765100)
Cream 0.025%, 45g = £15.04.

Bath additives
Balneum Plus® (Crookes 0115 968 8922)
Contains **soya** and **lauromacrogols**, 500ml = £7.50.

1 Smith E *et al.* (1984) Crotamiton lotion in pruritus. *International Journal of Dermatology.* **23**: 684–685.
2 Wasik F *et al.* (1996) Relief of uraemic pruritus after balneological therapy with a bath oil containing polidocanol (Balneum Hermal Plus). An open clinical study. *Journal of Dermatology Treatment.* **7**: 231–233.
3 Vieluf D *et al.* (1992) Dry and itching skin – therapy with a new preparation, containing urea and polidocanol. *Zeitschrift fur Hautkrankheiten.* **67**: 816–821.
4 Hauss H *et al.* (1993) Comparative study of a formulation containing urea and polidocanol and a greasy cream containing linoleic acid in the treatment of dry, pruritic skin lesions. *Dermatosen.* **41**: 184–188.
5 Freitag G and Hoppner T (1997) Results of a postmarketing drug monitoring survey with a polidocanol-urea preparation for dry, itching skin. *Current Medical Research Opinions.* **13**: 529–537.
6 Breneman D *et al.* (1992) Topical capsaicin for treatment of hemodialysis-related pruritus. *Journal of the American Academy of Dermatology.* **26**: 91–94.
7 Hahn G (1999) Strontium is a potent and selective inhibitor of sensory irritation. *Dermatology and Surgery.* **25**: 689–694.
8 Zhai H *et al.* (2000) Strontium nitrate decreased histamine-induced itch magnitude and duration in man. *Dermatology.* **200**: 244–246.
9 Zhai H *et al.* (2000) Strontium nitrate suppresses chemically-induced sensory irritation in humans. *Contact Dermatitis.* **42**: 98–100.

BARRIER PREPARATIONS BNF 13.2.2

Indications: Skin protection, napkin rash.

Pharmacology

Barrier preparations contain water-repellent substances which help to protect the skin. They can be used around stomas, and in the perineum and peri-anal areas in patients with urinary or faecal incontinence. Traditional formulations include **compound zinc ointments**. Morhulin® ointment (38% zinc oxide in cod-liver oil, wool fat and paraffin) is the barrier preparation of choice at Sir Michael Sobell House. A cream is less sticky and is sometimes preferable, e.g. Drapolene® (benzalkonium 0.01% and cetrimide 0.2% in white soft paraffin, cetyl alcohol and lanolin/wool fat). Some proprietary formulations include **dimeticone**, e.g. Siopel® (dimeticone 10%, cetrimide 0.3%, arachis/peanut oil) or other water-repellent silicone.

Cautions

It is important to ensure any signs of infection are treated promptly with antibiotics.

Dose and use

Protection around the stoma

The stomatherapists in Oxford use Comfeel® barrier cream prophylactically if the stoma effluent is liquid or if the appliance/flange is being changed more than o.d. It is gently rubbed in and any excess wiped off. If the skin becomes red and sore, Cavilon No-Sting Barrier Film® is used instead.

Incontinence

After cleansing and gentle drying, apply a barrier cream or ointment to the affected area whenever the dressing or padding is changed.

Supply

Morhulin® (Thornton & Ross 01484 842217)
Ointment 50g = £1.46.

Drapolene® (Parke-Davis 023 8062 0500)
Cream 100g = £1.37; 200g = £2.23; 350g = £3.66.

Siopel® (Bioglan 01426 438444)
Cream 50g = £0.86.

Comfeel® (Coloplast 01733 392000)
Barrier cream 60g = £4.23.

Cavilon No-Sting Barrier Film® (3M 01509 611611).
Foam applicator 5 × 1ml = £4.55; 5 × 3ml = £7.30.
Pump spray 28ml = £6.09.

TOPICAL CLEANSING AGENTS AND DISINFECTANTS — BNF 13.11

Indications: Cleansing skin and wounds.

Pharmacology

Antiseptics are used less often than in the past because many of them have undesirable effects (Table 12.3). **Sodium chloride solution** 0.9% (normal saline) is suitable for general cleansing of skin and wounds (or tap water if safe to drink). Useful disinfectants include **benzalkonium chloride, cetrimide** (also has detergent properties), **chlorhexidine** and **potassium permanganate solution** (1 in 10 000). **Povidone-iodine** is preferred to chlorinated solutions (e.g. dilute sodium hypochlorite solution) which are irritant. Astringent preparations, such as **potassium permanganate** solution are useful for oozing eczematous reactions. Because of a risk of carcinogenesis, **gentian violet** (**crystal violet**) and Bonney's blue (**brilliant green** and **crystal violet**) are available only on a named patient basis for marking skin before an operation.

Supply

Sodium chloride
Normasol® (SSL 01565 624000)
Solution 0.9% (*sterile*), 25 x 25ml sachet = £5.85.

Chlorhexidine (Baxter 01842 767189)
2000 solution (*pink*), 0.05%, 1L = £0.77.

Povidone-iodine
Betadine® (SSL 01565 624000)
Antiseptic solution 10%, 500ml = £1.75.
Dry powder spray 2.5%, pressurised aerosol 150g = £2.79.

---

1 Hatz R *et al.* (1994) *Wound Healing and Wound Management.* Springer-Verlag, London.

Table 12.3 Properties of antiseptics[1]

	Bactericidal (++) Bacteriostatic (+)	*Fungicidal (++) Fungistatic (+)*	*Virucidal (++) Virustatic (+)*	*Other characteristics*
Alcohols	++	++	+	Rapid onset of action at high concentrations; painful if skin broken
Phenol derivatives, e.g. hexachlorophane (Ster-Zac®) chloroxylenol (Dettol®)	++	++		Some absorption may occur
Iodine	++	++	++	Some iodine is absorbed; less effective in the presence of organic material; may cause contact dermatitis
Povidone-iodine	++	++	+	Some iodine is absorbed; has an inhibitory effect on wound healing
Chlorhexidene	++	+	+	
Cationic compounds e.g. benzalkonium chloride, cetrimide cetylpyridinium (Merocet®)	++	++		Adsorption at the surface; weak antibacterial action against Gram-negative bacteria
Quinoline derivatives e.g. dequalinium	+	+		
Heavy metals	+	+		Enzyme blocking; coagulatory action
Light metals	+			Astringent
Gentian (crystal) violet	+	+		Strong inhibition of wound healing *and risk of carcinogenesis*
Brilliant green	?	?		Strong inhibition of wound healing
Eosin	?	?		No inhibition of wound healing

13: ANAESTHESIA

Glycopyrronium

***Ketamine**

***Propofol**

GLYCOPYRRONIUM — BNF 15.1.3

Class: Antimuscarinic.

Indications: Drying secretions (e.g. †sialorrhoea, †drooling, †death rattle), †intestinal colic, †inoperable bowel obstruction.

Pharmacology

The secretory process is mainly under the control of the autonomic nervous system. Food in the mouth causes reflex secretion of saliva, and so does stimulation by acid of afferent vagal fibres in the lower oesophagus. Stimulation of the parasympathetic nerves causes profuse secretion of watery saliva, whereas stimulation of the sympathetic nerve supply causes the secretion from only the submaxillary glands of small quantities of saliva rich in organic constituents.[1] If the parasympathetic supply is interrupted, the salivary glands atrophy, whereas interruption of the sympathetic supply has no such effect. The muscarinic receptors in salivary glands are very responsive to antimuscarinics and inhibition of salivation occurs at lower doses than required for other antimuscarinic effects.[2] This reduces the likelihood of undesirable effects when antimuscarinics are given to reduce salivation. In some patients, a reduction in excess saliva results in improved speech.[3]

Glycopyrronium is a synthetic ionised quaternary ammonium antimuscarinic that penetrates biological membranes slowly and erratically.[4] In consequence it rarely causes sedation or delirium.[5,6] Absorption PO is poor and the IV to PO potency ratio is about 35:1.[7] Even so, glycopyrronium 200–400microgram PO t.d.s. produces plasma concentrations associated with an antisialogogic effect lasting up to 8h.[8–10] By injection, glycopyrronium is 2–5 times more potent than **hyoscine *hydrobromide*** as an antisecretory agent,[7] and may be effective in some patients who fail to respond to hyoscine. However, the efficacy of **hyoscine *hydrobromide***, **hyoscine *butylbromide*** and glycopyrronium as antisialogogues is generally similar, with death rattle reduced in 1/2–2/3 of patients.[11] The optimal parenteral single dose is 200microgram.[12] Compared to **hyoscine *hydrobromide***, the onset of action of glycopyrronium is slower.[13] It has less cardiac effects because of a reduced affinity for muscarinic-type 2 receptors.[14–16] Although at standard doses glycopyrronium does not change ocular pressures or pupil size, it can precipitate narrow-angle glaucoma. It is excreted by the kidneys and lower doses are effective in patients with renal dysfunction.[2,4] Inhaled or nebulised glycopyrronium is also used as a bronchodilator (not UK).[17]

Bio-availability <5% PO.
Onset of action 1min IV; 30–40min SC, PO.
Time to peak plasma concentration immediate IV; no data SC, PO.
Plasma halflife 1.7h.
Duration of action 7h.

Cautions

Glycopyrronium blocks the prokinetic effect of **metoclopramide**, **domperidone** and **cisapride**. Glycopyrronium decreases the effect of **levodopa** and phenothiazines; it increases the peripheral antimuscarinic toxicity of tricyclic antidepressants, phenothiazines and antihistamines.

Undesirable effects

For full list, see manufacturer's SPC.

Peripheral antimuscarinic effects, notably constipation, decreased sweating, dry mouth, nose and throat. Irritation/inflammation may occur at the site of injection.

Dose and use

Drooling

Glycopyrronium is an alternative to **hyoscine *hydrobromide***, **hyoscine *butylbromide*** and **atropine**.[3,18] It can be given PO or via a gastrostomy tube:[10]

- 200microgram stat and q8h
- if necessary, increase the dose progressively every 2–3 days to 600microgram q8h
- occasionally, doses of up to 2mg q8h are needed.

A subsequent reduction in dose is often possible, particularly when initial dose escalation has been rapid.

Death rattle

- 400microgram SC stat
- 1200microgram/24h CSCI
- 400microgram SC p.r.n.[19]

Some centres use **hyoscine *hydrobromide*** or **hyoscine *butylbromide*** instead.

Antispasmodic and inoperable intestinal obstruction

Glycopyrronium can be used as an alternative to **hyoscine *butylbromide***:[20]

- stat dose 200microgram SC
- followed by 600–1200microgram/24h CSCI.

For details of compatibility with other drugs, see Syringe drivers, p.297. *Glycopyrronium is immiscible with* ***dexamethasone, diazepam, dimenhydrinate, methylprednisolone, phenobarbital.***

Supply

Tablets 1mg, 2mg, 28 days @ 2mg t.d.s. = £84.17. (Unlicensed, available as a named patient supply from IDIS 020 8410 0700; see Special orders and named patient supplies, p.349).

Oral solution 1mg/10ml (0.01%), (prepared extemporaneously from glycopyrronium powder obtained from Antigen), 3g = £110. (The powder is licensed for use as a 5mg/10ml (0.05%) *topical* solution for the iontophoretic treatment of palmar and plantar hyperhydrosis.)[21]

Robinul® (Antigen 01704 562777)

Injection 200microgram/ml, 1ml amp = £0.60; 3ml amp = £1.01.

1 Ganong WF (1979) *Review of Medical Physiology* (9e). Lange Medical Publications, pp.177–181.

2 Ali-Melkkila T *et al.* (1993) Pharmacokinetics and related pharmacodynamics of anticholinergic drugs. *Acta Anaesthesiologica Scandinavica.* **37**: 633–642.

3 Rashid H *et al.* (1997) Management of secretions in esophageal cancer patients with glycopyrrolate. *Annals of Oncology.* **8**: 198–199.

4 Mirakhur R and Dundee J (1983) Glycopyrrolate pharmacology and clinical use. *Anaesthesia.* **38**: 1195–1204.

5 Gram D *et al.* (1991) Central anticholinergic syndrome following glycopyrrolate. *Anesthesiology.* **74**: 191–193.

6 Wigard D (1991) Glycopyrrolate and the central anticholinergic syndrome (letter). *Anesthesiology.* **75**: 1125.

7 Mirakhur R and Dundee J (1980) A comparison of the effects of atropine and glycopyrollate on various end organs. *Journal of the Royal Society of Medicine.* **73**: 727–730.

8 Ali-Melkkila T *et al.* (1989) Glycopyrrolate; pharmacokinetics and some pharmacodynamics findings. *Acta Anesthesiologica Scandinavica.* **33**: 513–517.

9 Blasco P (1996) Glycopyrrolate treatment of chronic drooling. *Archives of Paediatric and Adolescent Medicine.* **150**: 932–935.

10 Olsen A and Sjogren P (1999) Oral glycopyrrolate alleviates drooling in a patient with tongue cancer. *Journal of Pain and Symptom Management.* **18**: 300–302.

11 Hughes A *et al.* (2000) Audit of three antimuscarinic drugs for managing retained secretions. *Palliative Medicine.* **14**: 221–222.

12 Mirakhur R *et al.* (1978) Evaluation of the anticholinergic actions of glycopyrronium bromide. *British Journal of Clinical Pharmacology.* **5**: 77–84.

13 Back I *et al.* (2001) A study comparing hyoscine hydrobromide and glycopyrrolate in the treatment of death rattle. *Palliative Medicine.* **15**: 329–336.

14 Mirakhur R *et al.* (1978) Atropine and glycopyrronium premedication. A comparison of the effects on cardiac rate and rhythm during induction of anaesthesia. *Anaesthesia.* **33**: 906–912.

15 Warren J *et al.* (1997) Effect of autonomic blockade on power spectrum of heart rate variability during exercise. *American Journal of Physiology.* **273**: 495–502.
16 Scheinin H *et al.* (1999) Spectral analysis of heart rate variability as a quantitative measure of parasympatholytic effect – integrated pharmacokinetics and pharmacodynamics of three anticholinergic drugs. *Therapeutic Drug Monitoring.* **21**: 141–151.
17 Cydulka R and Emerman C (1995) Effects of combined treatment with glycopyrrolate and albuterol in acute exacerbation of chronic obstructive pulmonary disease. *Annals of Emergency Medicine.* **25**: 470–473.
18 Lucas V and Amass C (1998) Use of enteral glycopyrrolate in the management of drooling. *Palliative Medicine.* **12**: 207.
19 Bennett M *et al.* Using anti-muscarinic drugs in the management of death rattle: evidence based guidelines for palliative care. *Palliative Medicine.* **16**: In press.
20 Davis M and Furste A (1999) Glycopyrollate: a useful drug in the palliation of mechanical bowel obstruction. *Journal of Pain and Symptom Management.* **18**: 153–154.
21 Seukeran D and Highet A (1998) The use of topical glycopyrrolate in the treatment of hyperhidrosis. *Clinical and Experimental Dermatology.* **23**: 204–205.

*KETAMINE — BNF 15.1.1

Class: General anaesthetic.

Indications: Induction and maintenance of anaesthesia, †neuropathic, inflammatory, ischaemic and †myofascial pain unresponsive to standard therapies.[1,2]

Contra-indications: Raised intracranial pressure, epilepsy.

Pharmacology

The NMDA-glutamate receptor is a calcium channel closely involved in the development of central (dorsal horn) sensitisation (Figure 13.1).[3] At normal resting membrane potentials, the channel is

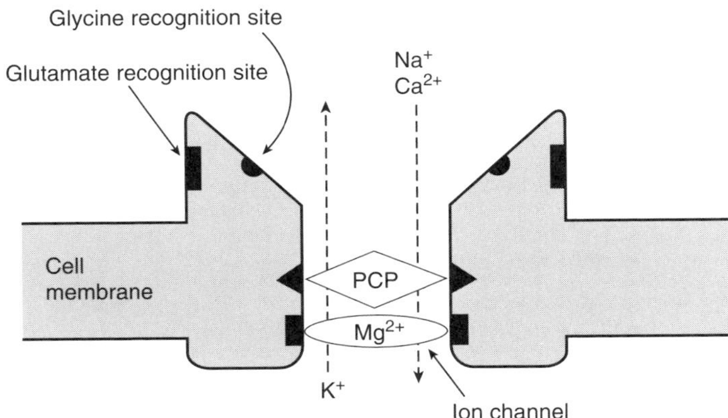

Figure 13.1 Diagram of NMDA (excitatory) receptor-channel complex. The channel is blocked by Mg^{2+} when the membrane potential is at its resting level (voltage-dependent block) and by drugs which act at the phencyclidine (PCP) binding site in the glutamate-activated channel, e.g. dextromethorphan, ketamine, methadone (use-dependent block).[3]

blocked by magnesium and inactive.[4] When the resting membrane potential is changed as a result of prolonged excitation, the channel unblocks with a reduction in opioid-responsiveness and the development of allodynia and hyperalgesia. These effects are probably mediated by the intracellular formation of nitric oxide.[5]

Ketamine is a dissociative anaesthetic which has analgesic properties in sub-anaesthetic doses.[6] Ketamine is the most potent NMDA-receptor-channel blocker available for clinical use, binding to the phencyclidine site when the channels are in the open activated state.[7] It also binds to a second membrane-associated site which does not require the channel to be open and thereby decreases the frequency of channel opening.[8] It is available clinically as a racemic mixture. Compared to the R-enantiomer, the S-enantiomer has greater affinity and selectivity for the NMDA-receptor and is more potent.[9] Ketamine has other actions which may also contribute to its analgesic effect, including interactions with other calcium and sodium channels, cholinergic transmission, noradrenergic and serotoninergic re-uptake inhibition (intact descending inhibitory pathways are necessary for analgesia) and μ, δ and κ opioid-like effects.[10] Ketamine also appears to have an antidepressant effect in patients with major depression.[11]

Evidence of ketamine's efficacy as an analgesic includes case reports and small retrospective surveys mainly in patients with neuropathic pain.[12–16] Several prospective studies have also been published including severe ischaemic limb pain and refractory pain in cancer.[17–20] Ketamine may be less effective in neuropathic pain of long duration (≥3 years).[21,22] Generally, ketamine is used in addition to **morphine** or alternative strong opioid when further opioid increments have been ineffective or precluded by unacceptable undesirable effects. When used in this way, ketamine is generally administered PO or SC.[15] It can also be administered IM, IV, SL, intranasally, PR and spinally (preservative-free formulation).[23–26] There is some evidence that short-term 'burst' treatment with ketamine may have long-term benefit.[19,20] For example, in patients taking regular strong opioids for ischaemic limb pain, a single 4h IV infusion of ketamine 0.6mg/kg reduced opioid requirements during a week-long period of observation.[20] In cancer, ketamine 100–500mg/24h by CSCI for 3–5 days relieved pain in 67% of patients and, in over 80% of these, the relief lasted for several weeks or more.

Oral ketamine undergoes extensive first-pass hepatic metabolism to norketamine. As an anaesthetic, norketamine is about 1/3 as potent as parenteral ketamine. However, as an analgesic it is equipotent. The maximum blood concentration of norketamine is greater after oral administration than after injection;[27] in chronic use norketamine may be the main analgesic agent. Less than 10% of ketamine is excreted unchanged, half in the faeces and half renally. Long-term use of ketamine leads to hepatic enzyme induction and enhanced ketamine metabolism.

Ketamine causes tachycardia and intracranial hypertension. Most patients experience vivid dreams, misperceptions, hallucinations and alterations in body image and mood as emergent phenomena after anaesthetic use, i.e. as the effects of a bolus dose wears off. These occur to a lesser extent with the sub-anaesthetic analgesic doses given PO or CSCI, and generally can be controlled by **diazepam**, **midazolam** or **haloperidol**.[26,28,29]

Bio-availability 93% IM; 20% PO.
Onset of action 5min IM; 15–30min SC; 30min PO.
Time to peak plasma concentration no data SC; 30min PO; 1h norketamine.[30]
Plasma halflife 1–3h IM; 3h PO; 12h norketamine.[31]
Duration of action 30min–2h IM; generally given by CSCI; 4–6h, sometimes longer PO.[32]

Cautions
Hypertension, cardiac failure, history of cerebrovascular accidents. Plasma concentration increased by **diazepam**.

Undesirable effects
For full list, see manufacturer's SPC.
Occur in about 40% of patients when given CSCI; less PO. Hypertension, tachycardia; psychotomimetic phenomena (euphoria, dsyphoria, blunted affect, psychomotor retardation, vivid dreams, nightmares, poor concentration, illusions, hallucinations, altered body image), delirium, dizziness, diplopia, blurred vision, nystagmus, altered hearing. Erythema and pain at injection site.

Dose and use
Dose recommendations vary considerably but ketamine is often started in a low dose PO (Box 13.A).[33] An oral solution is now available (see Supply) or can be extemporaneously

prepared by the pharmacy (Box 13.B). Alternatively, patients can be supplied with vials of ketamine and 1ml graduated syringes. Two needles (one as an air vent) should be inserted in the bung of the vial to facilitate withdrawing the ketamine; sterility is not necessary for PO administration. Use 10mg/ml or 50mg/ml; 100mg/ml is too bitter. Long-term success, i.e. both pain relief and tolerable undesirable effects, varies from <20% to about 50%.[22,24,34]

Box 13.A Dose recommendations for ketamine

PO[15,38]
Use direct from vial or dilute for convenience to 50mg/5ml (patient adds flavouring of choice, e.g. fruit cordial, to mask the bitter taste):

- starting dose 10–25mg t.d.s.–q.d.s and p.r.n.[39]
- increase dose in steps of 10–25mg up to 50mg q.d.s.
- maximum reported dose 200mg q.d.s.[40,41]
- give a smaller dose more frequently if psychotomimetic phenomena or drowsiness occurs which does not respond to a reduction in opioid.

SC[15]
≤500microgram/kg, typically 10–25mg p.r.n.

CSCI[12,15,28]
Because ketamine is irritant, dilute with sodium chloride 0.9% to the largest volume possible (i.e. for a Graseby syringe driver, 18ml in a 30ml luerlock syringe given over 12–24h):

- starting dose 1–2.5mg/kg/24h[13,39]
- increase by 50–100mg/24h; maximum reported dose 3.6g/24h.[42]

Alternatively, give as short-term 'burst' therapy:

- starting dose 100mg/24h
- increase after 24h to 300mg/24h if 100mg not effective
- increase after further 24h to 500mg/24h if 300mg not effective
- stop 3 days after last dose increment.[19]

Ketamine is miscible with dexamethasone (low-dose), diamorphine, haloperidol, levomepromazine (methotrimeprazine), metoclopramide, midazolam, morphine. Inflammation at infusion site may be helped by hydrocortisone 1% cream or by adding dexamethasone 0.5–1mg to the infusion (dilute in 5–10ml sodium chloride and then add ketamine).

Box 13.B Preparation of ketamine oral solution: pharmacy guidelines

Use ketamine 100mg/ml 10ml vials because this is the cheapest concentration.
Raspberry Syrup BP can be used for dilution but this is too sweet for some patients.
Alternatively, use purified water as the diluent and ask patients to add their own flavouring, e.g. fruit cordial, just before use to disguise the bitter taste.

To prepare 100ml of 50mg/5ml oral solution:

- 10ml vial of ketamine 100mg/ml for injection
- 90ml purified water.

Store in a refrigerator with an expiry date of 1 week from manufacture.

With higher doses by CSCI, the dose of **morphine** should be reduced if the patient becomes drowsy. If a patient experiences dysphoria or hallucinations, the dose of ketamine should be reduced and a benzodiazepine prescribed, e.g. **diazepam** 5mg PO stat & o.n., **midazolam** 5mg SC stat and 5–10mg CSCI, or **haloperidol**, e.g. 2–5mg PO stat & o.n., 2–5mg SC stat and 2–5mg CSCI.[29] In patients at greatest risk of dysphoria, i.e. those with high anxiety levels, these measures may be more effective if given before starting ketamine.[7] Ketamine has been used IV with **fentanyl** and **midazolam** to control intractable pain and agitation.[35,36]

Ketamine is used less in centres where spinal analgesia is readily available or where **methadone** is used as the NMDA-receptor-channel blocker of choice; the affinity of **methadone** and ketamine for the NMDA-receptor-channel binding site is approximately the same.[37]

Supply

Oral solution 50mg/5ml, 28 days @ 50mg q.d.s. = £58.78. (Unlicensed, available as a special order from Martindale 01708 386660; see Special orders and named patient supplies, p.349.)

Ketalar® (Pfizer 01304 616161)

Injection 10mg/ml, 20ml vial = £3.52; 50mg/ml, 10ml vial = £7.31; 100mg/ml, 10ml vial = £13.42.

Although use as an analgesic is unlicensed, ketamine injection can be prescribed both in hospitals and in the community. The procedure varies with the wholesaler the community pharmacist uses:

- if AHH, the pharmacist should contact Pfizer customer services (Tel: 01304 645262, Fax: 01304 655885) and provide the patient's name, dose of ketamine prescribed, quantity required, GP and pharmacist's details and wholesaler branch and account number; Pfizer will then contact AHH to initiate the supply
- if Unichem, the pharmacist should telephone their local Unichem customer services to receive a faxed form. This requires the same information as above and once returned to Unichem the supply is initiated.

---

1 Persson J *et al.* (1998) The analgesic effect of racemic ketamine in patients with chronic ischemic pain due to lower extremity arteriosclerosis obliterans. *Acta Anaesthesiologica Scandinavica.* **42**: 750–758.

2 Graven-Nielsen T *et al.* (2000) Ketamine reduces muscle pain, temporal summation, and referred pain in fibromyalgia patients. *Pain.* **85**: 483–491.

3 Richens A (1991) The basis of the treatment of epilepsy: neuropharmacology. In: M Dam (ed) *A Practical Approach to Epilepsy.* Pergamon Press, Oxford, pp.75–85.

4 Mayer M et *al.* (1984) Voltage-dependent block for Mg^{2+} of NMDA responses in spinal cord neurones. *Nature.* **309**: 261–263.

5 Elliott K et *al.* (1994) The NMDA receptor antagonists, LY274614 and MK-801, and the nitric oxide synthase inhibitor, NG-nitro-L-arginine, attenuate analgesic tolerance to the mu-opioid morphine but not to kappa opioids. *Pain.* **56**: 69–75.

6 Fallon MT and Welsh J (1996) The role of ketamine in pain control. *European Journal of Palliative Care.* **3**: 143–146.

7 Oye I (1998) Ketamine analgesia, NMDA receptors and the gates perception. *Acta Anaesthesiologica Scandinavica.* **42**: 747–749.

8 Orser B et *al.* (1997) Multiple mechanisms of ketamine blockade of N-methyl-D-aspartate receptors. *Anesthesiology.* **86**: 903–917.

9 Oye I et *al.* (1991) The chiral forms of ketamine as probes for NMDA receptor function in humans. In: T Kameyama (ed) *NMDA Receptor Related Agents: biochemistry, pharmacology and behavior.* NPP, Ann Arbor, Mich, pp.381–389.

10 Meller S (1996) Ketamine: relief from chronic pain through actions at the NMDA receptor? *Pain.* **68**: 435–436.

11 Berman R et *al.* (2000) Antidepressant effects of ketamine in depressed patients. *Biological Psychiatry.* **47**: 351–354.

12 Oshima E et *al.* (1990) Continuous subcutaneous injection of ketamine for cancer pain. *Canadian Journal of Anaesthetics.* **37**: 385–392.

13 Bell R (1999) Low-dose subcutaneous ketamine infusion and morphine tolerance. *Pain.* **83**: 101–103.

14 Cherry DA et *al.* (1995) Ketamine as an adjunct to morphine in the treatment of pain. *Pain.* **62**: 119–121.

15 Luczak J et *al.* (1995) The role of ketamine, an NMDA receptor antagonist, in the management of pain. *Progress in Palliative Care.* **3**: 127–134.

16 Mercadante S (1996) Ketamine in cancer pain: an update. *Palliative Medicine.* **10**: 225–230.

17 Lauretti G *et al.* (1999) Oral ketamine and transdermal nitroglycerin as analgesic adjuvants to oral morphine therapy and amitriptyline for cancer pain management. *Anesthesiology.* **90**: 1528–1533.
18 Lossignol D *et al.* (1999) Ketamine and morphine in cancer pain. In *Proceedings of the Ninth World Congress on Pain*, Vienna. IASP, Seattle.
19 Jackson K *et al.* (2001) 'Burst' ketamine for refractory cancer pain: an open-label audit of 39 patients. *Journal of Pain and Symptom Management.* **22**: 834–842.
20 Mitchell A *et al.* (2001) Does ketamine improve ischaemic limb pain? Results from a double blind, randomised controlled trial. *Poster abstract, Pain Society Annual Scientific Meeting, 27–30 March.* **Poster 42**: 50.
21 Mathisen L *et al.* (1995) Effect of ketamine, an NMDA receptor inhibitor, in acute and chronic orofacial pain. *Pain.* **61**: 215–220.
22 Haines D and Gaines S (1999) N of 1 randomised controlled trials of oral ketamine in patients with chronic pain. *Pain.* **83**: 283–287.
23 Lin T *et al.* (1998) Long-term epidural ketamine, morphine and bupivacaine attenuate reflex sympathetic dystrophy neuralgia. *Canadian Journal of Anaesthesia.* **45**: 175–177.
24 Batchelor G (1999) Ketamine in neuropathic pain. *The Pain Society Newsletter.* **1**: 19.
25 Beltrutti D *et al.* (1999) The epidural and intrathecal administration of ketamine. *Current Review of Pain.* **3**: 458–472.
26 Mercadante S *et al.* (2000) Analgesic effect of intravenous ketamine in cancer patients on morphine therapy: a randomized, controlled, double-blind, crossover, double-dose study. *Journal of Pain and Symptom Management.* **20**: 246–252.
27 Clements JA *et al.* (1982) Bio-availability, pharmacokinetics and analgesic activity of ketamine in humans. *Journal of Pharmaceutical Sciences.* **71**: 539–542.
28 Hughes A *et al.* (1999) Ketamine. *CME Bulletin Palliative Medicine.* **1**: 53.
29 Giannini A *et al.* (2000) Acute ketamine intoxication treated by haloperidol: a preliminary study. *American Journal of Therapeutics.* **7**: 389–391.
30 Grant IS *et al.* (1981) Pharmacokinetics and analgesic effects of IM and oral ketamine. *British Journal of Anaesthesia.* **53**: 805–810.
31 Domino E *et al.* (1984) Ketamine kinetics in unmedicated and diazepam premedicated subjects. *Clinical Pharmacology and Therapeutics.* **36**: 645–653.
32 Rabben T *et al.* (1999) Prolonged analgesic effect of ketamine, an N-methyl-D-aspartate receptor inhibitor, in patients with chronic pain. *Journal of Pharmacology and Experimental Therapeutics.* **289**: 1060–1066.
33 Hall E (1997) Personal communication.
34 Enarson M *et al.* (1999) Clinical experience with oral ketamine. *Journal of Pain and Symptom Management.* **17**: 384–386.
35 Berger J *et al.* (2000) Ketamine-fentanyl-midazolam infusion for the control of symptoms in terminal life care. *American Journal of Hospice and Palliative Care.* **17**: 127–132.
36 Enck R (2000) A ketamine, fentanyl, and midazolam infusion for uncontrolled terminal pain and agitation. *American Journal of Hospice and Palliative Care.* **17**: 76–77.
37 Gorman A *et al.* (1997) The d- and l- isomers of methadone bind to the non-competitive site on the N-methyl-D-aspartate (NMDA) receptor in rat forebrain and spinal cord. *Neuroscience Letters.* **223**: 5–8.
38 Broadley K *et al.* (1996) Ketamine injection used orally. *Palliative Medicine.* **10**: 247–250.
39 August Newsletter (2001) www.palliativedrugs.com
40 Clark JL and Kalan GE (1995) Effective treatment of severe cancer pain of the head using low-dose ketamine in an opioid-tolerant patient. *Journal of Pain and Symptom Management.* **10**: 310–314.
41 Vielvoye-Kerkmeer A (2000) Clinical experience with ketamine. *Journal of Pain and Symptom Management.* **19**: 3.
42 Lloyd-Williams M (2000) Ketamine for cancer pain. *Journal of Pain and Symptom Management.* **19**: 79–80.

*PROPOFOL **BNF 15.1**

Class of drug: General anaesthetic.

Indications: †Used at some centres for agitated delirium unresponsive to usual therapies.

Contra-indications: Children under 16. When used for sedation in children in intensive care, the death rate was increased 2–3 times compared to a control group.[1] Cases of metabolic acidosis, hyperlipaemia and hepatomegaly have also been reported.[1]

Pharmacology

Propofol is an ultrafast-acting IV anaesthetic agent. It is rapidly metabolised, mainly in the liver, to inactive compounds which are excreted in the urine. The incidence of untoward haemodynamic changes is low. Propofol reduces cerebral blood flow, intracranial pressure and cerebral metabolism. The reduction in intracranial pressure is greater if the baseline pressure is raised. Propofol also has an anti-emetic effect as evidenced by a reduced incidence of postoperative vomiting compared with other anaesthetic agents,[2] and by a reduction in nausea and vomiting during the first 24h after chemotherapy when given in subhypnotic doses.[3,4] Although short-acting, propofol has a long terminal halflife; this reflects redistribution from poorly perfused tissues.
Onset of action 0.5min.
Time to peak plasma concentration 4–8min.
Plasma halflife 30–60min initial elimination phase; 200min terminal elimination phase.
Duration of action 3–10min.

Cautions

There is a risk of seizures in epileptic patients. Propofol is an emulsion of oil-in-water. This gives it a white appearance and makes it a potential growth medium. Strict asepsis must be employed to prevent microbial contamination.

Undesirable effects

For full list, see manufacturer's SPC.
Uncommon: convulsions, myoclonus, opisthotonus, profound bradycardia, asystole, pulmonary oedema, nausea, vomiting, headache.
Rare: discolouration of urine, anaphylaxis, thrombosis, phlebitis.

Dose and use

Propofol is not used at Hayward House or Sir Michael Sobell House.
IV propofol should be used only if other measures have failed to relieve a patient's distress, such as a combination of SC **haloperidol** or **levomepromazine** (methotrimeprazine) with SC **midazolam**, or SC **phenobarbital**.[5,6] Propofol is given IV as a 1% solution (10mg/ml) in doses ranging from 5–70mg/h (0.5–7ml) using a computer-controlled volumetric infusion pump. The local pain which may occur when injected IV can be minimised by co-administration with **lidocaine** (lignocaine) and by using a large vein in the fore-arm or antecubital fossa. Propofol has no analgesic properties and therefore supplementary analgesic agents are required.

Propofol 10mg/h (1ml) is a typical starting dose with 10mg/h increments every 15min until a satisfactory level of sedation is achieved. Any change in rate has an effect in 5–10min. If it is necessary to increase the level of sedation quickly, boluses of 20–50mg can be given by increasing the rate to 1ml/min for 2–5min. If the patient is too sedated, the infusion should be turned off for 2–3min and then restarted at a lower rate. It is important to replenish the infusion quickly when a container empties, otherwise the sedation will wear off after a few minutes.

Supply

Diprivan® (AstraZeneca 0800 783 0033)
Injection (emulsion) 10mg/ml, 20ml amp =£3.88; 50ml vial = £9.70; 100ml vial = £19.40.
Injection (emulsion) 20mg/ml, 50ml vial = £19.40.

1 Anonymous (2001) Propofol (Diprivan) infusion: sedation in children aged 16 years or younger contraindicated. *Current Problems in Pharmacovigilance.* **27**: 10.
2 Korttila K (1993) Recovery from propofol: Does it really make a difference? *Journal of Clinical Anaesthesia.* **5**: 443–446.
3 Borgeat A *et al.* (1992) Propofol and chemotherapy emesis. *Canadian Journal of Anaesthesia.* **39**: 578–579.
4 Borgeat A *et al.* (1994) Adjuvant propofol enables better control of nausea and emesis secondary to chemotherapy for breast cancer. *Canadian Journal of Anaesthesia.* **41**: 1117–1119.
5 Mercadante S *et al.* (1995) Propofol in terminal care. *Journal of Pain and Symptom Management.* **10**: 639–642.
6 Moyle J (1995) The use of propofol in palliative medicine. *Journal of Pain and Symptom Management.* **10**: 643–646.

14: SYRINGE DRIVERS

Syringe drivers

Administering drugs by CSCI using a portable battery-powered syringe driver is common practice in palliative care in the UK.[1] The syringe driver can be used to deliver medication SC, ED or IT, generally over 24h. For most drugs, this method of administration is unlicensed. Two types of syringe driver manufactured by SIMS Graseby are widely used:

- **MS16A** with an *hourly* rate (mm/h) syringe driver and a *blue* front panel (Figure 14.1)

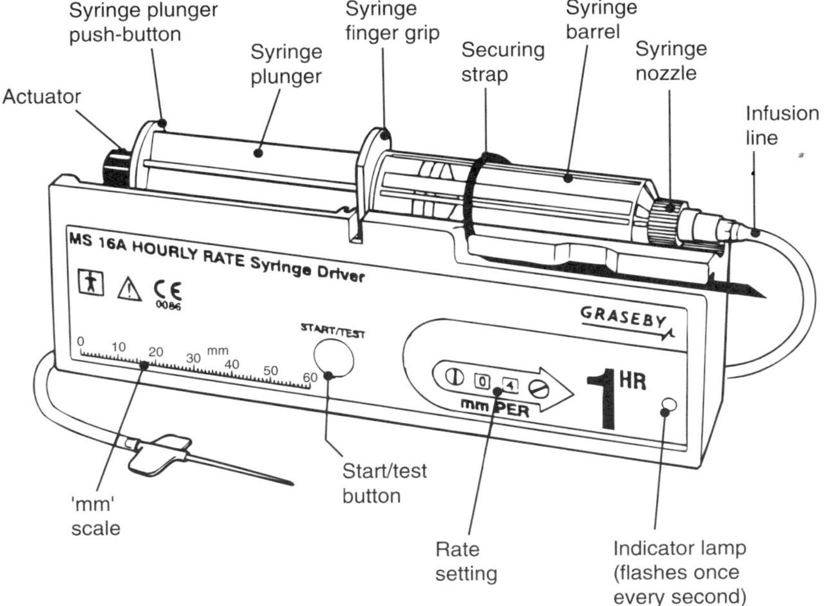

Figure 14.1 The SIMS Graseby MS16A.

• **MS26** with a *daily* rate (mm/24h) syringe driver and a *green* front panel (Figure 14.2).
The majority of centres use the MS26 because setting the rate is simpler and perhaps safer. However, the MS16A is more flexible, particularly when larger volumes are required, e.g. with **metoclopramide, midazolam** and **bupivacaine**. To reduce the likelihood of mistakes, it is best if only one or other type is used in a given locality.

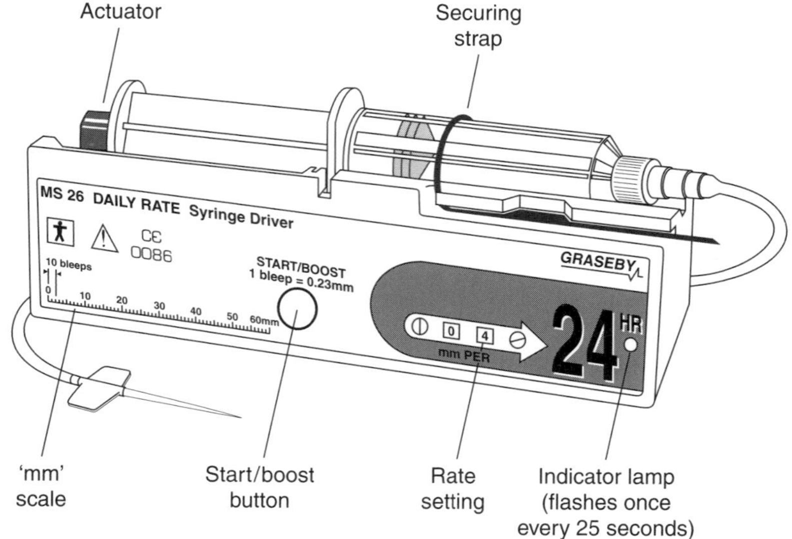

Figure 14.2 The SIMS Graseby MS26.

Rate setting

The rate of delivery is based upon a length of fluid in mm per unit time; this allows any brand of syringe to be used (Box 14.A). The MS16A and MS26 can deliver a maximum length of 60mm per syringe. There are several published reports about 'infusion confusion'[2,3] and a Department of Health Hazard 94(12) has been issued. Errors have arisen from confusion between the two different ways of determining the rate of drug delivery (hourly vs daily). Staff training is essential in order to highlight the differences and the potentially fatal hazards.[2,3] SIMS Graseby offer staff training, including a video, a manual and instruction by their local representatives.

Indications

Indications for use of a syringe driver include:

- persistent nausea and vomiting
- dysphagia
- intestinal obstruction
- coma
- poor absorption of oral drugs (rare)
- when SC, ED or IT route is used for drug administration.

Before setting up a syringe driver, it is important to explain its use with the patient and the family. Explanation is needed about what a syringe driver is, how it works, why it is planned to use one, together with comments about its advantages and possible disadvantages (Box 14.B). It is important that the syringe driver is not seen just as the last resort but as an effective method of relieving certain symptoms by injection. It is also important to appreciate that the syringe driver is merely a convenient alternative route of administration, and is not Step 4 on the analgesic ladder.

Box 14.A Setting the rate of a portable syringe driver

MS16A

rate = $\frac{\text{measured 'length of volume' in mm}}{\text{delivery time in hours}}$

e.g. $\frac{48\text{mm}}{24\text{h}}$ = 2mm/h (48mm is about 8ml in a 10ml BD plastipak syringe)

MS26

rate = $\frac{\text{measured 'length of volume' in mm}}{\text{delivery time in days}}$

e.g. $\frac{60\text{mm}}{1\text{ day}}$ = 60mm/day

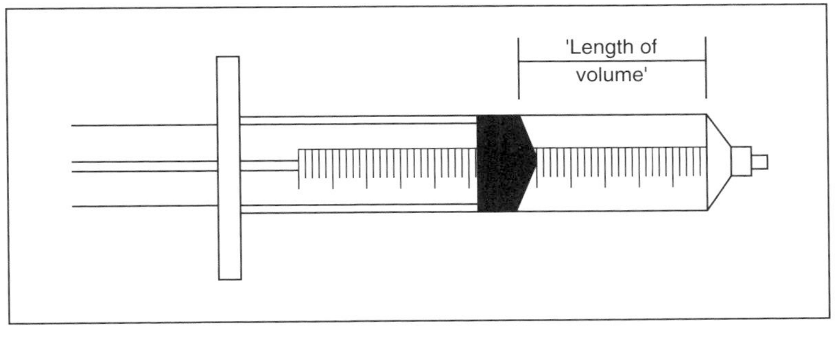

Box 14.B Advantages and disadvantages of a syringe driver

Advantages

Increased comfort for the patient because there is less need for repeated injections.
Control of multiple symptoms with a combination of drugs.
Round-the-clock comfort because plasma drug concentrations are maintained without peaks and troughs.
Independence and mobility maintained because the device is lightweight and can be worn in a holster under or over clothes.
Generally needs to be reloaded only o.d.

Disadvantages

Fear that it is a last resort.
Training necessary for staff.
Possible inflammation and pain at the infusion site (diazepam and chlorpromazine are too irritant to administer by CSCI).
Occasional technical problems with ED/IT infusions, e.g. a leaking connection causing a resurgence of symptoms and a risk of infection.
Lack of flexibility with o.d. prescription.

Drug compatibility

The prescription should be checked to determine whether the drug combination is physically compatible, i.e. miscible. Chart 1 (see p.370) and Chart 2 (see p.371) summarise the compatibility of the more commonly used two and three drug combinations with **alfentanil** and **diamorphine**.[4–23] Chart 3 (see p.372), Chart 4 (see p.373) and Chart 5 (see p.374) summarise the compatibility of the more commonly used two and three drug combinations with **morphine** ***sulphate*** and **morphine** ***tartrate***.[23–28] Some centres mix four drugs (Box 14.C). With few exceptions, these are all because of a decision to add **dexamethasone** or an antisecretory drug (for control of 'death rattle', i.e. **glycopyrronium**, **hyoscine** ***butylbromide***, **hyoscine** ***hydrobromide***. **Dexamethasone** should always be *the last to be added* to an already dilute combination of drugs in order to reduce the risk of incompatibility. However, it should be emphasised that **dexamethasone** is a long-acting drug and can be given as a bolus SC injection o.d. instead. The same holds true for **levomepromazine** (methotrimeprazine). Indeed, the combination of **cyclizine** and **haloperidol** can probably be circumvented by giving bolus SC **levomepromazine** (methotrimeprazine) o.d. or CSCI **promethazine** instead. Further information relating to drug compatibility can be obtained from hospital medical information pharmacists.[4–6]

Box 14.C Syringe driver compatibility: combinations of four drugs

Compatible[a]	**Incompatible**
Alfentanil +	*Alfentanil* +
Clonazepam, dexamethasone, haloperidol	Dexamethasone, haloperidol, midazolam
Clonazepam, glycopyrronium, haloperidol	
Cyclizine, glycopyrronium, midazolam	
Hyoscine butylbromide, levomepromazine, octreotide	
Diamorphine +	*Diamorphine* +
Clonazepam, cyclizine, glycopyrronium	Cyclizine, glycopyrronium, midazolam
Clonazepam, cyclizine, haloperidol	Cyclizine, haloperidol, hyoscine butylbromide
Clonazepam, dexamethasone, haloperidol	Cyclizine, hyoscine butylbromide, midazolam
Clonazepam, glycopyrronium, haloperidol	
Clonazepam, haloperidol, hyoscine hydrobromide	
Cyclizine, dexamethasone, haloperidol	
Cyclizine, dexamethasone, hyoscine butylbromide	
Cyclizine, dexamethasone, hyoscine hydrobromide	
Cyclizine, glycopyrronium, haloperidol	
Cyclizine, haloperidol, hyoscine hydrobromide	
Cyclizine, haloperidol, midazolam	
Cyclizine, haloperidol, octreotide	
Cyclizine, hyoscine hydrobromide, midazolam	
Dexamethasone, haloperidol, hyoscine butylbromide	
Dexamethasone, hyoscine hydrobromide, midazolam	
Glycopyrronium, haloperidol, midazolam	
Glycopyrronium, levomepromazine, octreotide	
Hyoscine butylbromide, levomepromazine, midazolam	

a. based on clinical experience in palliative care units in the UK.[4] Also see Chart 1 (p.370) and Chart 2 (p.371).

Many combinations have been successfully used in clinical practice without supporting laboratory data. When this is the case, regular monitoring of the contents of the syringe and the tubing has failed to detect evidence of physical incompatibility, e.g. crystallisation, precipitation, colour change. It would therefore help if details of any problems you encounter are registered at druginformation@palliativedrugs.com or use the red card inside the back cover of *PCF2*. Laboratory data about the drugs to be mixed, such as pH, can help in deciding whether to attempt to mix them (Table 14.1). As a general rule, drugs with similar pH are more likely to be compatible than those with widely differing pH. Alkaline drugs such as **ketorolac** and **dexamethasone** often cause compatibility problems because most drug solutions are acidic.

Table 14.1 The pH values of drugs delivered by syringe drivers[a]

Drug	*pH*	*Drug*	*pH*
Alfentanil	4–6	Hyoscine butylbromide	3.7–5.5
Bupivacaine	4–6.5	Hyoscine hydrobromide	5–7
Clonidine	4–4.5	Ketamine	3.5–5.5
Cyclizine lactate	3.3–3.7[b]	Ketorolac	6.9–7.9
Dexamethasone	7–8.5	Levomepromazine	4.5
Diamorphine	2.5–6	Methadone	3–6.5
Diclofenac	7.8–9	Metoclopramide	4.5–6.5
Glycopyrronium	2–3	Midazolam	3
Granisetron	4.7–7.3	Morphine	2.5–6
Haloperidol	3–3.8	Octreotide	3.9–4.5
Hyaluronidase	6.4–7.4	Ondansetron	3.3–4
Hydromorphone	4–5.5	Tropisetron	4.5–5.2

a. manufacturer's information
b. above pH 6.8, cyclizine base precipitates;[3] if diluted with 0.9% saline, cyclizine hydrochloride crystallises out.[10]

For most drug mixtures, the recommended diluent is WFI because there is less chance of precipitation, particularly at higher concentrations of drugs e.g. **diamorphine** (>450mg/ml). The choice between WFI and 0.9% saline as diluent is a matter of debate, as saline can in fact be used for most drugs, the main exception being **cyclizine**. Indeed, in an attempt to reduce site reactions with irritant drugs some suggest 0.9% saline as diluent (see Infusion site problems, p.302). However, further work is required and we do not recommend 0.9% saline as the routine diluent unless indicated by laboratory-based compatibility data as exists for **granisetron**, **ketamine**, **ketorolac**, **octreotide** and **ondansetron**. Even then it should be noted that there is generally no evidence that it is better than WFI for these drugs. (In any case, **granisetron** can be given as a bolus SC injection o.d.) Glucose 5% in water is commonly used as a diluent in some countries, e.g. USA.

Setting up a syringe driver

1 If symptoms are controlled, start the syringe driver 1–2h before the effect of the previous medication is due to wear off. If symptoms are uncontrolled, set up the syringe driver immediately, and give stat SC doses of the same drugs.

2 Volume permitting, many centres use a 10ml syringe. Others use a 20ml syringe as a minimum to allow greater dilution. Consistency of practice within individual units is important. Greater dilution reduces:
- the risk of incompatibility
- the impact of priming a line (less drug in the 'dead space')
- injection site skin reactions.

3 The syringe is filled with drugs and diluent up to a length of either 48mm (MS16A) or to the maximum length of 60mm (MS26), using the millimetre scale on the syringe driver.

4 Connect the syringe to the tubing attached to the butterfly cannula and prime the infusion line. Priming uses about 0.5ml and, with the MS16A set at 2mm/h, the contents of the syringe will be delivered short of 24h. However, subsequent infusions which do not involve priming of the line will last a full 24h. For the MS26, the tubing can be primed before measuring the length of the barrel and the rate set to ensure delivery over 24h.

5 After measuring the length of the barrel against the millimetre scale on the syringe driver, the delivery rate is set (see Box 14.A). With the MS16A, for safety reasons, the delivery rate is generally standardised at 2mm/h. With the MS26, for a 24h infusion, the delivery rate is equal to the length of fluid in the syringe. Fit the flange of the syringe into the slot provided on the syringe driver and secure with the rubber strap.

6 Insert the 9V battery and an audible alarm sounds. The syringe driver also makes this noise when:
- the syringe is empty

- the line is blocked
- the start/boost button is depressed for 5 seconds (MS16A) or 10 seconds (MS26).

7 Press the start/test (MS16A) or start/boost (MS26) button to silence the alarm and to activate the syringe driver. Replace the battery if the indicator light fails to flash every second (MS16A) or every 25 seconds (MS26). Each battery should last for about 50 full syringes; the light stops flashing 24h before the battery runs out.

Siting the CSCI

An 18 gauge butterfly needle should be inserted at an angle of 30–45° into SC tissue, avoiding oedematous areas, skin folds and breast tissue. Usual sites are the anterior chest wall or antero-lateral aspects of upper arms. Sometimes the anterior abdominal wall or anterior surface of the thighs are used. The tubing should be secured with a dressing (e.g. Tegaderm™) with a loop to minimise the possibility of pulling out the needle.

Checks in use

The use of specific charts for SC, ED and IT routes serve as a prescription chart and record of administration, and also reinforce training. The rate, condition of infusion site and remaining volume should be documented q4h. The calculation to determine whether the driver is running to time is based on the preceding 4h. The comments/action section is completed, e.g. if the infusion needs to be resited and hence reprimed. If so, record the time, the new site and the new syringe length. Comments might include details of incompatibility and mention any mishaps such as the syringe driver was found disconnected.

The MS26 boost facility

The MS26 boost facility is *not* recommended for the following reasons:

- the boost facility lacks a lock-out period. If the boost button is continually depressed, the MS26 will deliver 8 boluses before an alarm sounds and no further boosts are delivered. However, if the button is released, then continually depressed again, a further 8 bolus doses will be administered. Theoretically, this could be continued until the syringe is empty
- one boost delivers a length of fluid equivalent to 0.23mm that is unlikely to deliver an effective analgesic dose. Thus, a syringe containing **diamorphine** 100mg in 18ml would generally necessitate a p.r.n. dose of 15mg, whereas a boost of 0.23mm would only deliver 0.4mg
- analgesics are rarely infused alone and additional doses of the other drugs may be undesirable
- it may cause stinging at the infusion site.

Infusion site problems

A skin reaction at the infusion site is most commonly found with **cyclizine**, **levomepromazine** (methotrimeprazine) and **methadone**.[4] Excluding mixtures containing **cyclizine** or very high doses of **diamorphine** (>450mg/ml), 0.9% saline can be used as the diluent in an attempt to reduce site reactions with irritant infusions. Occasionally patients may be allergic to the nickel needles. Sites may last up to a week, depending on the drugs used. The site should be changed if painful or inflamed. Routine changing every 72h reduces the frequency of site problems. If frequent resiting is necessary, e.g. every 24–48h, consider the following strategies:

- use a larger syringe to enable a more dilute mixture to be used, thereby decreasing the final drug concentrations
- change to a q12h regimen, thereby permitting further dilution of the drugs
- change an irritant drug to a less irritant alternative, e.g. **cyclizine** to **haloperidol**
- **hyaluronidase** 1500units can be injected into the site *before* starting the infusion. Although its effect lasts only about 24h, if the site is rotated every 2–3 days, hyaluronidase generally needs to be injected only once per site and not daily. Do not add to the syringe because degradation of hyaluronidase may occur[4]
- add **hydrocortisone** 50–100mg or **dexamethasone** 0.5–1mg to the syringe
- use a plastic (Teflon™ or Vialon™) cannula instead of a butterfly needle.[29–31]

1 O'Doherty CA *et al.* (2001) Drugs and syringe drivers: a survey of adult specialist palliative care practice in the United Kingdom and Eire. *Palliative Medicine*. **15**: 149–154.

2 Carlisle D *et al.* (1996) Infusion Confusion. *Nursing Times*. **92**: 48–49.

3 Cousins DH and Upton DR (1995) Make infusion pumps safer to use. *Pharmacy in Practice*. **5**: 401–406.
4 Dickman A *et al*. (in press). The Syringe Driver: continuous subcutaneous infusions in palliative care. Oxford University Press, Oxford.
5 Trissel LA (2000) *Handbook on Injectable Drugs* (11e). American Society of Health-System Pharmacists.
6 Back I (2001) www.pallmed.net Syringe driver drugmix database.
7 Thorp SA Collection of in-house data. Hayward House, City Hospital, Nottingham.
8 French SA Collection of in-house data. Pharmacy Department, City Hospital, Nottingham.
9 Grassby PF (April 1995 and July 1997) UK Stability Database. Welsh Pharmaceutical Services, St. Mary's Pharmaceutical Unit, Corbett Road, Penarth, South Glamorgan.
10 Bradley K (1996) Swap data on drug compatibilities. *Pharmacy in Practice*. **6**: 69–72.
11 Allwood MC (1984) Diamorphine mixed with anti-emetic drugs in plastic syringes. *British Journal of Pharmacy Practice*. **6 (3)**: 88–90.
12 Allwood MC (1991) The stability of diamorphine alone and in combination with anti-emetics in plastic syringes. *Palliative Medicine*. **5**: 330–333.
13 Allwood MC *et al*. (1994) Stability of injections containing diamorphine and midazolam in plastic syringes. *International Journal of Pharmacy Practice*. **3**: 57–59.
14 Collins AJ *et al*. (1986) Stability of diamorphine hydrochloride with haloperidol in prefilled syringes for continuous subcutaneous administration. *Journal of Pharmacy and Pharmacology*. **38**: 51.
15 Fawcett JP *et al*. (1994) Compatibility of cyclizine lactate and haloperidol lactate. *American Journal of Hospital Pharmacy*. **51**: 292.
16 Grassby PF and Hutchings L (1997) Drug combinations in syringe drivers: the compatibility and stability of diamorphine with cyclizine and haloperidol. *Palliative Medicine*. **11**: 217–224.
17 Hutchinson HT *et al*. (1981) Continuous subcutaneous analgesics and anti-emetics in domiciliary terminal care. *Lancet*. **ii**: 1279.
18 Kyaterekera N *et al*. (1997) Stability of octreotide in the presence of diamorphine hydrochloride. *Journal of Pharmacy and Pharmacology*. **49 (suppl 4)**: 63.
19 Fielding H *et al*. (2000) The compatibility of octreotide acetate in the presence of diamorphine hydrochloride in polypropylene syringes. *Palliative Medicine*. **14**: 205–207.
20 Mehta AC (1996) Admixtures' storage is extended. *Pharmacy in Practice*. **6**: 113–118.
21 Regnard C *et al*. (1986) Anti-emetic/diamorphine mixture compatibility in infusion pumps. *British Journal of Pharmacy Practice*. **8**: 218–220.
22 Chandler SW *et al*. (1996) Combined administration of opioids with selected drugs to manage pain and other cancer symptoms: initial safety screening for compatibility. *Journal of Pain and Symptom Management*. **12**: 168–171.
23 Stewart J *et al*. (1998) Stability of ondansetron hydrochloride and 12 medications in plastic syringes. *American Journal of Health-Systems Pharmacy*. **55**: 2630–2634.
24 Schneider J (2001) Collection of in-house data. Division of Palliative Care, Newcastle Mater Hospital, NSW, Australia.
25 Bradshaw K (1992) Chemical compatibility and stability of morphine when mixed with various other injections. Therapeutic Goods Administration, Commonwealth Department of Health, Australia. *Laboratory Information Bulletin*. **4**: 1 (July).
26 Lawson W *et al*. (1991) Stability of hyoscine in mixtures with morphine for continuous subcutaneous administration. *Australian Journal of Hospital Pharmacy (Letter)*. **21**: 395–396.
27 Trissel L *et al*. (1994) Compatibility and stability of ondansetron hydrochloride with morphine sulphate and with hydromorphone hydrochloride in 0.9% sodium chloride injection at 4, 22 and 32°C. *American Journal of Hospital Pharmacy*. **51**: 2138–2141.
28 Peterson G *et al*. (1991) A preliminary study of the stability of midazolam in polypropylene syringes. *Australian Journal of Hospital Pharmacy*. **21**: 115–118.
29 Macmillan K *et al*. (1994) A prospective comparison study between a butterfly needle and a Teflon cannula for subcutaneous narcotic administration. *Journal of Pain and Symptom Management*. **9**: 82–84.
30 Dawkins L *et al*. (2000) A randomised trial of winged Vialon cannulae and metal butterfly needles. *International Journal of Palliative Nursing*. **6**: 110–111.
31 Ross JR *et al*. (2002) A prospective, within-patient comparison between metal butterfly needles and Teflon cannulae in subcutaneous infusion of drugs to terminally ill hospice patients. *Palliative Medicine*. **16**: 13–16.

Nottingham City Hospital NHS Trust

HAYWARD HOUSE

Macmillan Specialist Palliative Care Unit

SUBCUTANEOUS Syringe Driver Prescription Chart

Affix addressograph label here:

Name:	DOB:	Ward:
Hospital No:	Sex:	Consultant:

Address:

Instructions for setting up SUBCUTANEOUS syringe drivers

1 Check compatibility of drugs prescribed.

2 Make up all syringes to the volumes specified below.
Use **saline** for granisetron, ketamine, ketorolac, octreotide and ondansetron.
Use **water for injections** for all other drugs.

3 Set appropriate rate:

Graseby MS16A delivers in **millimetres per hour**.
Set at **02** to run at 2mm/h over **24** hours.
Set at **04** to run at 4mm/h over **12** hours.

Graseby MS26A delivers in **millimetres per 24 hours**.
Set at **48** to run at 2mm/h over **24** hours.
Set at **96** to run at 4mm/h over **12** hours.

For different syringes the appropriate volume that measures 48mm is:

10ml Plastipak ≈ 8ml. 20ml Plastipak ≈ 14ml. 30ml Plastipak ≈ 17.5ml.

4 Checks in use:

Check the contents of the syringe and tubing and the rate set.
Also measure the volume remaining every **four** hours.
If **not** running on time – refer to checklist and inform doctor.

Each prescription must be rewritten **daily**.

The dose of diamorphine must be written in words and figures for clarity, i.e. 15mg (fifteen).

If syringe driver is to be stopped, indicate clearly on prescription chart.

If the combination of drugs used is changed, prime and resite a new line to avoid problems with compatibility.

SUBCUTANEOUS SYRINGE DRIVER CHECKLIST

If fast (>30 minutes)

1 Check the rate setting is correct.

2 Change entire syringe driver for a new one and send for servicing.

3 Inform doctor if patient's clinical condition gives cause for concern.

If slow (>30 minutes)

1 Check the rate setting is correct.

2 Check syringe driver light is flashing.

3 Check that syringe is inserted correctly into the Graseby pump.

4 Check battery using meter – change if voltage is low.

5 Ascertain if syringe driver has been stopped and then restarted for any reason.

6 Check contents of syringe and line – is there any evidence of crystallisation?

7 Check site of subcutaneous needle – is this red/hard/lumpy/sore? Change if necessary. Consider further dilution of drugs to minimise irritation.

8 Inform a doctor if the patient's clinical condition warrants this, e.g. symptoms not relieved and patient needs p.r.n. drugs prescribing or has needed multiple p.r.n. doses.

At next four-hourly check

1 See steps 1–8.

2 If continuing to run through too slowly, change the syringe driver and send the faulty one for servicing.

Setting up a new driver

Always check:

1 The battery voltage using meter.

2 The rate set.

NAME: **HOSPITAL NO:**

	DRUGS	DOSE	Measurement in syringe at start		CHECKS IN USE Date and Time	Rate set / ? flashing	Site condition	Syringe line & contents	mm left	Slow/fast/ on time	Comments	Signature
Date			Start time	Rate set								
Route			Site	Syringe size								
Duration			Nurses signature (2 nurses to sign)									
Drs signature			Syringe driver pump Serial No:									

	DRUGS	DOSE	Measurement in syringe at start		CHECKS IN USE Date and Time	Rate set / ? flashing	Site condition	Syringe line & contents	mm left	Slow/fast/ on time	Comments	Signature
Date			Start time	Rate set								
Route			Site	Syringe size								
Duration			Nurses signature (2 nurses to sign)									
Drs signature			Syringe driver pump Serial No:									

	DRUGS	DOSE	Measurement in syringe at start		CHECKS IN USE Date and Time	Rate set / ? flashing	Site condition	Syringe line & contents	mm left	Slow/fast/ on time	Comments	Signature
Date			Start time	Rate set								
Route			Site	Syringe size								
Duration			Nurses signature (2 nurses to sign)									
Drs signature			Syringe driver pump Serial No:									

Twelve hourly drivers run at **4mm** per hour. **Twenty-four** hourly drivers run at **2mm** per hour.

Nottingham City Hospital NHS Trust

HAYWARD HOUSE

Macmillan Specialist Palliative Care Unit

EPIDURAL Syringe Driver Prescription Chart

Affix addressograph label here:

Name: DOB: Ward:

Hospital No: Sex: Consultant:

Address:

Instructions for setting up EPIDURAL syringe drivers

1 Always use a **luerlock** syringe.

2 All epidurals should be administered using a 20ml BD Plastipak luerlock syringe. The appropriate volume that measures 48mm is ≈ 14ml. **Saline** should always be used as a diluent.

3 Set appropriate rate:

Graseby MS16A delivers in **millimetres per hour**.
Set at **02** to run at 2mm/h over **24** hours.
Set at **04** to run at 4mm/h over **12** hours.

Graseby MS26A delivers in **millimetres per 24 hours**.
Set at **48** to run at 2mm/h over **24** hours.
Set at **96** to run at 4mm/h over **12** hours.

4 Checks in use:

Check the contents of the syringe and tubing and the rate set. Also measure the volume remaining every **four** hours. If **not** running on time – refer to checklist.

Examine the exit site if visible. *If red or inflamed, inform doctor – need for antibiotics?*

Each prescription must be rewritten **daily**.

The dose of diamorphine must be written in words and figures for clarity, i.e. 15mg (fifteen).

If syringe driver is to be stopped, indicate clearly on prescription chart.

When changing an epidural drug combination, consider changing the external line and priming it with the new combination as well, otherwise it may take up to 12 hours to detect any benefits of the new combination. Generally make up two syringes – one for priming and one for infusion. The doctor will decide whether this is necessary according to the patient's pain.

EPIDURAL CHECKLIST

If fast (>30 minutes)

1 Check the rate setting is correct.

2 Change entire syringe driver for a new one and send for servicing.

3 Inform doctor if patient's clinical condition gives cause for concern.

If slow (>30 minutes)

1 Check the rate setting is correct.

2 Check syringe driver light is flashing.

3 Check that syringe is inserted correctly into the Graseby pump.

4 Check battery using meter – change if voltage is low.

5 Ascertain if syringe driver has been stopped and then restarted for any reason.

6 Check contents of syringe and line – is there any evidence of crystallisation?

7 Check the exit site – is this red or inflamed? If so, inform doctor – patient may need antibiotics.

8 Inform a doctor if patient's clinical condition warrants this, e.g. symptoms not relieved and patient needs p.r.n. drugs prescribing or has needed multiple p.r.n. doses.

At next four-hourly check

1 See steps 1–8.

2 If continuing to run through too slowly change the syringe driver and send the faulty one for servicing.

Setting up a new driver

Always check:

1 The battery voltage using meter.

2 The rate set.

EPIDURAL INFORMATION

Drugs given by the epidural route must be *preservative-free*. A combination of diamorphine and bupivacaine is most commonly used with clonidine occasionally added.

Doses:

Bupivacaine: 0.25%, 0.5% and 0.75%; dose according to advice from an anaesthetist.

Diamorphine: starting dose generally 10–60mg (often one-tenth of previous 24-hour oral morphine dose).

Clonidine: 150–300microgram per 24 hours.

Dose increments should be small:

Bupivacaine usually 1–2ml.

Diamorphine usually 2.5–5mg.

p.r.n. doses of oral morphine should be calculated as one-sixth of the equivalent 24-hour oral morphine dose:

e.g. diamorphine 10mg epidurally daily = morphine 100mg PO daily.
p.r.n. dose = morphine 15mg PO (diamorphine 5mg SC).

Note: laxatives may need to be reduced when opioids are given by the epidural route.

NAME: **HOSPITAL NO:**

	DRUGS	DOSE	Measurement in syringe at start		CHECKS IN USE							
					Date and Time	Rate set / ? flashing	Site condition	Syringe line & contents	mm left	Slow/fast/ on time	Comments	Signature
Date			Start time	Rate set								
Route			Site	Syringe size								
Duration			Nurses signature (2 nurses to sign)									
Drs signature			Syringe driver pump Serial No:									

	DRUGS	DOSE	Measurement in syringe at start		CHECKS IN USE							
					Date and Time	Rate set / ? flashing	Site condition	Syringe line & contents	mm left	Slow/fast/ on time	Comments	Signature
Date			Start time	Rate set								
Route			Site	Syringe size								
Duration			Nurses signature (2 nurses to sign)									
Drs signature			Syringe driver pump Serial No:									

	DRUGS	DOSE	Measurement in syringe at start		CHECKS IN USE							
					Date and Time	Rate set / ? flashing	Site condition	Syringe line & contents	mm left	Slow/fast/ on time	Comments	Signature
Date			Start time	Rate set								
Route			Site	Syringe size								
Duration			Nurses signature (2 nurses to sign)									
Drs signature			Syringe driver pump Serial No:									

Twelve hourly drivers run at **4mm** per hour. **Twenty-four** hourly drivers run at **2mm** per hour.

Nottingham City Hospital NHS Trust

HAYWARD HOUSE

Macmillan Specialist Palliative Care Unit

INTRATHECAL Syringe Driver Prescription Chart

Affix addressograph label here:

Name: DOB: Ward:

Hospital No: Sex: Consultant:

Address:

Instructions for setting up INTRATHECAL syringe drivers

1 Always use a **luerlock** syringe.

2 All intrathecals should be administered using a 20ml BD Plastipak luerlock syringe. The appropriate volume that measures 48mm is ≈ 14ml. **Saline** should always be used as a diluent.

3 Set appropriate rate:

Graseby MS16A delivers in **millimetres per hour**.
Set at **02** to run at 2mm/h over **24** hours.
Set at **04** to run at 4mm/h over **12** hours.

Graseby MS26A delivers in **millimetres per 24 hours**.
Set at **48** to run at 2mm/h over **24** hours.
Set at **96** to run at 4mm/h over **12** hours.

4 Checks in use:

Check the contents of the syringe and tubing and the rate set. Also measure the volume remaining every **four** hours. If **not** running on time – refer to checklist.

Examine the exit site if visible. *If red or inflamed, inform doctor – need for antibiotics?*

Each prescription must be rewritten **daily**.

The dose of diamorphine must be written in words and figures for clarity, i.e. 15mg (fifteen).

If syringe driver is to be stopped, indicate clearly on prescription chart.

When changing an intrathecal drug combination, consider changing the external line and priming it with the new combination as well, otherwise it may take up to 12 hours to detect any benefits of the new combination. Generally make up two syringes – one for priming and one for infusion. The doctor will decide whether this is necessary according to the patient's pain.

INTRATHECAL CHECKLIST

If fast (>30 minutes)

1. Check the rate setting is correct.
2. Change entire syringe driver for a new one and send for servicing.
3. Inform doctor if patient's clinical condition gives cause for concern.

If slow (>30 minutes)

1. Check the rate setting is correct.
2. Check syringe driver light is flashing.
3. Check that syringe is inserted correctly into the Graseby pump.
4. Check battery using meter – change if voltage is low.
5. Ascertain if syringe driver has been stopped and then restarted for any reason.
6. Check contents of syringe and line – is there any evidence of crystallisation?
7. Check the exit site – is this red or inflamed? If so, inform doctor – patient may need antibiotics.
8. Inform a doctor if patient's clinical condition warrants this, e.g. symptoms not relieved and patient needs p.r.n. drugs prescribing or has needed multiple p.r.n. doses.

At next four-hourly check

1. See steps 1–8.
2. If continuing to run through too slowly change the syringe driver and send the faulty one for servicing.

Setting up a new driver

Always check:

1. The battery voltage using meter.
2. The rate set.

INTRATHECAL INFORMATION

Drugs given by the intrathecal route must be *preservative-free.* A combination of diamorphine and bupivacaine is most commonly used with clonidine occasionally added.

Doses:

Bupivacaine: 0.25% (only this strength is used); dose according to advice from an anaesthetist.

Diamorphine: starting dose can be as low as 0.5–1mg, but generally 5–20mg (often one-hundredth of previous 24-hour oral morphine dose).

Clonidine: 15–30microgram per 24 hours.

Dose increments should be small:

Bupivacaine usually 1ml.

Diamorphine usually 0.5–1mg, depending on total dose administered.

Clonidine usually 15microgram.

p.r.n. doses of oral morphine should be calculated as one-sixth of the equivalent 24-hour oral morphine dose:

e.g. diamorphine 5mg intrathecally daily = morphine 500mg PO daily.
p.r.n. dose = morphine 80mg PO (diamorphine 25mg SC).

Note: laxatives may need to be reduced when opioids are given by the intrathecal route.

NAME: **HOSPITAL NO:**

	DRUGS	DOSE	Measurement in syringe at start		CHECKS IN USE							
					Date and Time	Rate set / ? flashing	Site condition	Syringe line & contents	mm left	Slow/fast/ on time	Comments	Signature
Date			Start time	Rate set								
Route			Site	Syringe size								
Duration			Nurses signature (2 nurses to sign)									
Drs signature			Syringe driver pump Serial No:									

	DRUGS	DOSE	Measurement in syringe at start		CHECKS IN USE							
					Date and Time	Rate set / ? flashing	Site condition	Syringe line & contents	mm left	Slow/fast/ on time	Comments	Signature
Date			Start time	Rate set								
Route			Site	Syringe size								
Duration			Nurses signature (2 nurses to sign)									
Drs signature			Syringe driver pump Serial No:									

	DRUGS	DOSE	Measurement in syringe at start		CHECKS IN USE							
					Date and Time	Rate set / ? flashing	Site condition	Syringe line & contents	mm left	Slow/fast/ on time	Comments	Signature
Date			Start time	Rate set								
Route			Site	Syringe size								
Duration			Nurses signature (2 nurses to sign)									
Drs signature			Syringe driver pump Serial No:									

Twelve hourly drivers run at **4mm** per hour. **Twenty-four** hourly drivers run at **2mm** per hour.

Appendix 1: Anaphylaxis

Anaphylaxis is a potentially life-threatening systemic allergic reaction. It manifests as a constellation of features but there is disagreement over which are essential. The confusion about definition arises partly because systemic allergic reactions can be mild, moderate or severe. In practice, the term 'anaphylaxis' should be reserved for cases where there is:

- respiratory difficulty (related to laryngeal oedema and/or bronchoconstriction) *or*
- hypotension (presenting as fainting, collapse or loss of consciousness) *or*
- both.[1]

Urticaria, angioedema or rhinitis alone are best not described as anaphylaxis because neither respiratory difficulty nor hypotension is present.[1]

Causes

In anaphylaxis, an allergic reaction results from the interaction of an allergen with specific IgE antibodies bound to mast cells and basophils. This leads to activation of the mast cell with release of chemical mediators stored in granules (including histamine) as well as rapidly synthesised additional mediators. A rapid major systemic release of these mediators causes capillary leakage and mucosal oedema, resulting in shock and respiratory difficulty.[1]

In contrast, anaphylactoid reactions are caused by activation of mast cells and release of the same mediators, but without the involvement of IgE antibodies. For example, certain drugs act directly on mast cells. In terms of management it is not necessary to distinguish anaphylaxis from an anaphylactoid reaction. This difference is relevant only when investigations are being considered.

Common causes of this rare emergency include blood products, antibiotics, **aspirin**, another NSAID or **heparin**. A possible case has been recorded in a woman with known peanut allergy who received an **arachis** (peanut) **oil** enema.[2] Anaphylaxis is:

- specific to a given drug or chemically-related class of drugs
- more likely after parenteral administration
- more frequent in patients with aspirin-induced asthma or systemic lupus erythematosus.

Clinical features

Clinical manifestations of anaphylaxis typically develop within minutes of taking the causal drug (Box A1.A). Laryngeal oedema and/or bronchoconstriction occurs in only 10% of patients.[3]

Box A1.A Clinical features of anaphylaxis

Essential

Hypotension *and/or* respiratory difficulty (laryngeal oedema, bronchoconstriction)

Possible

Flushing	Tingling of the extremities
Urticaria	Weakness
Angioedema	Agitation

Management

Anaphylaxis requires urgent treatment with **adrenaline** (epinephrine) followed up with an antihistamine and **hydrocortisone** (Box A1.B). However, because their impact is not immediate, corticosteroids are only of secondary value.

Box A1.B Management of anaphylaxis in adults[3,4]

Adrenaline (epinephrine) 1 in 1000 (1mg/1ml), 500microgram (0.5ml) IM:
- if the patient is unconscious, double the dose
- repeat every 5min until blood pressure, pulse and breathing are satisfactory.

Oxygen administration is of primary importance.
Chlorphenamine (chlorpheniramine):
- 10–20mg IV over 1min
- 4–8mg PO t.d.s. for 24–48h to prevent relapse.

Hydrocortisone 200mg IV to prevent further deterioration.

If there is doubt about the adequacy of the circulation, the initial injection can be given as a dilute IV solution, i.e. *1 in 10 000 (1mg/10ml), 500microgram (5ml) over 5min.* However, because too rapid injection of IV adrenaline can cause ventricular arrhythmias, the IV route is generally discouraged unless intensive care facilities are available.

Continuing deterioration requires additional treatment with:
- a nebulised β_2-adrenoceptor stimulant, e.g. **salbutamol**, or IV **aminophylline**
- IV fluids.

Sometimes emergency tracheotomy and assisted respiration may be necessary.

1 Ewan P (1998) ABC of allergies: anaphylaxis. *British Medical Journal.* **316**: 1442–1445.
2 Pharmax (1998) Data on file.
3 Szczeklik A (1986) Analgesics, allergy and asthma. *Drugs.* **32**: 148–163.
4 Anonymous (2001) *British National Formulary* No. 41. British Medical Association and the Royal Pharmaceutical Society of Great Britain, London, pp.156–158.

Appendix 2: Synopsis of pharmacokinetic data

Table A2.1 contains selected pharmacokinetic data for most of the drugs featured in *PCF2*. The plasma halflives given in the table sometimes differ from those in the main text. This is because, for most drugs, several values have been published and here a single value has been chosen.[1,2]

It is important to remember that interindividual variability of pharmacokinetic parameters is generally considerable. For example, the typical range for the total clearance of various drugs is 4- to 5-fold. Further, bio-availability may vary according to formulation.

Key for Table A2.1

a. A = acid; Aa = amino acid; Alc = alcohol; Amf = ampholyte; B = base; B_4 = base with quaternary ammonium group; Gly = glycoside; Pep = peptide; S = steroid; Sa = substituted amide.
b. the pH at which the drug is 50% ionised.
c. the fraction of the drug eliminated by non-renal pathways in normal individuals; 1 – [fraction] gives an estimate of how much of the drug is excreted unchanged in the urine.
d. pharmacologically active metabolite(s).
e. metabolite(s) with possible pharmacological activity.
f. apparent volume of distribution at steady state.
g. after oral administration.

1 Holford NHG (ed) *Clinical Pharmacokinetics: drug data handbook* (3e). Adis International, Auckland.

2 Gelman CR *et al.* (eds) (2001) *Drugdex*® System Micromedex, Inc., Englewood, Colorado. Edition expires 12/2001.

Table A2.1 Pharmacokinetic drug data

	Nature[a]	*pKa*[b]	*Oral bio-availability (%)*	*Clearance (L/h)*	*Plasma halflife (h)*	*Volume of distribution (L)*	*Protein binding (%)*	*Non-renal elimination*[c]	*Comments*
Acetylcysteine			9	58#/8##	2#/5.5##	42#/35##[f]		0.7#	#Reduced acetylcysteine ##Total acetylcysteine
Alfentanil		6.5		20	1.5	49	90		
Amiloride[e]	B	8.7	50	≈31[g]	≈9.6	≈350[g]		0.25[e]	
Amitriptyline[d]	B	9.4	48	51	19	1085[f]	95	1.0[d]	
Aspirin[d]	A	3.5	68	39	0.25#	10.5	≈70	1.0#	#Active metabolite (salicylate) t½ = 2–30h
Atropine	B	9.25		70	2.2	231	50	0.45	
Baclofen[e]	A	3.9/9.6			3.5		30	0.15[e]	
Beclometasone dipropionate	S		60–90		15				
Betamethasone	S		72	11	6.5	126	6.4	0.95	
Bromocriptine[e]	Pep	4.9	6	56	3	≈238	90	1.0[e]	
Budesonide	S		10#	84	2.7	308	88		#High first-pass metabolism
Bumetanide[e]	A		90	12	1.75	16.8	96	0.35[e]	
Bupivacaine	B	8.1		35	2.7	70[f]	96	0.95	
Buprenorphine	B	8.49/10.03	30#	70	2.5	140	≈96	1.0	#Sublingual
Carbamazepine[d]	Sa		>70	1.1/4.5[g]	36/16#	84[g]	75	1.0[d]	#Single dose/long-term treatment
Cefradine	Amf	2.6/7.3	>90	17	0.8	17.5	10	0.15	
Cefuroxime	A	≈2.5		8	1.3	17.5	≈40	0.07	
Celecoxib				36	11	400	97		
Cetirizine				3	7–10	35	93	0.4	
Chlorpropamide[d]	A	4.8	>90	0.13[g]	40	≈10.5[g]	90	0.2[d]	
Chlordiazepoxide[d]	B	4.8	>86	1	20	28	96	1.0[d]	
Chlorphenamine[d] (chlorpheniramine)	B	9.2		7.2	20	238	72	0.8[d]	

Table A2.1 Continued

	Nature[a]	*pKa*[b]	*Oral bio-availability (%)*	*Clearance (L/h)*	*Plasma halflife (h)*	*Volume of distribution (L)*	*Protein binding (%)*	*Non-renal elimination*[c]	*Comments*
Chlorpromazine[d]	B	9.3	32#	38##	30	1470##	98	1.0[d]	#After PO administration ##After IM administration
Cimetidine	B	6.8	70#	36	2	91	20	0.3	#IM >90%
Cisapride			40–50		10	168	98	1.0	
Clindamycin[e]	B	7.45	87	12	3	56	93	0.9[e]	
Clonidine[e]	B	8.25	90	0.16–0.6#	6.2–12.8#	241.5	20	0.4[e]	#Dose-dependent
Clodronate disodium				6	2#			≈0.1	#Terminal elimination phase t½ = 13h
Clomipramine[d]	B			45	20	1162	98	1.0[d]	
Clonazepam	Amf	1.5/10.5	98	≈6[g]	25	210[g]	85	1.0	
Codeine[d]	B	7.95	55	98#	2.8	378#	≈7	1.0[d]	#After PO administration, corrected for bio-availability
Dantrolene[d]	A	7.5			≈9			0.95[d]	
Desipramine[d]	B	10.2	51	130[g]	22	1568[g]	80	1.0[d]	
Demeclocycline	Amf	3.3/7.2/9.4			12	126	≈70		
Dexamethasone	S		80	14.7	3	52.5	77	1.0	
Dextropropoxyphene	B	6.3		66	2.7	189	78	≈1.0	
Diazepam[d]	B	3.3	100	1.8	40#	140	98	1.0	#Active metabolite t½ = 30–200h
Diclofenac[e]	A		60	15.6	1.5	10.5	>99	1.0[e]	
Diflunisal	A		100	0.35–0.49#	5–20#	7.7	99	0.95	#Dose-dependent
Digoxin#	Gly		70	4.5	40	420	27	0.3	#Recommended therapeutic plasma concentration 0.8–2microgram/L
Diltiazem		7.7	41	60	5.1	315	98	1.0	
Diphenhydramine[e]	B	8.3	42	47	5	280	98.5	0.9[e]	
Diphenoxylate	B	7.07			2.5	322			
Dosulepin (dothiepin)			30	146	25	4900			

Table A2.1 Continued

	Nature[a]	pKa[b]	Oral bio-availability (%)	Clearance (L/h)	Plasma halflife (h)	Volume of distribution (L)	Protein binding (%)	Non-renal elimination[c]	Comments
Ethinylestradiol	S		40	23	13	203	97		
Erythromycin	B	8.8	35	26	1.3–2.4#	35–70#	73	0.8	#Dose-dependent
Erythropoietin	Pep		21.5	0.18#	8#	2.1#		0.9	#In dialysis patients after IV dose
Fentanyl[e]	B	8.43		47	3	≈210	83	0.95[e]	
Flecainide[d]			95	42.8#	12#/19.5##	588#	52	0.7[d]	Recommended therapeutic plasma concentration <800microgram/L #Healthy volunteers ##Arrhythmia patients
Flucloxacillin[d]	A	2.7		5	1.5	10.5	93	0.3[d]	
Fluconazole			90		30	56	11	0.3	
Fludrocortisone					0.5		75		
Flunitrazepam[e]	B	1.84	85	8[g]	29	259[g]		1.0[e]	
Fluoxetine				40(10)#	48(96)#	1400(2940)	94	0.97	#Multiple dose data in parenthesis
Flurbiprofen	A		>85	1.3[g]	3.5	7[g]	>99	0.9	
Fluticasone					8		91		
Fluvoxamine			77		20	1400		0.95	
Furosemide(frusemide)	A	3.9	65	8	1	21	97	0.35	
Gabapentin			60	7.5	5–7	49	0		
Glibenclamide[d]		5.3		5.5	1.5–10#	10.5	>99	1.0[d]	#Divergent values reported
Gliclazide	A	5.8		0.8	12	21	90	1.0	
Glyceryl trinitrate				≈1260	0.05	≈210			
Granisetron				14.7	11	231		0.9	Wide interindividual differences
Haloperidol	B	8.3	65	46	20	1400	90	1.0	
Heparin	A		0	2.5#	1.5#	4.9	95##	0.8	#Dose- and assay-dependent ##Lipoproteins

Table A2.1 Continued

	Nature[a]	*pKa*[b]	*Oral bio-availability (%)*	*Clearance (L/h)*	*Plasma halflife (h)*	*Volume of distribution (L)*	*Protein binding (%)*	*Non-renal elimination*[c]	*Comments*
Hydrocortisone	S			21–30#	1.3–1.9#	21–35#	75–95#		#Dose-dependent
Hyoscine hydrobromide	B	7.55	23	45	2.5	140		0.45	
Hyoscine butylbromide	B_4				14		11#		#Albumin
Ibuprofen	A	4.4/5.2	>80#	3.5[g]	2.5	9.8[g]	99	1.0	#Dose-dependent
Imipramine[d]	B	9.5	27	58	18	1470	89	1.0[d]	
Indoramin	B	7.8		66	5–15#	518	90	0.95	#Wide interindividual variability
Insulin	Pep			10–40#	0.25–2#		≈5	0.4	#Divergent values reported
Ipratropium bromide	B				≈3.5			0.3	
Isosorbide-5-mononitrate			93	7.6	4.4	49	0	0.8	
Itraconazole			40		30#		>99		#At steady rate
Ketamine[e]		7.5	20#	60	3	140	12	1.0[e]	#IM
Ketoconazole		2.9/6.5			8		99	1.0	
Ketorolac		3.49	80	2	5.6	17.5	99		
Lamotrigine			98	1.9	30	80.5	55	0.9	
Lansoprazole					2			1.0	
Levodopa[d]	Aa	2.3/8.7			1.4			1.0[d]	
Levomepromazine (methotrimeprazine)		7.7	50	2880	15–30				
Levothyroxine sodium				0.1	150	≈14	>99		
Lidocaine# (lignocaine)	B	7.86	35	40	3.9	210	60	0.95	#Recommended therapeutic plasma concentration 2–5mg/L
Lithium#			>85	1.6	27	56		1.02	#Therapeutic plasma concentration 0.4–1.2mmol/L
Lofepramine[d]			<10	686[g]	2.2		>99	1.0	Active metabolite desipramine

Table A2.1 Continued

	Nature[a]	*pKa*[b]	*Oral bio-availability (%)*	*Clearance (L/h)*	*Plasma halflife (h)*	*Volume of distribution (L)*	*Protein binding (%)*	*Non-renal elimination*[c]	*Comments*
Loperamide[e]	B	8.7			10		97	1.0[e]	
Lorazepam	Amf	1.3/11.5	93	3[g]	20	105[g]	90	1.0	
Medroxyprogesterone[e]	S			≈76#	≈36	≈42#	94	0.55[e]	#After PO and IM administration
Metformin			50	26–42#	1.5–4.5#†	70–280#	<5	0.01	#Divergent values reported; †terminal elimination t½ ≈ 10h
Methadone	B	8.25	92	7.5	29	280	80	0.6	
Methylphenidate			25/5#	28/51#	5.6/3.7#	186/126#[f]			#D/R enantiomer
Methylprednisolone	S	4.6	82	15	3	49		1.0	
Metoclopramide			85	38/23#	4/7#	210	30	0.7	#Possibly dose-dependent
Metronidazole[d]	B?	2.62	100#	3	8	49	<20	0.85[d]	#Rectal 70%
Mexiletine[e]#		8.75	85	27	10	350	70	0.8[e]	#Recommended therapeutic plasma concentration 0.8–2mg/L
Miconazole[e]		6.65	27	46	23	1400	99	1.0[e]	
Midazolam	B	6.1	35	20	3.0	84	95	1.0	
Misoprostol[d]					1.5#		85		#Active metabolite. Parent drug undetectable in plasma after oral dose
Morphine[e]	Amf	9.85/7.87	20–33	72	2.5#	245	35	0.9[e]	#Active metabolite (morphine-6-glucuronide) t½ = ≤7.5h in renal failure
Nabilone[d]			95		2#				#Halflife of active metabolites is 35h
Naloxone[e]	B	7.94	2	104	1.5	210		≈1.0[e]	
Naltrexone			5–60#	94	2.7	994	20	1.0	#Dose-dependent
Naproxen	A	4.15	99	0.3	14	7	99	0.9	
Nifedipine			50	42	1.8	98	97	1.0	
Nimesulide					4.8		99		
Nitrazepam	Amf	3.4/10.8	78	4	30	175	85	1.0	

Table A2.1 Continued

	Nature[a]	*pKa*[b]	*Oral bio-availability (%)*	*Clearance (L/h)*	*Plasma halflife (h)*	*Volume of distribution (L)*	*Protein binding (%)*	*Non-renal elimination*[c]	*Comments*
Nitrofurantoin[d]	A	7.2	87	41	1	56	≈40	0.7[d]	
Nordiazepam[d] (N-desmethyldiazepam)	Amf	11.65/3.35	50	1.5	80	175	97	1.0[d]	#Active metabolite of diazepam
Nortriptyline[d]	B	9.73	51	40	28	1470	93	1.0[d]	
Octreotide	Pep		<5	11.4	1.5	23.8		0.9	
Olanzapine				18.2	34	721–1288	93		
Omeprazole	Amf	3.97/8.8	67	35	0.5	24.5	95	1.0	
Ondansetron			60	29	3	161	70–76		
Orphenadrine	B	8.4			18		20		
Oxazepam	Amf	11.51/1.56	>90	8[g]	7	70[g]	>95	1.0	
Pamidronate disodium					27				
Paracetamol[d]	A	9.5	70–90	19.3	2.5	65.8	Low#	1.0[d]	#At therapeutic doses
Paroxetine			50		24		95	0.98	
Pethidine[d]	B	6.3	54	38	6.9	280	70	0.9[d]	
Phenobarbital#	A	7.2	100	0.3	100	49	50	0.7	#Recommended therapeutic plasma concentration 10–35mg/L
Phenoxymethylpenicillin	A	2.73			0.5	≈35	80	0.6	
Phenytoin#	A	8.33	98	##	9–40	56	90	1.0	#Recommended therapeutic plasma concentration 10–20mg/L ##Dose-dependent
Prednisolone			80	6.3–15#	3.6	28–91#	65–91#	1.0	#Concentration-dependent
Prochlorperazine	B	3.73/8.1			≈23				
Promethazine	B	9.1	25	68	12	910[f]			
Propantheline[e]	B_4			79	1.8			0.85[e]	
Propofol				104	0.05:0.5:4#	280[f]		1.0	#Tri-exponential
Propranolol[d]	B	9.45	≈30	63	4	196	93	1.0[d]	

Table A2.1 Continued

	Nature[a]	pKa[b]	Oral bio-availability (%)	Clearance (L/h)	Plasma halflife (h)	Volume of distribution (L)	Protein binding (%)	Non-renal elimination[c]	Comments
Quinine	B	4.3/8.4		5.5	14	112	90	0.8	
Ranitidine[d]	B	2.7	50	35	2	105	15	0.3[d]	
Risperidone[d]					3#	105	90		#Active metabolite (9-OH-risperidone) t½ = 24h
Rofecoxib			93		17	91	87	0.99	
Salbutamol	B	9.3	10.3		≈5				
Salmeterol					67		95–98		
Sertraline					26	>1400	99	1.0	
Sodium cromoglicate	A	2.0			0.1		7.0	0.6	
Spironolactone[d]	S		70		19#		98#	1.0[d]	#Active metabolite (canrenone)
Sufentanil		8.01		44	2.6	140	93		
Sulindac[d]	A	4.5	>88		7#		96	1.0#	#Active sulfide metabolite t½ = 18h
Temazepam	B	1.31	>80	4[g]	13	70[g]	97	1.0	
Tenoxicam				0.13	72	14	99	1.0	
Terazosin			82	3.3	12	21	90	0.9	
Terbutaline	Amf	10.1/11.2/8.8		13	15	112[f]	25	0.45	
Terfenadine[d]					20		97	1.0[d]	
Tetracycline	Amf	7.7/3.3/9.5	77	15[g]	6	140[g]		0.12	
Thalidomide[e]			67–93#	10	5–7	120		0.993	#In animals
Theophylline[d]#	Amf	8.6/3.5	96	3	8	35	50	0.9[d]	#Recommended therapeutic plasma concentration 10–20mg/L
Thioridazine[d]					≈20		99#	1.0[d]	#Concentration-dependent
Tinidazole			>90	3	13	45.5	12	0.75	
Tizanidine			40	120#	2.5	144#	30		#Based on a 60kg person
Tolbutamide	A	5.43		≈1[g]	7	10.5[g]	95#		#Concentration-dependent
Tramadol[d]				26	6	231	4	0.7[d]	

Table A2.1 Continued

	Nature[a]	*pKa*[b]	*Oral bio-availability (%)*	*Clearance (L/h)*	*Plasma halflife (h)*	*Volume of distribution (L)*	*Protein binding (%)*	*Non-renal elimination*[c]	*Comments*
Tranexamic acid	A	4.3/10.6	34	6.7	10			0.03	
Triamcinolone	S			45–70#	1.4	98–147#		1.0	#Dose-dependent
Trimethoprim	B	7.2	100	4.5[g]	11	91[g]	45	0.45	
Trimipramine[e]	B		41	67	23	2170	95	1.0[e]	
Tropisetron			52–66#	60/12##	8/35	546	59–71#	0.9	#Dose-dependent ##Two hydroxylation phenotypes
Valproic acid[d]#	A	4.95	100	0.5	13	10.5	90		#Recommended therapeutic plasma concentration 50–100mg/L
Vancomycin	B			4.0	10	42[f]	<10–55#	0.03	#Divergent values reported
Venlafaxine					4/10#	525/400#	27		#Parent drug/active metabolite
Vigabatrin				5.6	7	56	<1	0	
Warfarin[d]	A	5.0	100	0.2/0.15#[g]	35/50#	10.5[g]	99	1.0[d]	#S/R enantiomers
Zolpidem			70	18.2	2	37.8	90	1.0	
Zopiclone			80	14.8	4.9	98	45	1.0	

a. A = acid; Aa = amino acid; Alc = alcohol; Amf = ampholyte; B = base; B_4 = base with quaternary ammonium group; Gly = glycoside; Pep = peptide; S = steroid; Sa = substituted amide.
b. the pH at which the drug is 50% ionised.
c. the fraction of the drug eliminated by non-renal pathways in normal individuals; 1 – [fraction] gives an estimate of how much of the drug is excreted unchanged in the urine.
d. pharmacologically active metabolite(s).
e. metabolite(s) with possible pharmacological activity.
f. apparent volume of distribution at steady state.
g. after oral administration.

Appendix 3: Prolongation of the QT interval in palliative care

The QT interval lies on the electrocardiograph (ECG) between the beginning of the QRS complex (which marks the start of ventricular depolarisation) and the end of the T wave (which marks the end of ventricular repolarisation) (Figure A3.1).

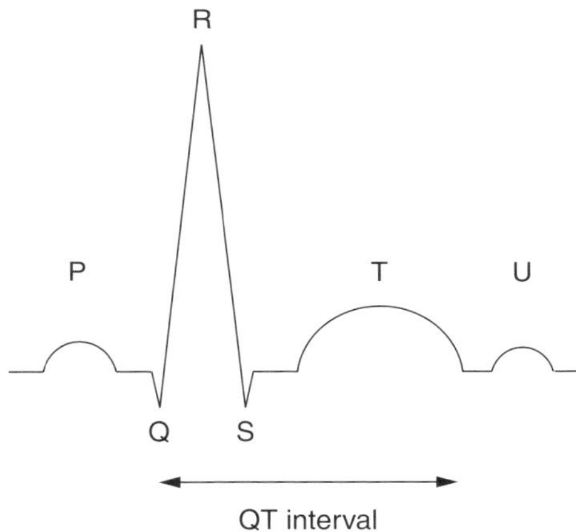

Figure A3.1 The QT interval.

The QT interval tends to be longer in females and with slower heart rates. A QTc interval (the QT interval corrected for heart rate) >450msec in males and >470msec in females is generally considered abnormal. A prolonged QT interval is associated with an increased risk of life-threatening ventricular tachyarrhythmia, particularly *torsades de pointes*, and of sudden death (Figure A3.2).[1] There is a risk of *torsades de pointes* with any prolongation of the QT interval, and the risk grows as the QT interval increases, particularly >500msec. A drug which increases an individual's QTc interval by 30–60msec should also raise concern and if by >60msec serious concern about the risk of arrhythmia.[2] The risk of *torsades de pointes* may be increased by other factors (Box A3.A). Classes of drugs commonly implicated include cardiac anti-arrhythmics, anti-psychotics, antihistamines and macrolides (Box A3.B).

The basic mechanism by which most drugs prolong the QT interval appears to be through potassium-channel blockade, interfering with potassium currents in (enhanced) and out (reduced) of the cardiac myocytes and thereby modifying the action potential duration.[3] The incidence of *torsades de pointes* appears greatest with the use of cardiac anti-arrhythmics, e.g. **quinidine** 2–9%, compared to other classes of drug, e.g. 1 in 120 000 patients treated with **cisapride**.[3] For some drugs, the risk is present only with plasma concentrations seen with:

- high doses
- IV administration
- a drug interaction, e.g. imidazole antifungals inhibit the P450 iso-enzyme CYP3A4 and thereby prevent the metabolism of **cisapride.**

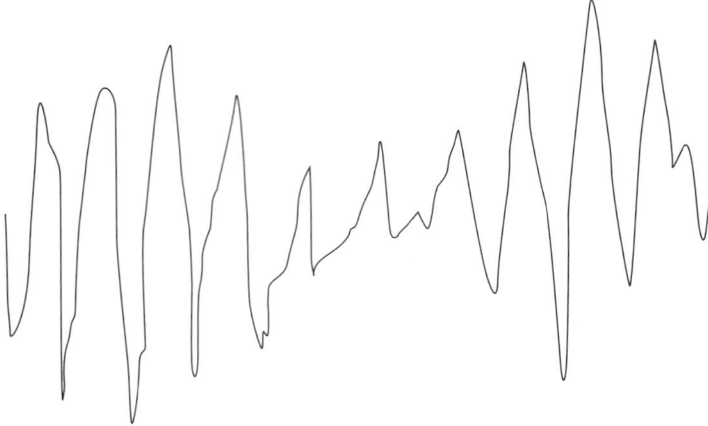

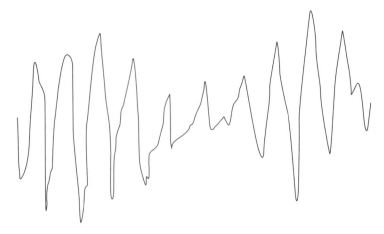

Figure A3.2 *Torsades de pointes*. Twisting complexes of ventricular tachycardia.

Box A3.A Risk factors for *torsades de pointes*	
Congenital long QT syndrome	Electrolyte imbalance
Female	hypokalaemia
History of	hypomagnesaemia
symptomatic arrhythmias	Liver and renal impairment
bradycardia <50 beats/min	reduced drug metabolism and excretion
hypertension	Hypothyroidism
other cardiac disease	Alcoholism
Drugs (see Box A3.2)	Malnutrition

However, the degree of QT prolongation is not always dose-related. Further, because many of the risk drugs are substrates for CYP2D6, the 5–10% of the white European population which are CYP2D6 poor metabolisers may be exposed to dangerously high plasma concentrations even with normal doses.[7] Also see Cytochrome P450, p.331.

Growing safety concerns in relation to drug-induced prolonged QT interval has seen several drugs withdrawn, e.g. **terodiline**, **astemizole**, **cisapride**, **droperidol**, or their licensed indications severely restricted, e.g. **thioridazine**. Some other commonly used antipsychotics, e.g. **haloperidol**, and tricyclic antidepressants, e.g. **amitriptyline**, also prolong the QT interval. Palliative care patients may be at particular risk of prolonged QT interval given the high prevalence of multiple drug use, malnutrition and metabolic disturbance.

In a survey of 100 patients referred to a specialist palliative care unit, who were not imminently dying, 15% had a prolonged QTc interval, but only one patient had a severely prolonged uncorrected QT of >500msec (Figure A3.3).[2,8] The demographics of patients with a normal or prolonged QTc interval were similar apart from the latter having a greater male:female ratio ($p = 0.001$) and more severe liver impairment ($p \leqslant 0.01$). There was no significant correlation between QTc interval and age, performance status, number of at risk drugs used, serum electrolytes or renal function. There was weak but significant correlation between QTc interval and alkaline phosphatase ($r = 0.24$, $p < 0.05$) and bilirubin ($r = 0.30$, $p < 0.01$). The only apparent risk factor in the patient with a QT of 560msec was ischaemic heart disease. Although a crude endpoint without post-mortem examination, there was no statistical difference in median survival and incidence of sudden death in patients with a prolonged QTc interval.

Box A3.B Commonly used drugs associated with prolonged QT interval [3–6]

Anti-arrhythmic drugs
Amiodarone
Bretylium
Disopyramide
N-acetyl-procainamide
Procainamide
Propafenone
Quinidine
Sotalol, d-sotalol

Psychiatric drugs
Amitriptyline
Chloral hydrate
Chlorpromazine
Citalopram
Clomipramine
Desipramine
Doxepin
Droperidol[a]
Fluoxetine
Fluphenazine
Haloperidol
Imipramine
Lithium
Maprotiline
Nortriptyline
Olanzapine
Pimozide[a]
Prochlorperazine
Risperidone
Sertindole[a]
Thioridazine[a]
Trifluoperazine
Venlafaxine

Antimicrobial and antimalarial drugs
Amantadine
Chloroquine
Clarithromycin
Clindamycin
Co-trimoxazole
Erythromycin
Ketoconazole
Pentamidine
Quinine
Spiramycin

Antihistamines
Astemizole[a]
Diphenhydramine
Fexofenadine
Hydroxyzine
Terfenadine[a]

Miscellaneous
β_2-receptor agonists (with hypokalaemia)
Cisapride[a]
Fos-phenytoin
Granisetron
Nicardipine
Octreotide
Ondansetron
Probucol
Sumatriptan
Tamoxifen
Terodiline[a]
Vasopressin

a. Drugs withdrawn, suspended or restricted because of safety concerns regarding prolonged QT interval.

Palliative medicine physicians need to be aware that prolonged QT interval is relatively common in their patients, although a severely prolonged QT interval is rare. These patients may be exposed to many risk factors for prolonged QT and *torsades de pointes*, including some of the drugs commonly used in palliative care. However, the risk of developing this arrhythmia is unknown.

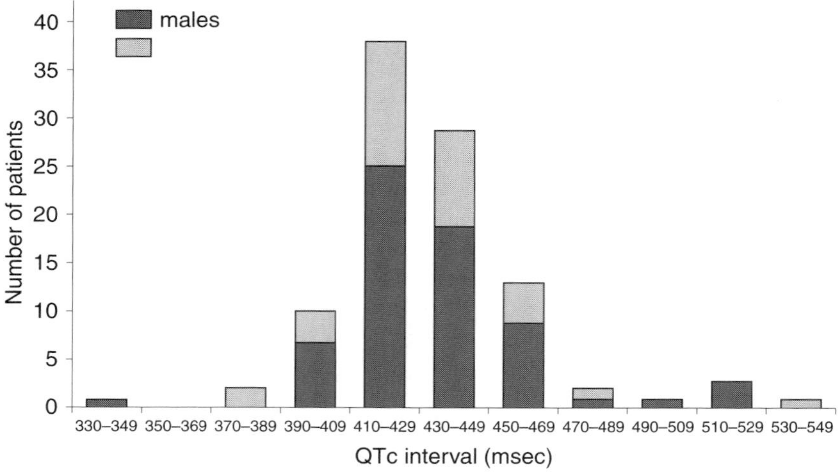

Figure A3.3 Distribution of QTc interval in 100 palliative care patients.

1 De Ponti F *et al.* (2000) QT-interval prolongation by non-cardiac drugs: lessons to be learned from recent experience. *European Journal of Clinical Pharmacology*. **56**: 1–18.

2 Anonymous (1996) Points to consider: the assessment of the potential for QT interval prolongation by non-cardiovascular medicinal products. European Agency for the Evaluation of Medicinal Products (EMEA); Committee for Proprietary Medicinal Products: CPMP/986/96.

3 Haverkamp W *et al.* (2000) The potential for QT prolongation and proarrhythmia by non-antiarrhythmic drugs: clinical and regulatory implications. *European Heart Journal*. **21**: 1216–1231.

4 Viskin S (1999) Long QT syndromes and torsade de pointes. *Lancet*. **354**: 1625–1633.

5 www.torsades.org

6 De Ponti F *et al.* (2001) Organising evidence on QT prolongation and occurrence of torsade de pointes with non-antiarrhythmic drugs: a call for consensus. *European Journal of Clinical Pharmacology*. **57**: 185–209.

7 Idle JR (2000) The heart of psychotropic drug therapy. *Lancet*. **355**: 1824.

8 Walker G *et al.* (2001) Hayward House, Nottingham, personal communication.

Appendix 4: Cytochrome P450

Polypharmacy (i.e. using more than one drug concurrently) introduces the possibility of clinically important drug interactions. In the past, concern about interactions focused mainly on changes in drug absorption, protein binding in the blood and renal excretion. There was also recognition of important metabolic interactions such as the serotonin syndrome observed with **pethidine** and MAOIs. However, studies over the last 20 years have shown that most of the potentially serious drug interactions involve hepatic biotransformation pathways catalysed by the cytochrome P450 mixed-function oxidase group of enzymes. These are the major drug metabolising enzymes involved in intramolecular biotransformation processes, principally *oxidation* and *reduction*.

The name cytochrome P450 is derived from the spectrometer characteristics of the group of enzymes; maximum absorbance is produced at or near 450nm. Cytochrome P450 enzymes exist in virtually all tissues but their highest concentration is in the liver. In mammals, the cytochrome P450 group of enzymes comprises at least 14 families (>40% identical gene content) with some 30 active subfamilies (>55% identical gene content) (Figure A4.1). Cytochrome P450 enzymes are identified by the root symbol CYP, followed by:

- a number designating the enzyme family
- a capital letter designating the subfamily
- a number designating the individual enzyme.

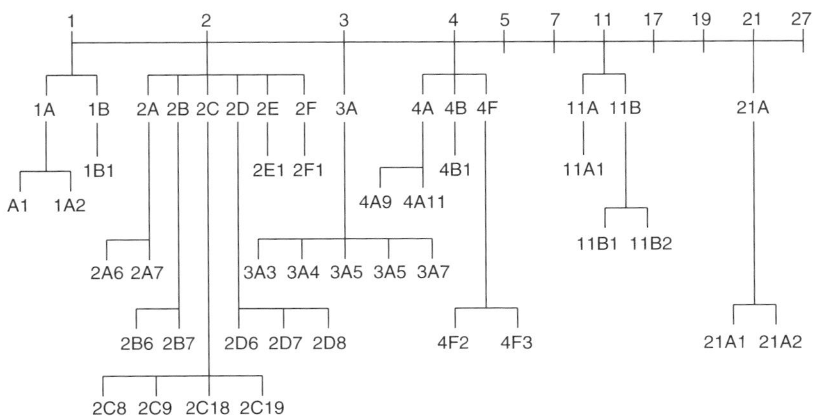

Figure A4.1 Cytochrome P450 enzyme tree.[1]

The mammalian P450 families can be divided into two major classes; those involved in the synthesis of steroids and bile acids and those which primarily metabolise foreign substances (xenobiotics). Enzymes of the CYP1, CYP2 and CYP3 families are responsible for many drug biotransformations and account for 70% of the total P450 content of the liver (Figure A4.2). Drugs responsible for interactions act either as *inhibitors* or *inducers*.

Inhibition

Inhibition of drug biotransformation begins within a few hours of the administration of the inhibitor drug, leading to an increase in the substrate drug plasma concentration, drug response and

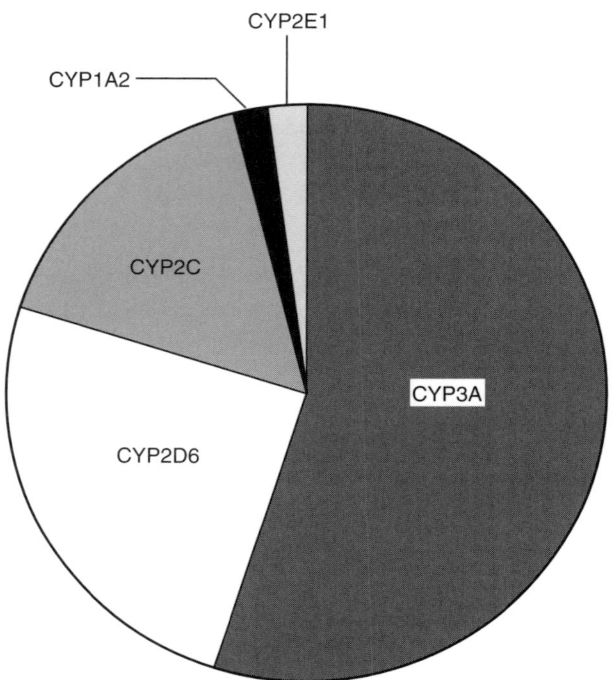

Figure A4.2 Proportion of drugs metabolised by different cytochrome P450 iso-enzymes. CYP2C includes all the 2C subfamily of enzymes.[1]

toxicity (*except pro-drugs which will have a corresponding reduced effect*).The mechanism of enzymatic inhibition is either competitive or non-competitive. In competitive inhibition, the inhibitor drug (e.g. **cimetidine**, **ketoconazole** and macrolide antibiotics) binds to the P450 enzyme and prevents the metabolism of the substrate drug. The extent of inhibition of one drug by another depends on their relative affinities for the P450 enzyme. In non-competitive inhibition the enzyme is destroyed or inactivated by the inhibitor drug or its metabolites (e.g. **chloramphenicol** and **spironolactone**). The occurrence of serious cardiac arrhythmias seen with the concurrent administration of **ketoconazole** (an inhibitor) and **terfenadine** is an example of a non-competitive inhibitory drug interaction involving CYP3A3/4[2] (Box A4.A).

Box A4.A Ketoconazole-induced terfenadine cardiotoxicity[3]

A 39 year-old woman began a course of terfenadine and after about 1 week started ketoconazole. Two days later she developed syncopal symptoms, prolongation of her QT interval on the ECG and *torsades de pointes*. Plasma assay showed high concentrations of terfenadine and reduced concentrations of its main metabolite suggesting inhibition of metabolism. It was concluded that ketoconazole-induced inhibition of terfenadine metabolism caused the cardiotoxicity.

A food–drug interaction has been highlighted involving grapefruit juice and substrates of CYP3A3/4 iso-enzymes such as **felodipine**, **nifedipine**, **ciclosporin** and **terfenadine**.[4] Grapefruit juice contains several bioflavonoids (naringenin, kaempferol and quercetin) which non-competitively inhibit oxidation reactions in the CYP3A3/4 enzymes in the gastro-intestinal wall.[5] The effect is variable because the flavonoids in grapefruit products vary up to 6-fold;[6] it is maximal when grapefruit juice is ingested 30–60min before the drug. In contrast, orange juice does not contain these bioflavonoids and does not inhibit drug metabolism. Box A4.B gives examples of enhanced drug effects resulting from enzyme inhibition. Table A4.1 gives numerous examples of cytochrome P450 enzyme inhibitors which may increase the plasma concentrations of various substrate drugs.[7,8]

Box A4.B Examples of drug interactions → increased effect

Cimetidine reduces diazepam clearance → increased effect.[9]
Ciprofloxacin reduces theophylline clearance by 18–113% → increased effect.[10]
Diltiazem prolongs the halflife of propranolol and metoprolol → increased effect.[11]
Erythromycin increases cisapride concentration → possible cardiac effects.
Fluvoxamine increases warfarin concentration by 65% → increased effect.[12]
Ketoconazole increases terfenadine concentration → possible life-threatening cardiac arrhythmias.[13]
Mexiletine reduces clearance of amitriptyline → increased effect.
SSRIs reduce clearance of tricyclic antidepressants → increased plasma concentrations by 50–350% → increased effect.[14–16]

Induction

Induction of the rate of drug biotransformation results in a decrease in the parent drug plasma concentrations and either decreased pharmacological effect or increased toxicity if active metabolites are formed or if the administered drug is an inactive pro-drug. The onset and offset of enzyme induction is gradual because:

- onset depends on drug-induced synthesis of new enzyme
- offset depends upon elimination of the enzyme-inducing drug and the decay of the increased enzyme stores.

Several molecular mechanisms for enzyme induction have been characterised, including increased DNA transcription (the most common), increased RNA processing and mRNA stabilisation.

Inducer drugs like **rifampicin**, **dexamethasone**, **griseofulvin** and anti-epileptics such as **carbamazepine**, **phenobarbital** and **phenytoin** induce members of the CYP3A subfamily. **Rifampicin** is the most potent inducer of cytochrome CYP3A in clinical use. Some oestrogens are metabolised by CYP3A3/4 and induction by **rifampicin** has caused oral contraceptive failure. In fact, any enzyme inducer can cause oral contraceptive failure. Box A4.C gives examples of decreased drug effects as a result of enzyme induction. Table A4.1 gives numerous examples of cytochrome P450 enzyme inducers which may decrease the plasma concentrations of various substrate drugs. **Carbamazepine** can potentially decrease the effect of many other drugs by decreasing their plasma concentrations (or can expedite the biotransformation of a drug to an active metabolite). For example, **carbamazepine** increases **diazepam** metabolism but, in this case, there may be no detectable clinical effect because of active metabolites.

Box A4.C Examples of drug interactions → decreased effect

Carbamazepine and phenytoin increase midazolam metabolism → decreased effect.[17]
Phenytoin increases carbamazepine metabolism → possible therapeutic failure.
Quinidine inhibits biotransformation of codeine to morphine → decreased analgesic effect.[18]
Rifampicin increases phenytoin clearance (halflife halved) → decreased effect.[19]

Table A4.1 Selected list of P450 drug interactions

Iso-enzyme	*Substrates*	*Inhibitors*	*Inducers*
CYP1A2	Amitriptyline Caffeine Clomipramine Clozapine Ethinylestradiol Imipramine Olanzapine Paracetamol Propranolol Theophylline Trimipramine	Cimetidine Ciprofloxacin[a] Diltiazem Enoxacin[a] Erythromycin (weak) Fluoxetine (weak)[b] Fluvoxamine[b] Grapefruit juice Mexiletine Norfloxacin (weak)[a] Paroxetine (weak)[b] Sertraline (weak)[b] Verapamil	Brassicas Charbroiled beef Smoking Omeprazole Phenobarbital Phenytoin
CYP2C9/10	Amitriptyline Diclofenac Fluvastatin Ibuprofen Imipramine Naproxen Phenytoin Piroxicam Tolbutamide Torasemide Warfarin Zafirlukast	Amiodarone Cimetidine Fluconazole[c] Fluvastatin (possibly) Metronidazole Miconazole Ritonavir Sulfamethoxazole Trimethoprim Zafirlukast	Carbamazepine Rifampicin
CYP2C18/19[d]	Amitriptyline Citalopram Clomipramine Diazepam Imipramine Lansoprazole Moclobemide Omeprazole Pentamidine Phenytoin Proguanil Propranolol	Cimetidine Fluoxetine[b] Fluvoxamine[b] Ketoconazole[c] Moclobemide Omeprazole	Phenytoin Rifampicin (possibly)
CYP2D6[e]	Amitriptyline Captopril Clomipramine Clozapine Codeine Desipramine Dextromethorphan Flecainide Fluoxetine Haloperidol Hydrocodone Imipramine Metoprolol Mexiletine	Amiodarone Cimetidine Flecainide Fluoxetine[b] Fluvoxamine (weak)[b] Haloperidol Levomepromazine Paroxetine[b] Perphenazine Propafenone Quinidine[f] Sertraline (weak)[b] Thioridazine Tramadol[g]	

continued

Table A4.1 Continued

Iso-enzyme	*Substrates*	*Inhibitors*	*Inducers*
CYP2D6[e] (cont)	Nortriptyline Ondansetron Oxycodone Paroxetine Perphenazine Propafenone Propoxyphene Propranolol Quinidine Risperidone Ritonavir Sertraline Thioridazine Timolol Tramadol Venlafaxine		
CYP2E1	Alcohol Caffeine Isoniazid Paracetamol Theophylline	Disulfiram Isoniazid	Alcohol Isoniazid
CYP3A4[h]/5	Alfentanil Alprazolam Amiodarone Amitriptyline Astemizole Carbamazepine Ciclosporin Cisapride Clomipramine Clozapine Codeine Corticosteroids Diazepam Diltiazem Erythromycin Ethinylestradiol Felodipine Imipramine Lidocaine Midazolam Nefazodone Nifedipine Paracetamol Phenytoin Pimozide Propafenone Quinidine Ritonavir Sertraline Simvastatin	Bromocriptine Ciclosporin Cimetidine Clarithromycin Danazol Diltiazem Erythromycin Ergotamine Ethinylestradiol Fluconazole[c] Fluoxetine[b] Fluvoxamine[b] Gestodene Grapefruit juice Indanivir Itraconazole[c] Ketoconazole[c] Miconazole Midazolam Nefazodone Nicardipine Nifedipine Omeprazole Paroxetine (weak)[b] Progesterone Propoxyphene Quinidine Ritonavir Sertraline (weak)[b] Testosterone	Carbamazepine Dexamethasone Phenobarbital Phenytoin Rifampicin Troglitazone

continued

Table A4.1 Continued

Iso-enzyme	*Substrates*	*Inhibitors*	*Inducers*
	Tamoxifen Terfenadine Triazolam Verapamil Warfarin	Verapamil Zafirlukast	

a. relative inhibitory potency of fluoroquinolones: enoxacin>ciprofloxacin>norfloxacin>ofloxacin (almost none)
b. *in vitro* data suggest only moderate inhibition of SSRIs. CYP1A2 inhibition: Fluvoxamine>all other SSRIs; CYP2D6 inhibition: paroxetine and fluoxetine>sertraline>fluvoxamine (almost none); CYP3A4 inhibition: fluvoxamine>fluoxetine>paroxetine and sertraline (almost none)
c. relative inhibitory potency of imidazoles: ketoconazole≈itraconazole>fluconazole (and possibly clotrimazole)
d. genetic polymorphism. Autosomal recessive inheritance: 2% of white Caucasians and 20% of orientals do not express this enzyme and are 'slow metabolisers'
e. genetic polymorphism. Autosomal recessive inheritance: 7% of white Caucasians and 1–2% of blacks and orientals do not express this enzyme and are 'slow metabolisers'
f. most potent CYP2D6 inhibitor
g. significant competitive inhibition of quinidine and propafenone metabolism has been documented with tramadol administration
h. expressed in gastro-intestinal mucosa resulting in substantial first-pass metabolism during absorption of some drugs.

General polymorphism

Genetic differences in the amount of drug metabolised by an enzymatic pathway has resulted in the classification of individuals into slow (poor) metabolisers and rapid (extensive) metabolisers.[20] Recent data suggest that, for some pathways, there may also be ultra-rapid metabolisers. Inevitably, even within the general population of rapid metabolisers, there is a normal distribution ranging from well below-average to well above-average. However, the slow metabolisers (and ultra-rapid ones) form a discontinuous genetically distinct group – they are not merely one end of a spectrum. Slow metaboliser status is generally linked to only one enzyme in any one individual, and is inherited as an autosomal recessive trait (Table A4.2).

Table A4.2 Genetic polymorphism and slow metaboliser status[1]

Pathway	*Drugs affected*	*Population affected*
N-acetylation	Caffeine Dapsone Hydralazine Isoniazid Procainamide	North European 60–70% American whites and blacks 50% Asians 5–10%
CYP2D6 (debrisoquine hydroxylase)	β-blockers Codeine Debrisoquine Flecainide Oxycodone Phenothiazines SSRIs (some) Tricyclic antidepressants (some)	Whites 5–10% Asians 1%
CYP2C19	Diazepam PPIs S-mephenytoin	Whites 3–5% Asians 20%

Non-genetic circumstances in which drug metabolism may become relatively slower include liver damage (with an associated decrease in cytochrome P450 enzyme activity) and old age. In general, age-related decreases in liver mass, hepatic enzyme activity and hepatic blood flow result in a decrease in the overall metabolic capacity of the liver in the elderly. This is of particular importance in relation to drugs which have a high 'hepatic extraction ratio', e.g. **amitriptyline**, **lidocaine** (lignocaine), **propranolol**, **verapamil**.

1 Riddick DS (1997) Drug biotransformation. In: Kalant H and Roschlau W (eds) *Principles of Medical Pharmacology* (6e). Oxford University Press, New York.
2 Honig PK *et al.* (1993) Terfenadine-ketoconazole interaction: pharmacokinetic and electrocardiographic consequences. *Journal of the American Medical Association*. **269**: 1513–1518.
3 Monaham BP *et al.* (1990) Torsades de Pointes occurring in association with terfenadine. *Journal of the American Medical Association*. **264**: 2788–2790.
4 Benton R *et al.* (1996) Grapefruit juice alters terfenadine pharmacokinetics, resulting in prolongation of repolarization on the electrocardiogram. *Clinical Pharmacology and Therapeutics*. **59**: 383–388.
5 Gibaldi M (1992) Drug interactions. Part II. *Annals of Pharmacotherapy*. **26**: 829–834.
6 Tailor S *et al.* (1996) Peripheral oedema due to nifedipine-itraconazole interaction: a case report. *Archives of Dermatology*. **132**: 350–352.
7 Aeschlimann JR and Tyler LS (1996) Drug interactions associated with cytochrome P-450 enzymes. *Journal of Pharmaceutical Care in Pain and Symptom Control*. **4**: 35–54.
8 Johnson MD *et al.* (1999) Clinically significant drug interactions. *Postgraduate Medicine*. **105**: 193–222.
9 Klotz U *et al.* (1980) Delayed clearance of diazepam due to cimetidine. *New England Journal of Medicine*. **302**: 1012–1014.
10 Nix DE *et al.* (1987) Effect of multiple dose oral ciprofloxacin on the pharmacokinetics of theophylline and indocyanine green. *Journal of Antimicrobial Chemotherapy*. **19**: 263–269.
11 Tateishi T *et al.* (1989) Effect of diltiazem on the pharmacokinetics of propranolol, metoprolol and atenolol. *European Journal of Clinical Pharmacology*. **36**: 67–70.
12 Tatro DS (1995) Fluvoxamine drug interactions. *Drug Newsletter*. **14**: 20ff.
13 Eller MG *et al.* (1991) Pharmacokinetic interaction between terfenadine and ketoconazole. *Clinical Pharmacology and Therapeutics*. **49**: 130.
14 Vandel S *et al.* (1992) Tricyclic antidepressant plasma levels after fluoxetine addition. *Neuropsychobiology*. **25**: 202–207.
15 Finley PR (1994) Selective serotonin reuptake inhibitors: Pharmacologic profiles and potential therapeutic distinctions. *Annals of Pharmacotherapy*. **28**: 1359–1369.
16 Pollock BG (1994) Recent developments in drug metabolism of relevance to psychiatrist. *Harvard Review of Psychiatry*. **2**: 204–213.
17 Backman JT *et al.* (1996) Concentrations and effect of oral midazolam were greatly reduced in patients treated with carbamazepine or phenytoin. *Epilepsia*. **37**: 253–257.
18 Sindrup HS *et al.* (1992) The effect of quinidine on the analgesic effect of codeine. *European Journal of Clinical Pharmacology*. **42**: 587–591.
19 Kay L *et al.* (1985) Influence of rifampicin and isoniazid on the kinetics of phenytoin. *British Journal of Clinical Pharmacology*. **20**: 323–326.
20 Meyer UA (1991) *Pharmacogenetics*. **1**: 66–67.

Appendix 5: Drug-induced movement disorders

Drug-induced movement disorders encompass:

- extrapyramidal reactions
  - parkinsonism
  - acute dystonia
  - acute akathisia
  - tardive dyskinesia
- neuroleptic (antipsychotic) malignant syndrome.

The features of the various syndromes are listed in Box A5.A.[1] Most extrapyramidal reactions are caused by drugs which block dopamine receptors in the CNS; these include all antipsychotics and **metoclopramide**.[2] Extrapyramidal reactions are dose-related. There is probably also a genetic factor. In essence, extrapyramidal reactions are a consequence of an imbalance between two or more neurotransmitters. The imbalance varies between different causal agents. With the typical antipsychotics (i.e. phenothiazines and butyrophenones), a high potency drug like **haloperidol** possesses a much greater affinity for D_2-receptors than for cholinergic receptors. The degree of imbalance between dopamine and acetylcholine increases the likelihood of extrapyramidal reactions. With atypical antipsychotics (e.g. **olanzapine** and **risperidone**) there is generally a much lower propensity for causing drug-induced movement disorders. This is probably because the antagonism of D_2-receptors is balanced by antagonism of serotonin (5HT).[3,4] Other drugs have been implicated (Box A5.B),[5,6] including antidepressants and **ondansetron**.[7,8] A link between extrapyramidal reactions and the serotoninergic system is seen in the propensity of SSRIs to induce such disorders, including akathisia.[9] A 'four neurone model' has been proposed, embracing dopamine, muscarinic, 5HT and GABA receptors, to help explain how all these drugs cause extrapyramidal reactions.[10]

Parkinsonism

Parkinsonism develops in up to 40% of patients treated long-term with antipsychotics.[11] It is most common in those over 60 years of age. It develops at any stage but generally not before the second week. There may be asymmetry in the early stages. The tremor of drug-induced parkinsonism typically:

- has a frequency of <8 cycles per second (cps)
- is worse at rest
- is suppressed during voluntary movements
- is associated with rigidity and bradykinesia (Box A5.A).

This is different from drug-induced tremors of the hands, head, mouth or tongue which have a frequency of 8–12cps, and are best observed with hands held outstretched or mouth held open (Box A5.C).

Treatment

- prescribe an antimuscarinic antiparkinsonian drug
  - **benzatropine** 1–2mg IV/IM → 2mg PO o.d.–b.d. *or*
  - **procyclidine** 5–10mg IV/IM → 2.5–5mg PO t.d.s. *or*
  - **orphenadrine** 50mg PO b.d.–t.d.s.
- if possible, reduce or stop causal drug.

Acute dystonia

Acute dystonias occur in up to 10% of patients treated with antipsychotics.[11] They are most common in young adults. They develop abruptly within days of starting treatment, and are accompanied by anxiety (Box A5.A).

Box A5.A Movement disorders associated with dopamine-receptor antagonists[1]

Parkinsonism
Coarse resting tremor of limbs, head, mouth and/or tongue
Muscular rigidity (cogwheel or leadpipe)
Bradykinesia, notably of face
Sialorrhoea (drooling)
Shuffling gait

Acute dystonias
one or more of
Abnormal positioning of head and neck (retrocollis, torticollis)
Spasms of jaw muscles (trismus, gaping, grimacing)
Tongue dysfunction (dysarthria, protrusion)
Dysphagia
Laryngo-pharyngeal spasm
Dysphonia
Eyes deviated up, down or sideways (oculogyric crisis)
Abnormal positioning of limbs or trunk

Acute akathisia
one or more of
Fidgety movements or swinging of legs
Rocking from foot to foot when standing
Pacing to relieve restlessness
Inability to sit or stand still for several minutes

Tardive dyskinesia
Exposure to antipsychotic medication for >3 months (>1 month if >60 years of age)
Involuntary movement of tongue, jaw, trunk or limbs:
choreiform (rapid, jerky, non-repetitive)
athetoid (slow, sinuous, continual)
rhythmic (stereotypic)

Neuroleptic (antipsychotic) malignant syndrome
Severe muscle rigidity *and*
Pyrexia
with two or more of
Tremor
Sweating
Muteness
Dysphagia
Incontinence
Drowsiness
Tachycardia
Elevated/labile blood pressure
Leucocytosis
Evidence of muscle injury, e.g. myoglobinuria, raised plasma creatine kinase

Treatment
- **benzatropine** 1–2mg or **procyclidine** 5–10mg IV/IM for immediate relief. Benefit is seen within 10min; peak effect within 30min. If necessary, repeat after 30min
- continue treatment with a standard oral antimuscarinic antiparkinsonian drug, e.g. **orphenadrine**
- some centres use IV/IM **diphenhydramine** 20–50mg, followed by 25–50mg b.d.–q.d.s.
- consider discontinuing or reducing dose of causal drug
- if caused by **metoclopramide**, substitute **domperidone**.

Box A5.B Drugs which may cause extrapyramidal effects[5,6]

Palliative care
Antidepressants[a]
- tricyclics
- SSRIs

Antipsychotics
Carbamazepine
Metoclopramide
Ondansetron
Sodium valproate

General
Diltiazem
Fenfluramine
5-hydroxytryptophan
Lithium
Methyldopa
Methysergide
Reserpine

a. all classes of antidepressants have been implicated except RIMAs.

Box A5.C Drug-induced (non-parkinsonian) tremor[12]

Anti-epileptics
- sodium valproate

Antidepressants
- SSRIs
- tricyclics

Antipsychotics
- butyrophenones
- phenothiazines

β-adrenoceptors
- salbutamol
- salmeterol

Lithium
Methylxanthines
- caffeine
- aminophylline
- theophylline

Psychostimulants
- dexamfetamine
- methylphenidate

Acute akathisia

Akathisia is a form of motor restlessness in which the subject is compelled to pace up and down or to change the body position frequently (Box A5.A). It occurs in up to 20% of patients receiving antipsychotics.[11] It is most common in the 16–50 age range. It can develop within days of starting treatment. If the drug is continued, it may progress to parkinsonism. **Haloperidol** and **prochlorperazine** carry the highest risk.[13] It is uncommon for **metoclopramide** to cause akathisia. Concurrent administration of **morphine** or **sodium valproate** may be additional risk factors.[12] Akathisia is thought to be a risk factor for the development of tardive dyskinesia.

Treatment

Antimuscarinic antiparkinsonian drugs are not helpful unless the akathisia is associated with drug-induced parkinsonism:[14]

- if possible, discontinue or reduce the dose of the causal drug
- switch to an atypical antipsychotic or to a typical antipsychotic with more antimuscarinic activity
- if necessary, add an anti-akathisia agent, preferably a *lipophilic* β-adrenoceptor antagonist; i.e. **propranolol** 20–60mg b.d.[15] or **metoprolol** 50–100mg b.d.
- alternatively, prescribe a $5HT_{2a}$ antagonist, e.g. **mianserin** 15–30mg/day, **cyproheptadine** 8–16mg/day, **ritanserin** 5–20mg/day.[15]

Propranolol, a highly *lipophilic* non-selective β-adrenoceptor antagonist, and **metoprolol**, a *lipophilic* β_1–adrenoceptor antagonist, are equally effective. In contrast, **atenolol**, a *hydrophilic* β_1-adrenoceptor antagonist, is ineffective.

If the patient is very distressed, a benzodiazepine can be prescribed in addition for a few days, e.g. **diazepam** 5–10mg/day, **clonazepam** 0.5–1mg/day, **lorazepam** 1–2mg/day.[15]

Tardive dyskinesia

Tardive (late) dyskinesia is caused by the long-term administration of drugs that block dopamine receptors, particularly D_2-receptors.[16] It occurs in 20% of patients receiving a typical antipsychotic for more than 3 months. It is most common in women, the elderly and those on high doses, e.g. **chlorpromazine** 300mg/24h or more.[17,18] Tardive dyskinesia typically manifests as involuntary stereotyped chewing movements of the tongue and orofacial muscles (Box A5.A). The involuntary movements are made worse by anxiety and reduced by drowsiness and during sleep.

Tardive dyskinesia is associated with akathisia in 25% of cases. In younger patients, tardive dyskinesia may present as abnormal positioning of the limbs and tonic contractions of the neck and trunk muscles causing torticollis, lordosis or scoliosis. In younger patients, tardive dyskinesia may occur if antipsychotic treatment is stopped abruptly.

Early diagnosis

'Open your mouth and stick out your tongue.'

The following indicate a developing tardive dyskinesia:

- worm-like movements of the tongue
- inability to protrude tongue for more than a few seconds.

Treatment

- withdrawal of the causal agent leads to resolution in 30% in 3 months and a further 40% in 5 years; sometimes irreversible, particularly in the elderly
- often responds poorly to drug therapy; antimuscarinic antiparkinsonian drugs may exacerbate
- **tetrabenazine**, depletes presynaptic dopamine stores and blocks postsynaptic dopamine receptors; best not used in depressed patients; start with 12.5mg t.d.s. → 25mg t.d.s., increasing the dose slowly to avoid troublesome hypotension
- **reserpine**, depletes presynaptic dopamine stores; may be used in place of **tetrabenazine** but causes similar adverse effects
- **levodopa**, may produce long-term benefit after causing initial deterioration
- **baclofen**, **clonazepam**, **diazepam** and **sodium valproate** have all been tried with inconsistent results (all drugs which act by potentiating GABA-ergic inhibition)
- increase the dose of the causal drug; paradoxically, this may help but should be considered only in desperation.

Neuroleptic (antipsychotic) malignant syndrome

Neuroleptic (antipsychotic) malignant syndrome is a potentially life-threatening reaction which occurs in about 0.2% of patients prescribed an antipsychotic.[19,20] Most cases occur within 2 weeks of starting treatment or a dose increase.[16] It is more likely to occur in patients also receiving **lithium**. Symptoms indistinguishable from neuroleptic (antipsychotic) malignant syndrome have also been reported in patients with Parkinson's disease.[21,22] The classic features are fever, tachycardia, sweating, delirium, rigidity, tremulousness and muteness (Box A5.A). Clinical features overlap with those of serotonin syndrome (Box 4.F; see p.89), suggesting a common pathophysiology.[23] The syndrome typically develops over 2–3 days but the onset can be more insidious. Death occurs in up to 20% of cases, most commonly as a result of respiratory failure. The use of a dopamine agonist, e.g. **bromocriptine**, halves the mortality to about 10%.[24] Subsequent prescription of an antipsychotic carries a 30–50% risk of recurrence.[25]

Treatment

Neuroleptic (antipsychotic) malignant syndrome is a self-limiting condition once the causal drug is discontinued, and generally resolves in 1–2 weeks unless it is the result of a depot antipsychotic, when it may take a month to resolve. Supportive treatment typically comprises:

- discontinuation of the causal drug
- prescription of a muscle relaxant, e.g. a benzodiazepine
- in severe cases, **bromocriptine** (a dopamine agonist).

Although **dantrolene** is used in treating malignant hyperthermia during anaesthesia, its acute use is generally not practical in palliative care.[24,26] Likewise, the use of electroconvulsive therapy (ECT) is not a realistic option.[27]

1 American Psychiatric Association (1994) Neuroleptic-induced movement disorders. In: *Diagnostic and Statistical Manual of Mental Disorders* (4e) *(DSM-IV)*. American Psychiatric Association, New York, pp.736–751.

2 Tonda M and Guthrie S (1994) Treatment of acute neuroleptic-induced movement disorders. *Pharmacotherapy.* **14**: 543–560.
3 Hoes M (1998) Recent developments in the management of psychosis. *Pharmacy and World Science.* **20**: 101–106.
4 Geddes J *et al.* (2000) Atypical antipsychotics in the treatment of schizophrenia: systematic overview and meta-regression analysis. *British Medical Journal.* **321**: 1371–1376.
5 Zubenko G *et al.* (1987) Antidepressant-related akathisia. *Journal of Clinical Psychopharmacology.* **7**: 254–257.
6 Anonymous (1994) Drug-induced extrapyramidal reactions. *Current Problems in Pharmacovigilance.* **20**: 15–16.
7 Arya D (1994) Extrapyramidal symptoms with selective serotonin reuptake inhibitors. *British Journal of Psychiatry.* **165**: 728–733.
8 Matthews H and Tancil C (1996) Extrapyramidal reaction caused by ondansetron. *The Annals of Pharmacotherapy.* **30**: 196.
9 Lane R (1998) SSRI-induced extrapyramidal side-effects and akathisia: implications for treatment. *Journal of Psychopharmacology.* **12**: 192–214.
10 Hamilton M and Opler L (1992) Akathisia, suicidality, and fluoxetine. *Journal of Clinical Psychiatry.* **53**: 401–406.
11 Launer M (1996) Selected side-effects: 17. Dopamine-receptor antagonists and movement disorders. *Prescribers' Journal.* **36**: 37–41.
12 American Psychiatric Association (1994) Medication-induced postural tremor. In: *Diagnostic and Statistical Manual of Mental Disorders* (4e) *(DSM-IV)*. American Psychiatric Association, New York, pp.749–751.
13 Gattera J *et al.* (1994) A retrospective study of risk factors of akathisia in terminally ill patients. *Journal of Pain and Symptom Management.* **9**: 454–461.
14 Fleischhacker W *et al.* (1990) The pharmacologic treatment of neuroleptic-induced akathisia. *Journal of Clinical Psychopharmacology.* **10**: 12–21.
15 Poyurovsky M and Weizman A (1997) Serotonergic agents in the treatment of acute neuroleptic-induced akathisia: open-label study of buspirone and mianserin. *International Clinical Psychopharmacology.* **12**: 263–268.
16 American Psychiatric Association (1992) *Tardive dyskinesia: a task force report of the American Psychiatric Association.* American Psychiatric Association, Washington, DC.
17 Woerner M *et al.* (1998) Prospective study of tardive dyskinesia in the elderly: rates and risk factors. *American Journal of Psychiatry.* **155**: 1521–1528.
18 Jeste D (2000) Tardive dyskinesia in older patients. *Journal of Clinical Psychiatry.* **61 (suppl 4)**: 27–32.
19 Caroff S and Mann S (1993) Neuroleptic malignant syndrome. *Medical Clinics of North America.* **77**: 185–202.
20 Adnet P *et al.* (2000) Neuroleptic malignant syndrome. *British Journal of Anaesthesia.* **85**: 129–135.
21 Mann S *et al.* (1991) Pathogenesis of neuroleptic malignant syndrome. *Psychiatry Annals.* **21**: 175–180.
22 Ong K *et al.* (2001) Neuroleptic malignant syndrome without neuroleptics. *Singapore Medical Journal.* **42**: 85–88.
23 Kontaxakis V *et al.* (2000) Olanzapine-associated neuroleptic malignant syndrome: Is there any overlap with the serotonin syndrome? *Journal of the European College of Neuropsychopharmacology.* **10 (suppl 3)**: S313.
24 Sakkas P *et al.* (1991) Pharmacotherapy of neuroleptic malignant syndrome. *Psychiatry Annals.* **21**: 157–164.
25 Wells A *et al.* (1988) Neuroleptic rechallenges after neuroleptic malignant syndrome: case report and literature review. *Drug Intelligence and Clinical Pharmacy.* **22**: 475–479.
26 Rosenberg M and Green M (1989) Neuroleptic malignant syndrome: Review of response to therapy. *Archives of Internal Medicine.* **149**: 1927–1931.
27 Caroff S *et al.* (1998) Specific treatment of the neuroleptic malignant syndrome. *Biological Psychiatry.* **44**: 378–381.

Appendix 6: Discoloured urine

There are many causes of discoloured urine (Box A6.A). If the urine is red, it is often assumed to be haematuria.

Box A6.A Common causes of discoloured urine

Orange/yellow
Nitrofurantoin

Red/pink
Beetroot
Dantron (in co-danthramer and co-danthrusate)
Doxorubicin
Nefopam
Phenolphthalein (in alkaline urine) present in several proprietary laxatives, e.g. Agarol®
Rhubarb
Rifampicin

Blue
Methylene blue; present in some proprietary urinary antiseptic mixtures, e.g. Urised® (USA)
Pseudomonas aeruginosa (pyocyanin) in alkaline urine

Dark
Metronidazole

Appendix 7: Taking controlled drugs abroad

Some patients receiving palliative care travel abroad, and they will need to take their medicines with them. Practitioners can help ensure a trouble-free trip by advising them, if relevant, about controlled drugs.[1,2] Although Schedule 2, 3, and 4 Part I controlled drugs are normally subject to stringent import and export licensing requirements, the Home Office has an open general licence which lists controlled drugs and permitted quantities which can be taken out of and brought into the UK for personal use without a licence (Table A7.1).[3] Thus, in many cases a letter from the patient's general practitioner or other involved doctor, stating the patient's drug regimen, is sufficient. Advice should be sought from the Home Office when higher doses are prescribed, as a *drugs export licence* is likely to be required. Advice and/or the licence is obtainable from:

Action Against Drugs Unit
Room 239
Home Office
50 Queen Anne's Gate
London SW1H 9AT

Telephone: 020 7273 3147
Fax: 020 7273 2157

There is no standard form but applications must be supported by a letter from a doctor stating:
- the patient's name and address
- names and quantities of drugs to be taken abroad
- strength and form in which the drugs will be dispensed
- dates of travel to and from UK.

Two weeks should be allowed for processing the application.
Licences are issued to comply with the Misuse of Drugs Act and facilitate passage through UK customs control. Covering letters or licences should be carried in the patient's hand luggage in case the UK customs want to examine them. Medicines should be contained in their original packaging.

However, drugs export licences have no legal status outside the UK. Before travelling, patients should check with the relevant Embassy or High Commission about any requirements relating to the import of controlled drugs into that country. Similarly, drugs listed in Schedule 4 Part I, and Schedule 5 are not subject to import or export licences in the UK but patients should check about any requirements for taking them into the country concerned. (Schedule 4 Part I includes most benzodiazepines.)

Table A7.1 Some of the controlled drugs and their permitted quantities on the Open General Licence list[a]

Amfetamine	300mg
Buprenorphine	24mg
Dexamfetamine	900mg
Dextromoramide tartrate	900mg
Diamorphine hydrochloride ampoules[b]	1350mg
Diazepam	900mg
Dihydrocodeine[c]	3600mg
Dipipanone	600mg
Fentanyl	45mg
Hydromorphone	360mg
Methadone[d]	500mg
Methylamfetamine	900mg
Methlyphenidate	900mg
Morphine	1200mg
Oxycodone	900mg
Phenobarbital	2700mg
Phenobarbital sodium	12000mg
Temazepam	900mg

a. the maximum quantities which may be carried by patients without a licence from the UK Home Office, provided they carry with them a covering letter from their prescribing doctor
b. permission will be needed from the relevant country's Ministry of Health because medicinal diamorphine is illegal in countries other than the UK. Australia, Greece, Italy, Germany, France, Japan, South Africa, Netherlands, USA and Zimbabwe will not allow anyone to bring in medicinal diamorphine from the UK
c. not controlled if not injectable or <100mg by injection
d. if >2000mg, the Home Office requires confirmation of travel from the doctor, e.g. the air tickets have been seen.

1 Anonymous (2001) Controlled drugs and drug dependence. *British National Formulary* No. 41. p.8.
2 Myers K (1999) Flying home: Helping patients to arrange international air travel. *European Journal of Palliative Care*. **6**: 158–161.
3 Home Office (2002) Personal communication.

Appendix 8: Special orders and named patient supplies

Special order and named patient supplies are unlicensed products.

Special order

'Special order' refers to the fact that the manufacturer holds a 'specials' licence which enables them to manufacture extemporaneous preparations on a large-scale basis. These are drug formulations unavailable under full licence, but can be prepared from other ingredients or formulations, e.g. oral solutions of some diuretics, alternative strengths of creams. Certain hospitals have pharmaceutical manufacturing units which can supply 'special order' products (see *BNF* index of 'special order' manufacturers for the list of such hospitals).

The following companies manufacture 'special order' products (list not exhaustive). Details of products and prices are available on request.

AAH Specials (Tel: 0191 261 1709, Fax: 0191 261 1709)
BCM Specials (Tel: 0800 952 1010, Fax: 0800 085 0673)
Eldon Laboratories (Tel: 0191 286 0446, Fax: 0191 286 0455)
Mandeville (Tel: 01296 394142, Fax: 01296 397223)
Martindale Pharmaceuticals Ltd (Tel: 01708 386660, Fax: 01708 384032)
Oxford Pharmaceuticals (Tel: 020 8861 0788, Fax: 020 8427 1994)
Rosemont Pharmaceuticals Ltd (Tel: 0113 244 1999, Fax: 0113 246 0738)
The Specials Laboratory (Tel: 0191 261 0555, Fax: 0191 261 0555)

Named patient supply

'Named patient' supply refers to the supply of products, unlicensed in the UK, that have been prescribed by a doctor for an individual patient. Records of patient details need to be retained by the supplier. Named patient (unlicensed) products may be available from UK manufacturers even if a licence has been withdrawn, e.g. **cisapride**. Alternatively products may need to be imported from other countries.

Companies which will obtain information and organise the supply of drugs licensed in other countries include:

IDIS (International Drug Information Service) Ltd World Medicines (Tel: 020 8410 0700, Fax: 020 8410 0800)

John Bell and Croyden (Tel: 020 7935 5555, Fax: 020 7935 9605)

Appendix 9: Nebulised drugs

Nebulisers are used in asthma and COPD for both acute exacerbations and long-term prophylaxis.[1] Other uses include the pulmonary delivery of antimicrobial drugs for cystic fibrosis, bronchiectasis and AIDS-related pneumonia. Nebulisers are also used in palliative care. The aim is to deliver a therapeutic dose of a drug as an aerosol in particles small enough to be inspired within 5–10min. A nebuliser is preferable to a hand-held inhaler when:

- a large drug dose is needed
- co-ordinated breathing is difficult
- hand-held inhalers are ineffective
- a drug is unavailable in an inhaler.

Commonly used nebulisers are:

Jet: the aerosol is generated by a flow of gas from, for example, an electrical compressor or an oxygen cylinder. At least 50% of the aerosol produced at the recommended driving gas flow should be particles small enough to inhale (British standard BS7711).

Ultrasonic: the aerosol is generated by ultrasonic vibrations of a piezo-electric crystal.

Aerosol output (the mass of particles in aerosol form produced/min) is not necessarily the same as drug output (the mass of drug produced/min as an aerosol). Ideally, the drug output of a nebuliser should be known for each of the different drugs given. Various factors affect the drug output and deposition:

- gas flow rate (generally air at 6–8L/min but oxygen if treating acute asthma)
- chamber design
- volume (commonly 2–2.5ml, up to 4ml)
- residual volume (commonly 0.5ml)
- physical properties of the drug in solution
- breathing pattern of the patient.

The choice of nebuliser can be crucial, particularly when trying to produce an aerosol small enough to deliver a drug to the alveoli. Ideally, a nebuliser should be prescribed in co-operation with the local nebuliser service which can generally provide an assessment, information and education service for staff, patients and their families. Information should include:

- a description of the equipment and its use
- drugs used, doses and frequencies
- equipment maintenance/cleaning
- action to take if treatment becomes less effective
- action to take and emergency telephone number to use if equipment breaks down.

Written information should also be given to patients (Box A9.A). Patients should be instructed to take steady normal breaths (interspersed with occasional deep ones) and nebulisation time should be less than 10min or 'to dryness'. Because there is always a residual volume, 'dryness' should be taken as 1min after spluttering starts. In general, whereas a mask can be used for bronchodilators, a mouthpiece should be used for other drugs to limit environmental contamination and/or contact with the patient's eyes. However, a mask may be preferable in patients who are acutely ill, fatigued or very young, regardless of the nature of the drug.

Nebulisers in palliative care

Nebulisers are used to ease cough and breathlessness in advanced cancer (Tables A9.1 and A9.2); they should be reviewed after 2 days to check efficacy. When using **lidocaine** (lignocaine) or **bupivacaine** for a dry cough (not recommended for breathlessness), pretreat with **salbutamol** because of the risk of bronchospasm. After treatment with a local anaesthetic, patients should be advised not to eat or drink for 1h because the reduced gag/cough reflex increases the risk of aspiration. Comparative pharmacokinetic data for inhaled corticosteroids are given in Table A9.3.

Box A9.A Advice about using a nebuliser at home

To help your breathing, your doctor has prescribed a drug to be used with a nebuliser. The nebuliser converts the drug into a fine mist which you inhale.

The apparatus

Your nebuliser system consists of the following parts:

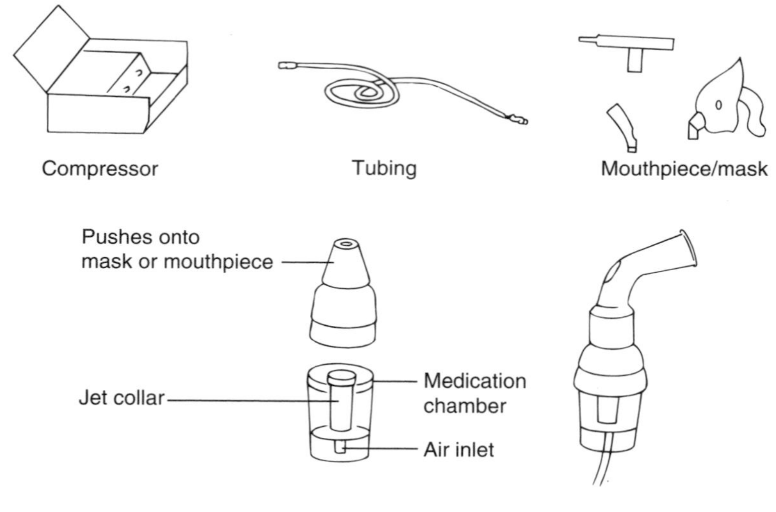

The compressor is the portable pump which pumps air along the tubing into the nebuliser. The nebuliser is a small chamber for the liquid medicine, through which air is blown to make a mist.

The nebuliser has a screw-on top onto which the mask or mouthpiece is attached.

How to use your nebuliser

Place the medication in the nebuliser, replace the screw-on top and turn the compressor on. Inhale by mouthpiece or mask while breathing at a normal rate. Stop 1 minute after the nebuliser contents start spluttering or after a maximum of 10 minutes.

General advice

If you have a cough, the nebuliser may help you to expectorate, so have some tissues nearby.

You may wish to use the nebuliser before attempting an activity which makes you feel out of breath.

If the effects of the nebuliser wear off or you have any questions or concerns about it, please speak to your doctor or nurse.

Cleaning

Wash the mouthpiece/mask and nebuliser in warm water and detergent, then rinse and dry well. Ideally this should be done after every use, but *once a day as a minimum*. Attach the tube and run the nebuliser empty for a few moments after cleaning it to make sure the equipment is dry. Once a week, unplug and wipe the compressor and tubing with a damp cloth.

Table A9.1 Nebulised drugs and cancer-related cough or breathlessness[2]

Class of drug	*Indications*	*Scientific evidence*	*Comments*
Normal saline	Loosening of tenacious secretions	None	Probably underused in this setting; may also help breathlessness
Mucolytic agents e.g. hypertonic saline, acetylcysteine	To thin viscous sputum	Conflicting evidence	May result in copious liquid sputum which the patient may still not be able to cough up
Corticosteroids e.g. budesonide	Stridor, lymphangitis, radiation pneumonitis, cough after the insertion of a stent	None	Very limited clinical experience only; may not be more beneficial than use of inhaler or oral routes
Local anaesthetics e.g. lidocaine, bupivacaine	Cough, particularly if caused by lymphangitis carcinomatosa	Conflicting evidence for both dyspnoea[3,4] and cough[5]	Risk of bronchospasm; reduces gag reflex
Opioids e.g. morphine, diamorphine, fentanyl	Breathlessness associated with diffuse lung disease	Anecdotal evidence supportive,[6] but controlled trials indicate that no better than 0.9% saline[7,8]	Not recommended; risk of bronchospasm
Bronchodilators e.g. salbutamol	Treatment of reversible airway obstruction	Extrapolated from patients with asthma and COPD	Use only if trial of therapy demonstrates real benefit

Table A9.2 Recommended uses of nebulised drugs in palliative care

Indication	*Drug*	*Initial regimen*	*Dose titration*	*Comments*
Tenacious secretions	Saline 0.9%	5ml q6h	Up to q2h	
Reversible airway obstruction	Salbutamol Terbutaline	2.5mg q4h–q6h 5mg q4h–q6h	Up to 5mg q4h Up to 10mg q4h	Risk of sensitivity to cardiac stimulant effects
Cough	*†Lidocaine 2% *†Bupivacaine 0.25%	5ml p.r.n. 5ml p.r.n.	Up to q6h Up to q8h	Risk of bronchospasm; fast for 1h after nebulisation

Table A9.3 Pharmacokinetic details of inhaled corticosteroids[9]

	Anti-inflammatory activity[a]	*Affinity for lung tissue*[b]	*Human lung GR complex halflife (h)*	*Systemic bio-availability (%)*		*Plasma halflife (h)*
				Inhaled	*Oral*	
Beclometasone	3.5	0.4	?	20	<20	15
Budesonide	1	9.4	5.1	25	11	2.8
Fluticasone	?	18.0	10.5	20	<1	3.1
Triamcinolone	5.3	3.6	3.9	21	22	1.5

a. thymic involution assay
b. compared to dexamethasone.

1 BTS and others (1997) Current best practice for nebuliser treatment. *Thorax*. **32: (suppl 2).**
2 Ahmedzai S and Davis C (1997) Nebulised drugs in palliative care. *Thorax*. **52**: S75–S77.
3 Winning A *et al.* (1988) Ventilation and breathlessness on maximal exercise in patients with interstitial lung disease after local anaesthetic aerosol inhalation. *Clinical Science*. **74**: 275–281.
4 Wilcock A *et al.* (1994) Safety and efficacy of nebulized lignocaine in patients with cancer and breathlessness. *Palliative Medicine*. **8**: 35–38.
5 Howard P *et al.* (1977) Lignocaine aerosol and persistent cough. *British Journal of Diseases of the Chest*. **71**: 19–24.
6 Young IH *et al.* (1989) Effect of low dose nebulized morphine on exercise endurance in patients with chronic lung disease. *Thorax*. **44**: 387–390.
7 Davis C *et al.* (1993) *The pharmacokinetics of nebulized morphine*. Proceedings of International Association for the Study of Pain. IASP Publications, Seattle, pp.379 (abstract 995).
8 Noseda A *et al.* (1997) Disabling dyspnoea in patients with advanced disease: lack of effect of nebulized morphine. *European Respiratory Journal*. **10**: 1079–1083.
9 Demoly P and Chung K (1998) Pharmacology of corticosteroids. *Respiratory Medicine*. **97**: 385–394.

Appendix 10: Administering drugs via feeding tubes

Administering drugs via feeding tubes is an unlicensed activity. There is little published data and most recommendations are theoretical and/or based on local policy. An alternative licensed option may therefore be preferable, e.g. rectal or parenteral formulations. However, if given by tube, there is a range of possibilities (Figure A10.1). Guidance should be sought from a pharmacist regarding which option is feasible or most appropriate.

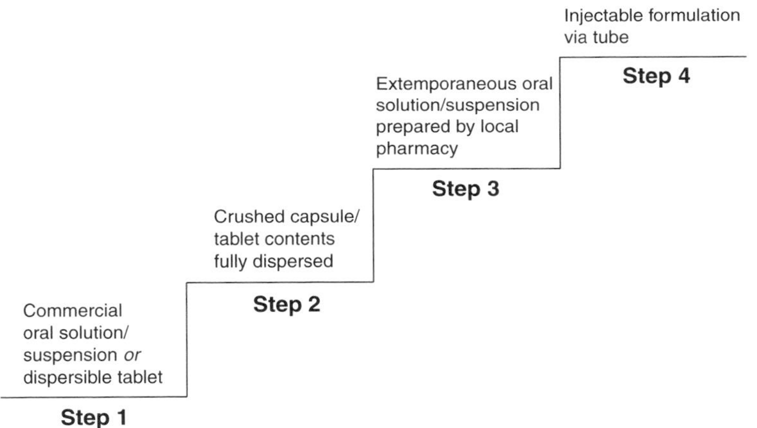

Figure A10.1 4-step ladder for drug administration by feeding tubes. Step 1 is the preferred option; for further explanation, see Choosing a suitable formulation p.356.

There are several types of feeding tubes (Box A10.A). These can be further classified according to lumen size (French gauge), number of lumens (single or multiple) and length of use (short-term, long-term/fixed).

Box A10.A Main types of feeding tubes

Nasogastric (NG), inserted into the stomach via the nose.
Nasojejunal (NJ), inserted into the jejunum via the nose.
Percutaneous endoscopic gastrostomy (PEG), inserted into the stomach via the abdominal wall.
Percutaneous endoscopic jejunostomy (PEJ), inserted into the jejunum via the abdominal wall.
Percutaneous endoscopic gastro-jejunostomy (PEGJ), inserted into the jejunum via the abdominal wall and through the stomach.

In addition to the general guidance (Box A10.B), the following should be considered when giving drugs via feeding tubes:

- *sterility with jejunal tube*, use sterile water because the acid barrier in the stomach is bypassed;[1] some centres use an aseptic technique to reduce the risk of infective diarrhoea
- *site of drug delivery with jejunal tubes*, absorption may be unpredictable because the tube may extend beyond the main site of absorption of the drug, e.g. **cefalexin**, **ketoconazole**;[2] care should also be taken with drugs that have a narrow therapeutic range, e.g. **digoxin**, **warfarin**, **phenytoin** and other anti-epileptics[2]
- *size of lumen*, narrow lumen tubes are more likely to block, particularly with thick oral syrups; dilute with 30–60ml water before administration; the internal diameter of equivalent French gauge tubes varies between manufacturers
- *number of lumens*, ensure the correct lumen is used with multilumen tubes; *do not use an aspiration gastric decompression port for drug administration*; some tubes have one lumen terminating in the stomach and another in the jejunum
- *function of the tube*, drugs should not be administered by tube if it is on free-drainage or suction.[3]

Box A10.B General guidelines for administration of drugs via feeding tubes

Drug charts should state the route of administration, e.g. NJ, and specify the lumen to be used.

Ensure the siting of the tube has been medically confirmed.

Oral syringes (i.e. a syringe to which a needle cannot be attached) should be used to prevent accidental parenteral administration.[4,5]

Stop the infusion of the feed when administering drugs.

Flush the tube slowly with at least 15ml of water, *sterile if jejunal tube*; use either a 30ml or 50ml oral syringe.

Administer each drug separately (by gravity flow) as a sediment-free liquid (Figure A10.1); flush in between and afterwards with at least 15ml of water, *sterile if jejunal tube*; use either a 30ml or 50ml oral syringe.

Document the total volume of fluid given (including flushes) on a fluid balance chart.

Monitor the clinical response if:
- changing from m/r to normal-release preparations
- a drug has a narrow therapeutic range
- the bio-availability of the drug differs between tablet and liquid.

Do not administer bulk-forming laxatives because they may block the tubes; use an enteral feed with a high fibre content instead.[3]

Do not add drugs to feeds; this increases the risk of incompatibility, microbial contamination, tube blockage, and underdosing or overdosing if the feed rate is altered.[6]

Choosing a suitable formulation

Guidance is given in Table A10.1 (see p.360) on the formulations available for many drugs used in palliative care. However, commercially available oral solutions/suspensions/syrups are not always suitable because of:

- *osmotic diarrhoea* due to high osmolality and sorbitol content; the normal osmolality of gastrointestinal secretions is 100–400mosm/kg, whereas many liquid formulations are >1000mosm/kg;[1–3] reduce osmolality by diluting with as much water as is practical. Sorbitol in cumulative doses of >7.5g generally causes diarrhoea; often severe with doses >20g
- *altered bio-availability and/or pharmacokinetics* when converting from tablets to oral solution, e.g. **digoxin**, **phenytoin**, **sodium fusidate**, or from m/r preparations to oral solution; the dose and/or frequency may need to be changed according to the clinical response
- *tube blockage/caking* caused by high viscosity preparations, e.g. **co-amoxiclav**; minimise by diluting with 30–60ml water or use suspensions rather than syrups[3]
- *clumping of the feed*, particularly if the formulation is acidic, i.e. pH <4[3]

- *bezoar formation* causing indigestible concretions, e.g. **sucralfate**
- *binding to the plastic tubing*, e.g. **carbamazepine**, **clonazepam**, **diazepam**, **phenytoin**; reduce by diluting with 30–60ml water.

Many tablets and capsule contents will disperse completely when crushed and mixed with water, even though they are not marketed as dispersible. *Do not administer crushed tablets or capsule contents which have not completely dispersed in water; sediment increases the risk of blocking the tube*[3,7] (Box A10.C). The liquid contents of some capsules can be drawn out with a syringe, but should be administered immediately in case of light sensitivity.

Box A10.C Guidelines for administering crushed tablets and capsule contents

Administer each drug separately.[2]

Crush tablet(s) or capsule contents using a mortar and pestle; alternatively use two metal spoons to crush and a clean empty medicine bottle to mix.

Add 10ml of tap water and mix well; *use sterile water for jejunal tubes.*

Ensure the drug is completely dispersed with no sediment, then draw up using a 30ml or 50ml oral syringe and administer via the feeding tube, flushing before and after according to guidelines (Box A10.B).

Rinse the mortar with water and administer the rinsings through the tube to ensure the patient receives the whole dose.

Avoid plastic containers as the drug may adhere to the plastic.[8]

Do not crush

E/c preparations (including e/c coated capsule contents) as this will destroy the properties of the formulation, may alter bio-availability and/or block the tube.[7,9,10]

M/r preparations (including m/r coated capsule contents) as this may cause dangerous dose peaks and troughs.[3,7,10]

Cytotoxics, prostaglandin analogues, hormone antagonists or antibiotics as there are risks to the staff through inhalation and/or topical absorption.[3,7,10]

Buccal or sublingual preparations as their bio-availability may be dramatically reduced if absorbed via the gastro-intestinal tract.[3,7,10]

Before administering an injectable formulation via a feeding tube, check the osmolality. Many injections are hypertonic and therefore unsuitable. Some injections may also contain additives unsuitable for oral administration, e.g. polyethylene glycol in **amiodarone**.[13] Further, this is generally an expensive option and should be considered only short-term. All injections should be further diluted with 30–60ml water before administration.

Flushing feeding tubes

Flushing tubes before and after medication reduces the risk of blocking.[11,12] A minimum of 15ml before, in between and after medications is recommended. Using 30ml or 50ml oral syringes reduces the risk of rupturing the tube.[13] Tubes should be flushed *slowly* to prevent a coating of the previous drug being left around the inside of the tube.

Drug interactions

A number of specific drug interactions can occur when drugs are administered via feeding tubes (Box A10.D). The most important clinically are with drugs with a narrow therapeutic range, e.g. **digoxin**, **phenytoin**, **warfarin**. Following the guidance in Box A10.B and Box A10.D will reduce the risk of dangerous interactions. Clinical response should be monitored, and appropriate precautionary measures taken if the feed is discontinued at any time, particularly if dose adjustments have been made.

Box A10.D Drug interactions and preventive action when giving drugs by tubes

Binding of drugs to tubes
e.g. carbamazepine, diazepam, phenytoin[3]
Dilute the drug with at least 30–60ml of water and flush well; monitor clinical response.

Direct interaction of drug and feed causing coagulation in the tube
e.g. acidic solutions (chlorphenamine (chlorpheniramine), promethazine, thioridazine) and antacids[6,14]
Find alternative route/preparation if possible; dilute the drug as much as possible to minimise drug-feed contact and flush with 30–60ml of water.

Documented drug/enteral feed incompatibilities affecting drug absorption
e.g. carbamazepine, ciprofloxacin, hydralazine, phenytoin, theophylline, warfarin[3,6]
Stop the feed for 1h before and 1–2h after administering the drug (phenytoin 2h before and after);[3] dilute the drug as much as possible, and flush with 30–60ml water.

Drugs requiring administration on an empty stomach
e.g. penicillins, ketoconazole, tetracyclines[3]
Balance the risk of reduced absorption against practicality of stopping feed for 1h before and after each dose; consider alternative route/drug; not applicable in jejunal feeding because the stomach is bypassed,[7] just ensure efficient flushing.

Drug-feed indirect interaction
e.g. warfarin and vitamin K in feed[15]
Monitor INR and adjust anticoagulant dose if necessary.

Drug-drug direct interaction
e.g. iron or zinc and ciprofloxacin
Alter drug timings.

Unblocking tubes

Do not use a guidewire for unblocking a tube because of the danger of perforation.[13] Various agents have been used to unblock tubes (Box A10.E).[3] Their use is based on anecdote. Acidic solutions, e.g. **cranberry juice** and carbonated drinks, could make the situation worse by causing feed coagulation.[3]

Box A10.E Preparations used to unblock feeding tubes[3]

Warm water
Soda water
Cola
Pineapple juice
Cranberry juice
Pancreatin granules removed from capsule
Meat tenderiser, contains papain, a mixture of proteolytic enzymes
Clogg Zapper, a commercial powder for breaking up food formula clogs in enteral feeding devices

1 Nottingham City Hospital/University Hospital/Nottingham Healthcare NHS Trusts (1999) Care of a patient receiving jejunal feeding. *Nursing practice guidelines.*
2 Adams D (1994) Administration of drugs through a jejunostomy tube. *British Journal of Intensive Care.* **4**: 10–17.
3 Thomson FC *et al.* (2000) Enteral and parenteral nutrition. *Hospital Pharmacist.* **7**: 155–164.
4 Cousins DH and Upton DR (1997) Medication errors. *Pharmacy in practice.* **7**: 597–598.

5 Cousins DH and Upton DR (1998) Medication errors. *Pharmacy in practice.* **8**: 209–210.

6 Engle KK and Hannawa TE (1999) Techniques for administering oral medications to critical care patients receiving continuous enteral nutrition. *American Journal of Health-System Pharmacists.* **56**:1441–1444.

7 Gilbar PJ (1999) A guide to drug administration in palliative care (review). *Journal of Pain and Symptom Management.* **17**: 197–207.

8 Naysmith M and Nicholson J (1998) Nasogastric drug administration. *Professional Nurse.* **13**: 424–427.

9 Beckwith MC *et al.* (1997) Guide to drug therapy in patients with enteral feeding tubes: dosage form selection and administration methods. *Hospital Pharmacist.* **32**: 57–64.

10 Mitchell JF (1998) Oral dosage forms that should not be crushed: 1998 update. *Hospital Pharmacist.* **33**: 399–415.

11 Bengmark S (1988) Progress in perioperative enteral tube feeding. *Clinical Nutrition.* **17**: 145–152.

12 Brennan-Krupp K and Heximer B (1998) Going with the flow. *Nursing.* **28**: 54–55.

13 Shaw JE (1994) A worrying gap in knowledge. Nurses' knowledge of enteral feeding practice. *Enteral feeding.* **July**: 656–666.

14 Valli C *et al.* (1986) Interaction of nutrients with antacids: a complication during enteral tube feeding. *Lancet.* **i**: 747–748.

15 Stockley IH (1996) *Drug Interactions* (4e). The Pharmaceutical Press, London.

16 Mid Essex Hospital services NHS Trust Pharmacy services (1998) *Administration of medication via a percutaneous endoscopic gastrostomy (PEG) tube.*

17 Southern General Hospital, Victoria Infirmary, South Glasgow University Hospitals NHS Trust, University of Strathclyde/GGHB Pharmacy Practice Unit, Western General Hospital, Lothian University Hospitals NHS Trust, University of Strathclyde/Lothian Pharmacy Practice Unit (2001) *A to Z guide to administration of drugs via nasogastric/PEG tube.*

18 AstraZeneca (1999) Personal communication.

19 Leicestershire Health Authority (1994) Pharmacy technical services (NOVA Laboratories). *Information Bulletin: Suspension Diluents used in Leicestershire.*

20 Nottingham City Hospital NHS Trust Pharmacy (1998) *Administering drugs to patients by artificial enteral methods.*

Table A10.1 Information on formulations available for administering drugs down feeding tubes.[2,6,7,16–20]

Drug	*Oral solution/ suspension/ dispersible preparation available*	*Crushed tablet/ capsule contents disperse completely*[a]	*Oral solution/ suspension prepared by local pharmacy*	*Injection can be diluted and administered down feeding tube*	*Comments*
Amitriptyline[a]	Yes	Yes (APS®)	Yes (C)[b]		
Aminophylline					Change to theophylline or use IV route
Amoxycillin	Yes			Yes	
Antacids	Yes				Not recommended as can coagulate with feed; not needed with jejunal tube
Ascorbic acid	Yes				
Aspirin	Yes				
Baclofen	Yes	Yes (Lioresal®) Takes 5min	Yes (K)[c]		Commercial oral solution not recommended as too viscous
Carbamazepine[a]	Yes	Yes (Tegretol®)			Dilute to reduce adherence to the tube; stop feed for 1h before and 1–2h after dose. Jejunal administration not recommended because may cause plasma levels to decrease
Chlorpromazine	Yes	Yes (Largactil®) Takes 5min	Yes (K)		
Cimetidine	Yes	Yes (Dyspamet®, Tagamet®)		Yes (Tagamet® 100mg/ml)	Commercial oral solution may cause diarrhoea
Ciprofloxacin	Yes	Yes (Ciproxin®)	Yes (C)		Commercial oral solution not recommended as too viscous. Use sterile water not tap water (to avoid ion chelation) and dilute with 30–60ml water. Stop feed for 1h before and 1–2h after dose. Do not administer with iron or zinc
Cisapride	Yes	Yes (Prepulsid®)	Yes (K)		

Table A10.1 Continued

Drug	*Oral solution/ suspension/ dispersible preparation available*	*Crushed tablet/ capsule contents disperse completely*[a]	*Oral solution/ suspension prepared by local pharmacy*	*Injection can be diluted and administered down feeding tube*	*Comments*
Clonazepam		Yes (Rivotril®)	Yes (K)		Dilute with 30–60ml to reduce binding to the tube
Clonidine		Yes (Catapres®)	Yes (K)	Yes (Catapres®)	
Co-danthramer	Yes				No information on suitability via feeding tube
Co-danthrusate	Yes				No information on suitability via feeding tube
Codeine phosphate	Yes	Yes Takes 5min	Yes (K)		Dilute viscous commercial oral solution
Co-amoxiclav	Yes				Dilute to half-strength (to avoid caking)
Cyclizine		Yes (Valoid®) Takes 5min	Yes (C)	Yes	
Cyproterone			Yes (K)		
Dantrolene			Yes (K)		
Dexamethasone	Yes[d]	Yes (Organon®)	Yes (K)	Yes	
Diamorphine			Yes		
Diazepam	Yes	Yes	Yes (K)		Dilute with 30–60ml to reduce binding to the tube
Diclofenac[a]	Yes				
Digoxin	Yes	Yes (Lanoxin®)			50microgram Lanoxin® oral solution = 62.5microgram tablet; commercial oral solution may cause diarrhoea
Dihydrocodeine[a]	Yes				No information on suitability via feeding tube
Docusate	Yes				No information on suitability via feeding tube

Table A10.1 Continued

Drug	*Oral solution/ suspension/ dispersible preparation available*	*Crushed tablet/ capsule contents disperse completely*[a]	*Oral solution/ suspension prepared by local pharmacy*	*Injection can be diluted and administered down feeding tube*	*Comments*
Domperidone	Yes	Yes (Motilium®)	Yes (K)		
Erythromycin	Yes				No information on suitability via feeding tube
Etamsylate			Yes (K)		
Ferrous sulphate					Convert to ferrous fumarate oral syrup. Ferrous sulphate 200mg = ferrous fumarate 7ml oral syrup 140mg/5ml; no information on suitability
Flecainide		Yes (Tambocor®)	Yes (C)	Yes	Use sterile water (not tap). Do not mix injection with alkaline solutions, e.g. chlorides, phosphates, sulphates
Flucloxacillin	Yes			Yes	Stop feed for 1h before and after dose
Fluconazole	Yes		Yes (K)		
Furosemide (frusemide)	Yes	Yes (Lasix®)	Yes (K)		
Gabapentin		Yes			
Glibenclamide		Yes (Daonil®)	Yes (K)		
Gliclazide		Yes (Diamicron®) Takes 5min	Yes (K)		
Granisetron	Yes				No information on suitability via feeding tube
Haloperidol	Yes	Yes (Serenace®) Takes 5min			Commercial oral solution may cause diarrhoea
Ibuprofen[a]	Yes	Yes (Brufen®) Takes 5min			

Table A10.1 Continued

Drug	*Oral solution/ suspension/ dispersible preparation available*	*Crushed tablet/ capsule contents disperse completely*[a]	*Oral solution/ suspension prepared by local pharmacy*	*Injection can be diluted and administered down feeding tube*	*Comments*
Imipramine[a]	Yes	Yes (Tofranil®) Takes 5min	Yes (C)		
Itraconazole	Yes				No information on suitability via feeding tube
Ketoconazole	Yes				Stop feed for 1h before and after dose. *Jejunal administration not recommended; low pH needed for absorption*
Lansoprazole	Yes	Yes (special procedure)			Commercial oral suspension not recommended as too viscous. Capsule contents may be mixed with sodium bicarbonate 8.4% and water using a specific procedure. Contact pharmacy or Lederle for full details
Levomepromazine (methotrimeprazine)		Yes (Nozinan® 25mg, 100mg)	Yes (K)		
Loperamide	Yes	Yes			Commercial oral solution may cause diarrhoea
Lorazepam		Yes (Ativan®)	Yes (K)		
Medroxyprogesterone		Yes (Provera® 5mg,10mg,100mg, Farlutal® 500mg) Takes 5min	Yes (K)	Yes	
Megestrol acetate		Yes Takes 5min	Yes (K)		
Menadiol sodium phosphate			Yes (K)		

Table A10.1 Continued

Drug	*Oral solution/ suspension/ dispersible preparation available*	*Crushed tablet/ capsule contents disperse completely* [a]	*Oral solution/ suspension prepared by local pharmacy*	*Injection can be diluted and administered down feeding tube*	*Comments*
Metformin		Yes (Glucophage®) Takes 5min	Yes (K)		
Methadone	Yes				No information on suitability via feeding tube
Metoclopramide	Yes	Yes (Maxolon®) Takes 5min			Commercial oral solution may cause diarrhoea
Metronidazole	Yes		Yes (K)	Yes	
Midazolam			Yes	Yes	
Morphine[a]	Yes				The m/r granules in Zomorph® capsules and MST Continus® suspension can be used in *larger* bore tubes; mix (do not crush) m/r granules with 30ml water to form the suspension and flush with 30–60ml. Contact Link for full details of procedure for Zomorph®. Otherwise convert to normal-release liquid
Nabilone		Yes			
Naproxen[a]	Yes	Yes (Naprosyn®, Synflex®) Takes 5min			Do not crush e/c formulations
Nifedipine[a]					Contents of liquid capsules may be drawn up using large bore needle and syringe and flushed down tube using saline (NOT water) immediately (light sensitive). May need more than one capsule to obtain the correct volume; 5mg = 0.17ml, 10mg = 0.34ml. Risk of profound hypotension particularly if converting from m/r preparation

Table A10.1 Continued

Drug	*Oral solution/ suspension/ dispersible preparation available*	*Crushed tablet/ capsule contents disperse completely*[a]	*Oral solution/ suspension prepared by local pharmacy*	*Injection can be diluted and administered down feeding tube*	*Comments*
Nitrofurantoin[a]			Yes (K)		
Olanzapine	Yes				No information on suitability via feeding tube
Omeprazole	Yes				Losec MUPS® may be dispersed in 25ml water, 15ml syrup simplex, or 5ml full-cream yoghurt, using a specific procedure specified by the company. Contact pharmacy or AstraZeneca for details. Not recommended for tubes below 7 French gauge
Ondansetron	Yes	Yes (Zofran®) Takes 5min		Yes	
Orphenadrine	Yes	Yes (Disipal®) Takes 5min	Yes (C)		
Oxybutynin	Yes	Yes (Ditropan®) Takes 5min	Yes (K)		
Oxycodone[a]	Yes				No information on suitability via feeding tube
Paracetamol	Yes				
Phenobarbital	Yes	Yes	Yes (K)		
Phenoxymethylpenicillin (Penicillin V)	Yes				Stop feed for 1h before and after dose

Table A10.1 Continued

Drug	*Oral solution/ suspension/ dispersible preparation available*	*Crushed tablet/ capsule contents disperse completely* [a]	*Oral solution/ suspension prepared by local pharmacy*	*Injection can be diluted and administered down feeding tube*	*Comments*
Phenytoin	Yes				Phenytoin oral suspension 30mg/5ml; 90mg (15ml) = 100mg phenytoin sodium tablet/capsule. Convert to once daily dose. Stop feed for 2h before and after administration, and flush tube with 60ml water, *shake liquid well*, then dilute dose with 30–60ml water, administer and flush. May cause diarrhoea
Phytomenadione		Yes (Konakion®) Takes 5min		Yes (Konakion MM®)	
Pilocarpine			Yes		
Potassium supplements	Yes				Commercial oral syrup may cause diarrhoea
Prednisolone	Yes		Yes (K)	Yes	
Prochlorperazine	Yes	Yes (Stemetil®)			Commercial oral solution may cause diarrhoea
Propantheline			Yes		
Ranitidine	Yes	Yes (Zantac®) Takes 5min	Yes (K)	Yes	Commercial oral solution may cause diarrhoea
Risperidone	Yes				No information on suitability via feeding tube
Rofecoxib	Yes				No information on suitability via feeding tube
Senna	Yes	Yes (Senokot®)	Yes (K)		
Sodium fusidate	Yes				Sodium fusidate tablets 500mg = 750mg oral suspension

Table A10.1 Continued

Drug	*Oral solution/ suspension/ dispersible preparation available*	*Crushed tablet/ capsule contents disperse completely*[a]	*Oral solution/ suspension prepared by local pharmacy*	*Injection can be diluted and administered down feeding tube*	*Comments*
Sodium valproate[a]	Yes	Yes (Epilim® Crushable) Takes 5min		Yes	Commercial oral solution may cause gastro-intestinal irritation. Do not crush e/c formulations
Spironolactone	Yes[d]	Yes (Aldactone®) Takes 5min	Yes (K)		
Sucralfate	Yes	Yes			Not recommended due to high viscosity, bezoar formation and binding with feed; likely to block tube. Need to stop feed for 1h before and after dose; impractical for q4h schedule
Temazepam	Yes				No information on suitability via feeding tube
Theophylline[a]	Yes				Care converting from m/r. Need to stop feed for 1h before and 1–2h after dose; impractical for q.d.s. schedule
Thioridazine	Yes	Yes (Melleril®) Takes 5min	Yes (C)		Avoid if possible as causes coagulation with feed. Dilute drug well and flush with 30–60ml water to minimise contact. Commercial oral suspensions may cause diarrhoea
Tolbutamide		Yes (Rastinon®)	Yes (K)		
Tramadol[a]	Yes	Yes		Yes	
Tranexamic acid	Yes	Yes (Cyklokapron®)	Yes (K)		
Trimethoprim	Yes		Yes (K)		

Table A10.1 Continued

Drug	*Oral solution/ suspension/ dispersible preparation available*	*Crushed tablet/ capsule contents disperse completely*[a]	*Oral solution/ suspension prepared by local pharmacy*	*Injection can be diluted and administered down feeding tube*	*Comments*
Vancomycin			Yes	Yes	
Warfarin		Yes (Marevan®)	Yes (K)		INR may be affected by the varying content of Vitamin K in feeds. Need to stop feed for 1h before and 1–2h after dose

a. Do not crush m/r preparations. Take care if converting from m/r to normal-release preparations because dose, frequency and clinical effect may be different
b. C = Diluent C suspending agent
c. K = Keltrol (Diluent A) suspending agent
d. Unlicensed product, available from e.g. Rosemont (see Special orders and named patient supplies, p.349).

Appendix 11: Syringe driver compatibility charts

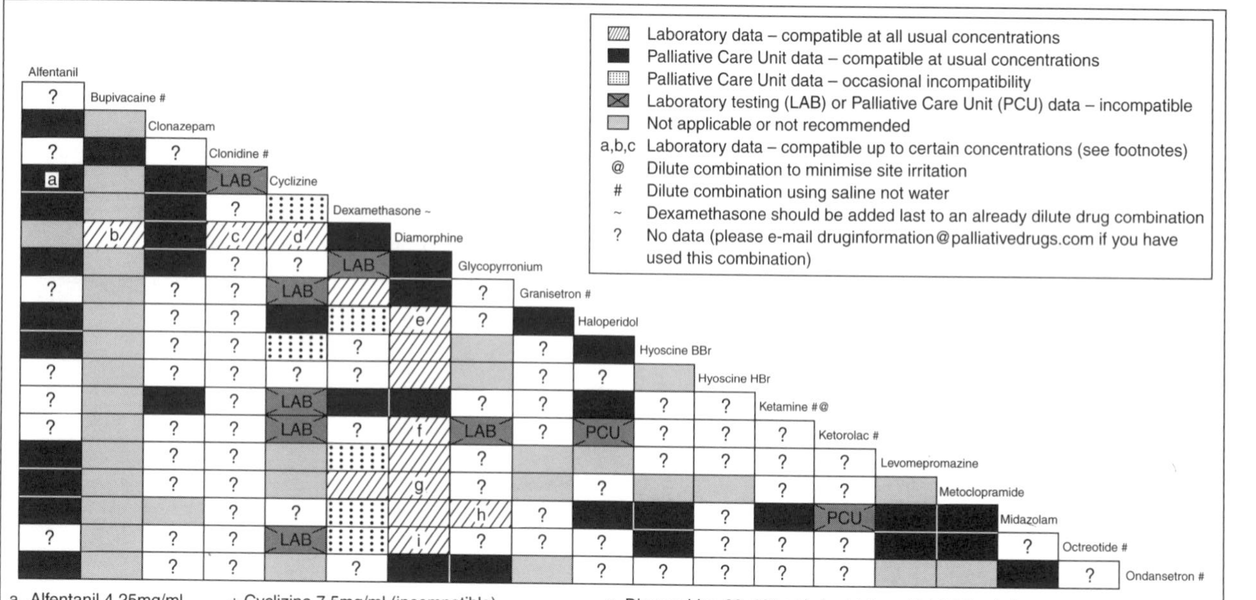
Alfentanil
Bupivacaine #
Clonazepam
Clonidine #
Cyclizine
Dexamethasone ~
Diamorphine
Glycopyrronium
Granisetron #
Haloperidol
Hyoscine BBr
Hyoscine HBr
Ketamine #@
Ketorolac #
Levomepromazine
Metoclopramide
Midazolam
Octreotide #
Ondansetron #
Laboratory data – compatible at all usual concentrations
Palliative Care Unit data – compatible at usual concentrations
Palliative Care Unit data – occasional incompatibility
Laboratory testing (LAB) or Palliative Care Unit (PCU) data – incompatible
Not applicable or not recommended
a,b,c Laboratory data – compatible up to certain concentrations (see footnotes)
@ Dilute combination to minimise site irritation
# Dilute combination using saline not water
~ Dexamethasone should be added last to an already dilute drug combination
? No data (please e-mail druginformation@palliativedrugs.com if you have used this combination)
a. Alfentanil 4.25mg/ml + Cyclizine 7.5mg/ml (incompatible)
b. Diamorphine 10mg/ml + Bupivacaine 0.5% (stable for 4 weeks)
c. Diamorphine 0.6mg/ml + Clonidine 60microgram/ml (stable for 21 days)
d. Diamorphine any strength + Cyclizine 6.7mg/ml
Diamorphine 15mg/ml + Cyclizine 15mg/ml
Diamorphine 20mg/ml + Cyclizine 10mg/ml
e. Diamorphine 20–100mg/ml + Haloperidol 0.75mg/ml
Diamorphine 50mg/ml + Haloperidol 1.5mg/ml
f. Diamorphine 100mg + Ketorolac 90mg (stable for 24h in saline)
g. Diamorphine 25mg/ml + Metoclopramide 5mg/ml
h. Glycopyrronium 0.2mg/ml + Midazolam 5mg/ml (stable for 4h test)
i. Diamorphine 25mg/ml + Octreotide 75microgram/ml (stable for 24h in WFI)
Note: Usual diluent is water unless otherwise specified. This chart summarises information about 24h CSCI drug combinations used in Palliative Care Units. 'Compatible in PCUs' means that no obvious physical signs of incompatibility were observed, i.e. crystallisation, precipitation, discolouration and that the desired clinical effect was achieved.

Chart I Syringe driver compatibility chart for diamorphine and alfentanil: combination of *two* drugs. For larger, colour charts *see* www.palliativedrugs.com.

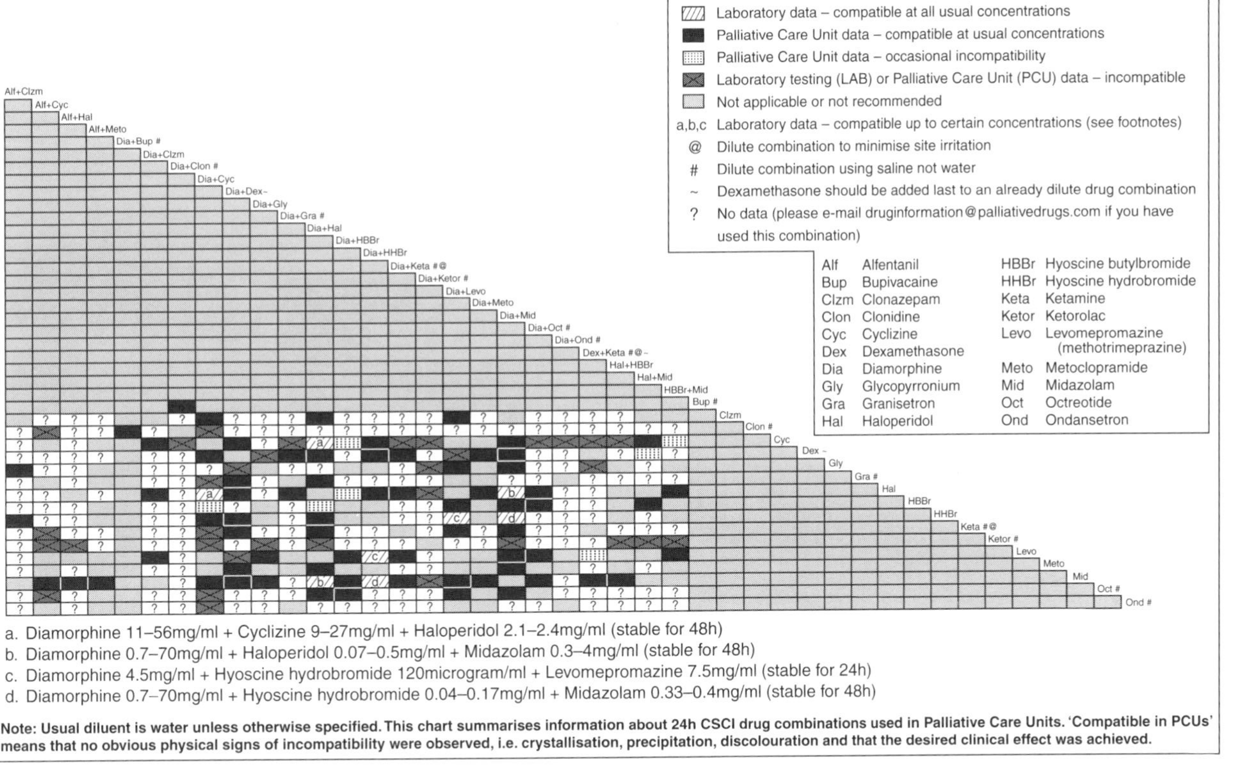
Laboratory data – compatible at all usual concentrations
Palliative Care Unit data – compatible at usual concentrations
Palliative Care Unit data – occasional incompatibility
Laboratory testing (LAB) or Palliative Care Unit (PCU) data – incompatible
Not applicable or not recommended
a,b,c Laboratory data – compatible up to certain concentrations (see footnotes)
@ Dilute combination to minimise site irritation
# Dilute combination using saline not water
~ Dexamethasone should be added last to an already dilute drug combination
? No data (please e-mail druginformation@palliativedrugs.com if you have used this combination)
Alf Alfentanil
Bup Bupivacaine
Clzm Clonazepam
Clon Clonidine
Cyc Cyclizine
Dex Dexamethasone
Dia Diamorphine
Gly Glycopyrronium
Gra Granisetron
Hal Haloperidol
HBBr Hyoscine butylbromide
HHBr Hyoscine hydrobromide
Keta Ketamine
Ketor Ketorolac
Levo Levomepromazine (methotrimeprazine)
Meto Metoclopramide
Mid Midazolam
Oct Octreotide
Ond Ondansetron
Alf+Clzm
Alf+Cyc
Alf+Hal
Alf+Meto
Dia+Bup #
Dia+Clzm
Dia+Clon #
Dia+Cyc
Dia+Dex~
Dia+Gly
Dia+Gra #
Dia+Hal
Dia+HBBr
Dia+HHBr
Dia+Keta #@
Dia+Ketor #
Dia+Levo
Dia+Meto
Dia+Mid
Dia+Oct #
Dia+Ond #
Dex+Keta #@~
Hal+HBBr
Hal+Mid
HBBr+Mid
Bup #
Clzm
Clon #
Cyc
Dex ~
Gly
Gra #
Hal
HBBr
HHBr
Keta #@
Ketor #
Levo
Meto
Mid
Oct #
Ond #
a. Diamorphine 11–56mg/ml + Cyclizine 9–27mg/ml + Haloperidol 2.1–2.4mg/ml (stable for 48h)
b. Diamorphine 0.7–70mg/ml + Haloperidol 0.07–0.5mg/ml + Midazolam 0.3–4mg/ml (stable for 48h)
c. Diamorphine 4.5mg/ml + Hyoscine hydrobromide 120microgram/ml + Levomepromazine 7.5mg/ml (stable for 24h)
d. Diamorphine 0.7–70mg/ml + Hyoscine hydrobromide 0.04–0.17mg/ml + Midazolam 0.33–0.4mg/ml (stable for 48h)
Note: Usual diluent is water unless otherwise specified. This chart summarises information about 24h CSCI drug combinations used in Palliative Care Units. 'Compatible in PCUs' means that no obvious physical signs of incompatibility were observed, i.e. crystallisation, precipitation, discolouration and that the desired clinical effect was achieved.

Chart 2 Syringe driver compatibility chart for diamorphine and alfentanil: combination of *three* drugs. For larger, colour charts *see* www.palliativedrugs.com.

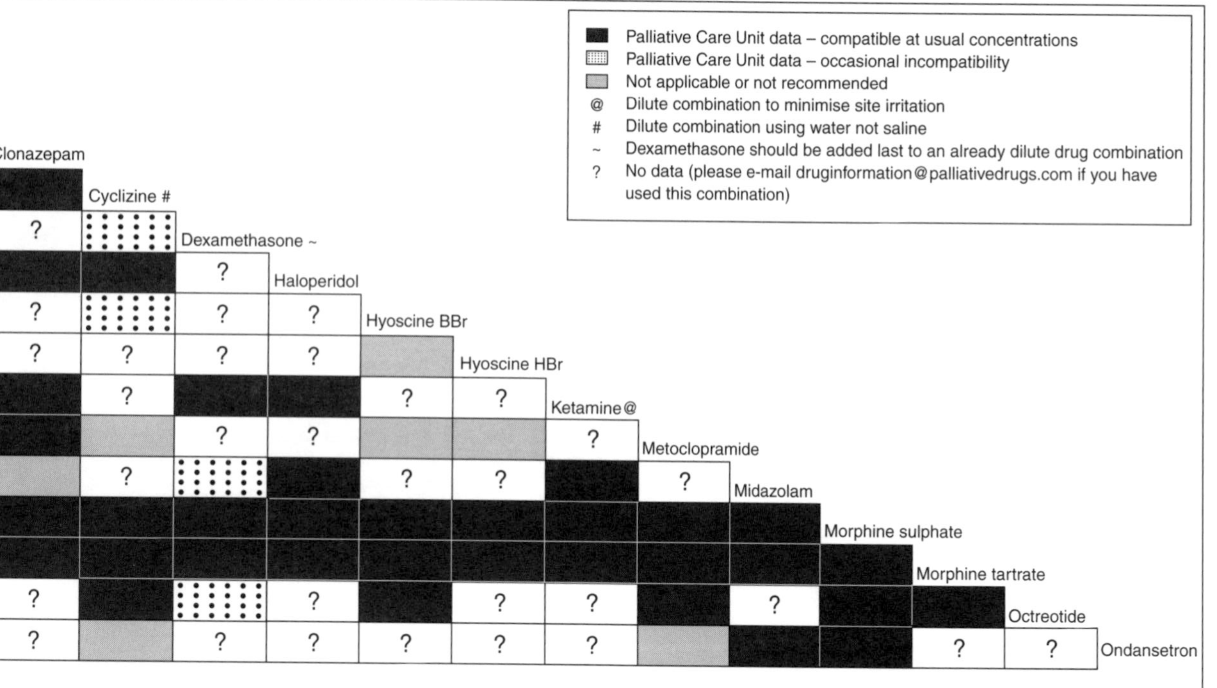

Note: Usual diluent is normal saline unless otherwise specified. This chart summarises information about 24h CSCI drug combinations used in Palliative Care Units. 'Compatible in PCUs' means that no obvious physical signs of incompatibility were observed, i.e. crystallisation, precipitation, discolouration and that the desired clinical effect was achieved.

Chart 3 Syringe driver compatibility chart for morphine sulphate and tartrate: combination of *two* drugs. For larger, colour charts *see* www.palliativedrugs.com.

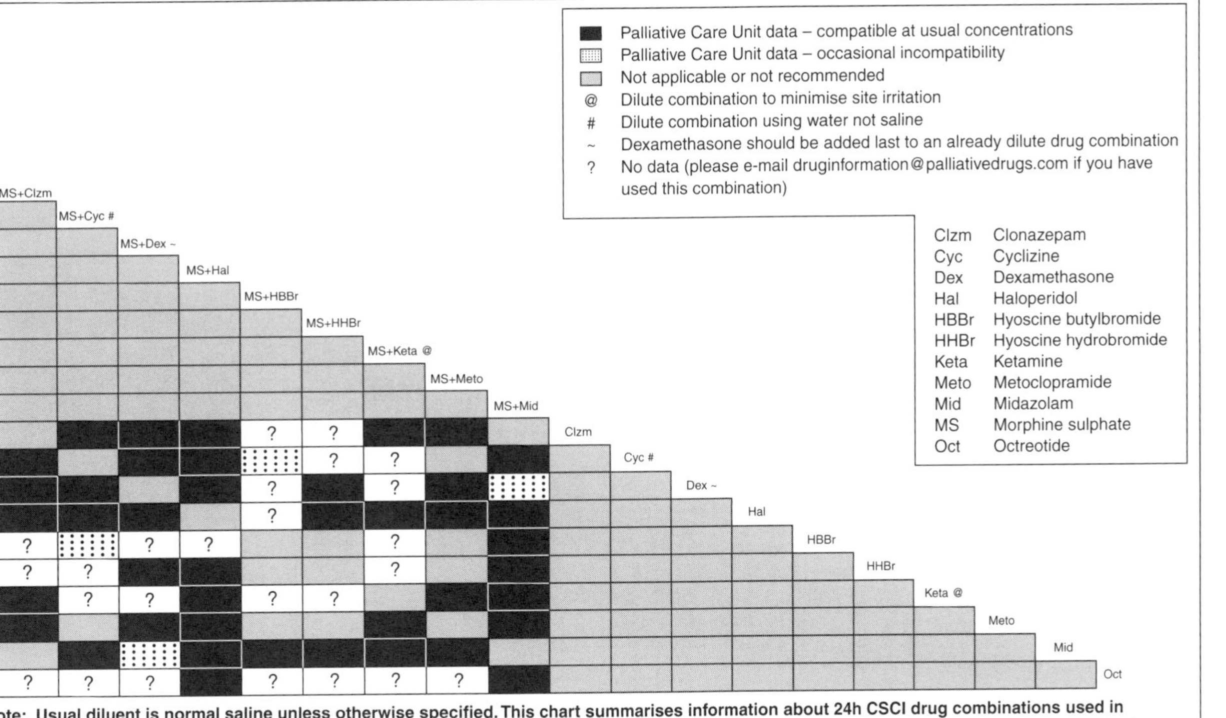

Note: Usual diluent is normal saline unless otherwise specified. This chart summarises information about 24h CSCI drug combinations used in Palliative Care Units. 'Compatible in PCUs' means that no obvious physical signs of incompatibility were observed, i.e. crystallisation, precipitation, discolouration and that the desired clinical effect was achieved.

Chart 4 Syringe driver compatibility chart for morphine sulphate: combination of *three* drugs. For larger, colour charts *see* www.palliativedrugs.com.

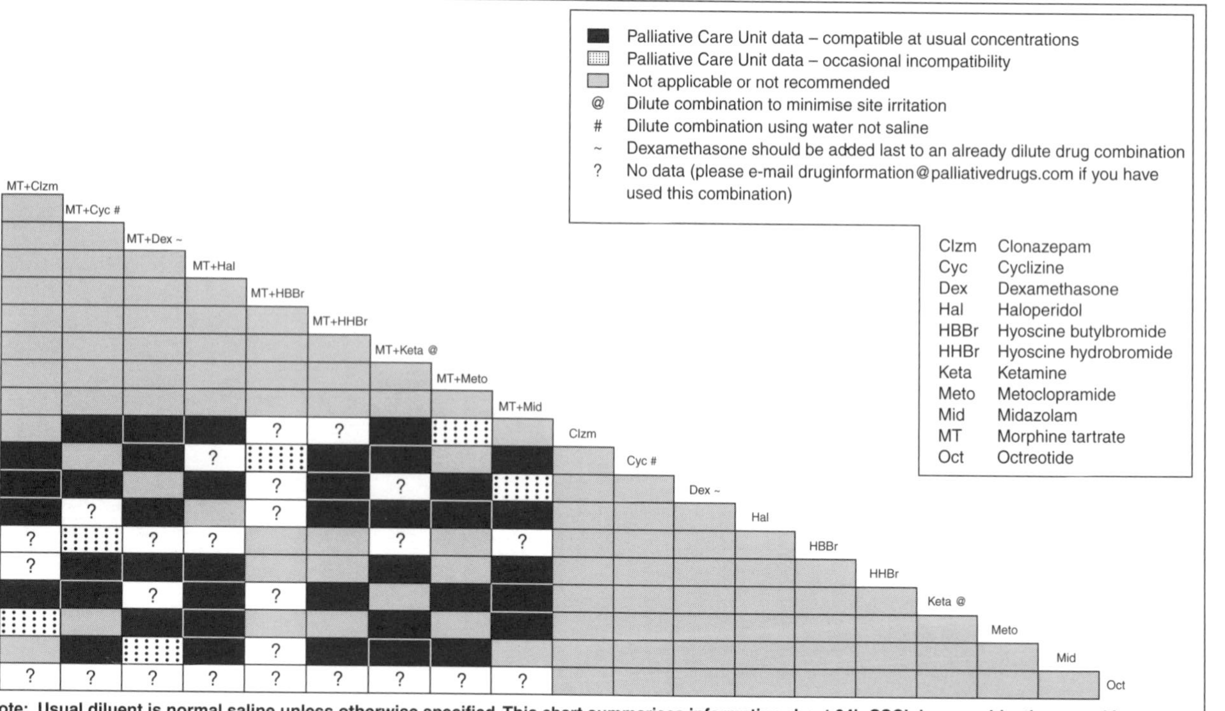

Chart 5 Syringe driver compatibility chart for morphine tartrate: combination of *three* drugs. For larger, colour charts see www.palliativedrugs.com.

Index

Note: Main references are in **bold**.

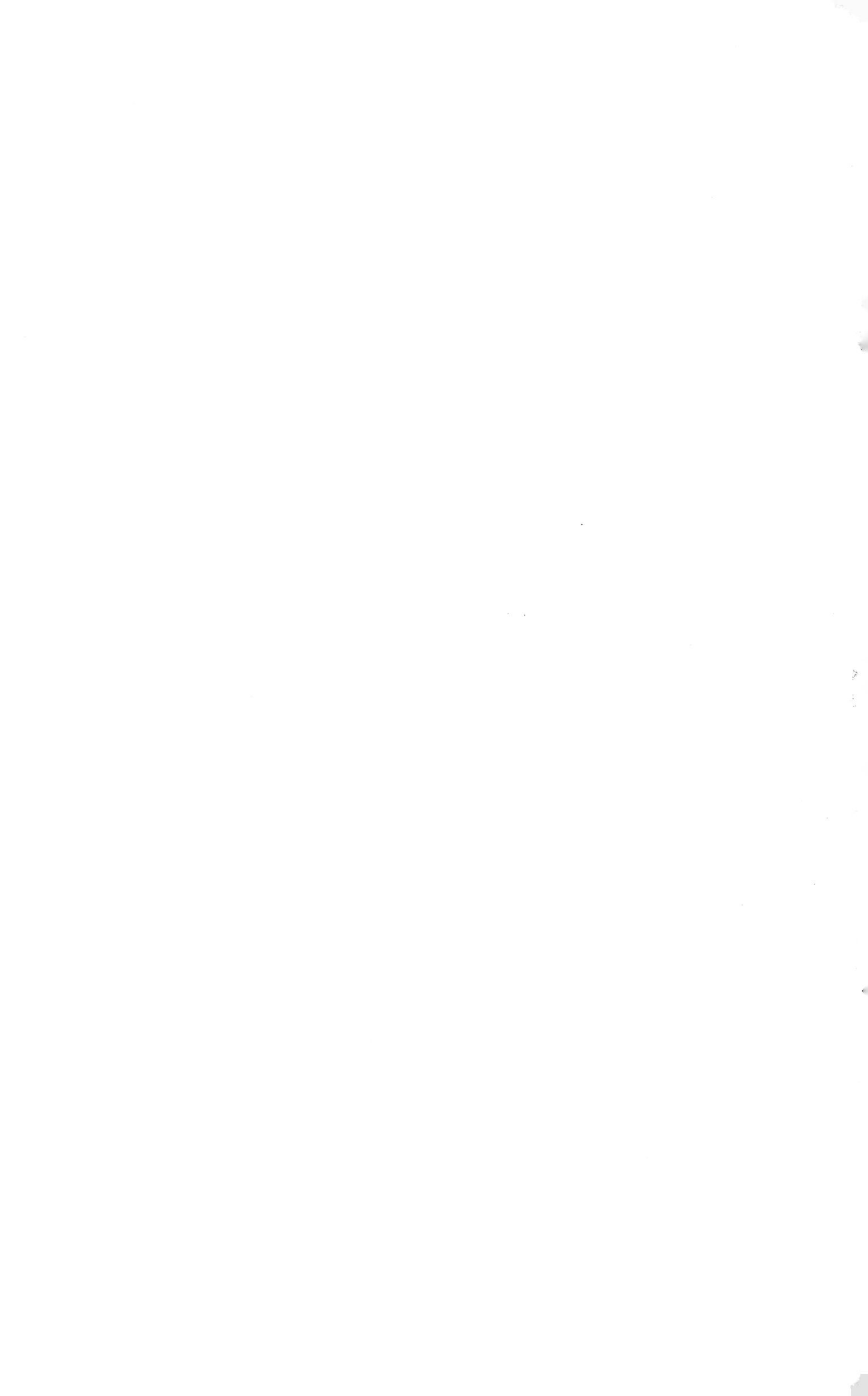